eureka

General Surgery & Urology

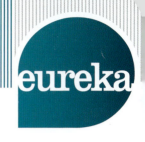

General Surgery & Urology

Stephen Parker BSc MS DipMedEd
FRCS
Consultant Breast and General
Paediatric Surgeon
St Mary's Hospital
Newport, UK

Series Editors

Janine Henderson MRCPsych
MClinEd
MB BS Programme Director
Hull York Medical School
York, UK

David Oliveira PhD FRCP
Professor of Renal Medicine
St George's, University of London
London, UK

Stephen Parker BSc MS DipMedEd
FRCS
Consultant Breast and General
Paediatric Surgeon
St Mary's Hospital
Newport, UK

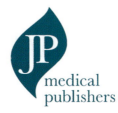

JP
medical
publishers

London • Philadelphia • New Delhi • Panama City

ISBN: 978-1-909836-04-4

British Library Cataloguing in Publication Data
A catalogue record for this book is available from the British Library

Library of Congress Cataloging in Publication Data
A catalog record for this book is available from the Library of Congress

Publisher:	Richard Furn
Development Editors:	Thomas Fletcher, Paul Mayhew, Alison Whitehouse
Editorial Assistants:	Sophie Woolven, Katie Pattullo
Copy Editor:	Carrie Walker
Graphic narratives:	James Pollitt
Cover design:	Forbes Design
Page design:	Designers Collective

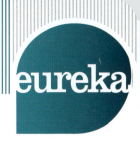

Series Editors' Foreword

Today's medical students need to know a great deal to be effective as tomorrow's doctors. This knowledge includes core science and clinical skills, from understanding biochemical pathways to communicating with patients. Modern medical school curricula integrate this teaching, thereby emphasising how learning in one area can support and reinforce another. At the same time students must acquire sound clinical reasoning skills, working with complex information to understand each individual's unique medical problems.

The *Eureka* series is designed to cover all aspects of today's medical curricula and reinforce this integrated approach. Each book can be used from first year through to qualification. Core biomedical principles are introduced but given relevant clinical context: the authors have always asked themselves, 'why does the aspiring clinician need to know this'?

Each clinical title in the series is grounded in the relevant core science, which is introduced at the start of each book. Each core science title integrates and emphasises clinical relevance throughout. Medical and surgical approaches are included to provide a complete and integrated view of the patient management options available to the clinician. Clinical insights highlight key facts and principles drawn from medical practice. Cases featuring unique graphic narratives are presented with clear explanations that show how experienced clinicians think, enabling students to develop their own clinical reasoning and decision making. Clinical SBAs help with exam revision while Starter questions are a unique learning tool designed to stimulate interest in the subject.

Having biomedical principles and clinical applications together in one book will make their connections more explicit and easier to remember. Alongside repeated exposure to patients and practice of clinical and communication skills, we hope *Eureka* will equip medical students for a lifetime of successful clinical practice.

Janine Henderson, David Oliveira, Stephen Parker

About the Series Editors

Janine Henderson is the MB BS undergraduate Programme Director at Hull York Medical School (HYMS). After medical school at the University of Oxford and clinical training in psychiatry, she combined her work as a consultant with postgraduate teaching roles, moving to the new Hull York Medical School in 2004. She has a particular interest in modern educational methods, curriculum design and clinical reasoning.

David Oliveira is Professor of Renal Medicine at St George's, University of London (SGUL), where he served as the MBBS Course Director between 2007 and 2013. Having trained at Cambridge University and the Westminster Hospital he obtained a PhD in cellular immunology and worked as a renal physician before being appointed as Foundation Chair of Renal Medicine at SGUL.

Stephen Parker is a Consultant Breast and General Paediatric Surgeon at St Mary's Hospital, Isle of Wight. He trained at St George's, University of London, and after service in the Royal Navy was appointed as Consultant Surgeon at University Hospital Coventry. He has a particular interest in e-learning and the use of multimedia platforms in medical education.

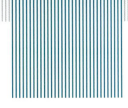

Preface

Surgical and anaesthetic techniques have rapidly evolved over the last two decades, yet despite improvements in outcome surgery remains inherently risky, particularly in the emergency setting. Irrespective of speciality, all clinicians need to understand the principles and practice of surgery, and the role that medical and surgical treatments play in the integrated care of the patient. Such understanding enables clinicians to make appropriate and timely referrals and keep their patients fully informed.

Eureka General Surgery & Urology provides the knowledge and skills to understand the general principles common to all types of surgery, as well as describing the specific presentations and management of conditions requiring both elective and emergency surgery.

The first two chapters cover themes common to all surgical conditions. Chapter 1 describes the appropriate manner in which to prepare patients for surgery; the steps required to ensure the safety of the patient during surgery; and the principles of postoperative management necessary for a rapid recovery. Chapter 2 discusses the clinical features common to many surgical conditions and the range of investigative options available to the clinician.

Each of the following chapters covers the most important surgical conditions affecting the organ systems that fall under the broad umbrella of general surgery and urology. The relevant core sciences underpinning these conditions are described at the start of each chapter, and serve as an introduction to the subsequent discussion of the diseases and their management. Two final chapters include, firstly, descriptions of the presentation and management of common surgical emergencies and secondly, SBA questions with detailed answers.

The importance of performing the correct operation, on the right patient, in a timely fashion and with the safest possible outcome should never be under-estimated. I hope *Eureka General Surgery & Urology* provides all medical students with an appreciation of these principles, and a solid basis for all those who proceed into surgical training.

Stephen Parker
April 2015

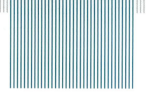

Contents

Series Editors' Foreword	v
About the Series Editors	v
Preface	vii
Glossary	x
Acknowledgements	xi

Chapter 1 First principles

Preoperative issues	1
Perioperative issues	8
Postoperative issues	13

Chapter 2 Clinical essentials

Introduction	23
Common symptoms of surgical diagnoses	23
Common signs of surgical diagnoses	26
Investigations	35
Screening programmes	38
Surgical techniques	39

Chapter 3 Breast disease

Introduction	45
Case 1 Breast lump	46
Core sciences	47
Triple assessment	50
Disorders of breast development	54
Benign breast disease	54
Breast pain	57
Breast cancer	57
Gynaecomastia	62

Chapter 4 Endocrine surgery

Introduction	65
Case 2 Neck lump	66
Core sciences	68
History, examination and investigation	73
Altered thyroid states	76
Thyroglossal cysts	78
Solitary thyroid nodules	79
Thyroid neoplasms	80
Thyroiditis	82
Parathyroid conditions	83
Adrenal conditions	85
Carcinoid tumours	89

Chapter 5 Upper gastrointestinal surgery

Introduction	91
Case 3 Epigastric pain and weight loss	92
Core sciences	94
History, examination and investigation	98
Gastro-oesophageal reflux	100
Achalasia	101
Peptic ulcer disease	102
Oesophageal cancer	104
Gastric cancer	106

Chapter 6 Colorectal surgery

Introduction	111
Case 4 Groin lump	112
Case 5 Change in bowel habit	113

Core science 115
History, examination and investigation 118
Abdominal wall hernias 121
Intestinal stomas 124
Enterocutaneous fistulae 124
Inflammatory bowel disease 125
Diverticular disease 129
Colorectal polyps 130
Colorectal cancer 131
Perianal conditions 134

Chapter 7 Hepatobiliary surgery

Introduction 139
Case 6 Jaundice 140
Core science 141
History and examination 145
Obstructive jaundice 148
Gallstone disease 150
Pancreatic cancer` 152
Liver and biliary cancer 155
Portal hypertension and ascites 157
Splenic disorders 160

Chapter 8 Urology

Introduction 163
Case 7 Abdominal pain and microscopic haematuria 164
Case 8 Urinary frequency 165
Case 9 Painless haematuria and a loin mass 166
Core science 167
History and examination 172
Urinary tract infection 176
Ureteric and bladder calculi 178
Renal cancer 180
Bladder cancer 182
Bladder outflow obstruction 183
Prostate cancer 185
Testicular disorders 186
Penile disorders 189

Chapter 9 Vascular surgery

Introduction 193
Case 10 Cold painful foot 194
Core science 195
History, examination and investigation 198
Intermittent claudication and chronic limb ischaemia 203
Acute limb ischaemia 205
Diabetic foot 207
Carotid artery disease 208
Abdominal aortic aneurysm 210
Vascular trauma 212
Varicose veins 213
Venous hypertension and leg ulceration 215
Lymphatic conditions 216
Raynaud's disease 218

Chapter 10 Surgical emergencies

Introduction 221
Acute appendicitis 222
Acute mesenteric ischaemia 224
Upper gastrointestinal haemorrhage 225
Lower gastrointestinal haemorrhage 227
Intestinal obstruction 229
Sigmoid volvulus 231
Gastrointestinal perforation 232
Acute pancreatitis 234

Chapter 11 Self-assessment

SBA questions 239
SBA answers 247

Index 255

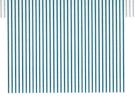

Glossary

ACTH	adrenocorticotrophic hormone
ADH	antidiuretic hormone
ADH	antidiuretic hormone
APACHE	Acute Physiology and Chronic Health Evaluation
APUD	amine precursor uptake and decarboxylation
5-ASA	5-aminosalicylic acid
ASA	American Society of Anesthiologists
BMI	body mass index
CT	computed tomography
DCIS	ductal carcinoma in situ
DMSA	dimercaptosuccinic acid
DTPA	diethylene triamine pentacetic acid
DVT	deep vein thrombosis
ERCP	endoscopic retrograde cholangiopancreatography
ERV	expiratory reserve volume
FEV_1	forced expiratory volume in 1 second
FSH	follicle-stimulating hormone
FVC	forced vital capacity
GORD	gastro-oesophageal reflux disease
HbA_{1c}	glycosylated haemoglobin
HCC	hepatocellular carcinoma
HER2	human epidermal growth factor receptor 2
IRV	inspiratory reserve volume
KUB	kidney–ureter–bladder
LH	luteinising hormone
MAG3	mercaptoacetyltriglycine
MEN	multiple endocrine neoplasia
MRA	magnetic resonance angiography
MRCP	magnetic resonance cholangiopancreatography
MRI	magnetic resonance imaging
MSU	midstream specimen of urine
RR	respiratory rate
SIRS	systemic inflammatory response syndrome
T3	tri-iodothyronine
T4	thyroxine
TIA	transient ischaemic attack
TIPPS	transjugular intrahepatic portosystemic shunting
TSH	thyroid-stimulating hormone
TURP	transurethral prostatectomy
TV	tidal volume
UTI	urinary tract infection

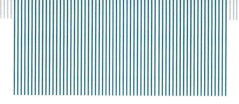

Acknowledgements

Thanks to the following medical students for their help reviewing chapters: Jessica Dunlop, Aliza Imam, Roxanne McVittie, Daniel Roberts and Joseph Suich.

Figure 6.5 is copyright of Sam Scott-Hunter and is reproduced from Tunstall R, Shah N. *Pocket Tutor Surface Anatomy.* London, JP Medical, 2012.

Figures 2.6–2.10, 3.7, 4.13 and 9.8 are reproduced from Cartledge P, et al. *Pocket Tutor Clinical Examination.* London: JP Medical, 2014.

Chapter 1
First principles

Preoperative issues 1   Postoperative issues 13
Perioperative issues. 8

Starter questions

Answers to the following questions are on page 21-22.

1. Why is surgery inherently dangerous?
2. What is informed consent?
3. Can children give consent for operations?
4. Why is asepsis crucial during surgery?
5. Why are antibiotics important during surgery?
6. Why does postoperative pain vary between patients?

Preoperative issues

An admission to hospital for a surgical procedure is divided into three phases: preoperative, operative and postoperative. Preoperative preparation, particularly for elective surgery, is vital to achieve the safest outcome for the patient. It begins with the decision to treat and ends with the admission for surgery. Important steps include a preoperative anaesthetic assessment, providing the patient with information and obtaining the patient's consent.

Consent for surgery

Informed consent is the process of getting the patient's permission to undertake a procedure on them (**Figure 1.1**). The patient's autonomy must be respected at all times. Most patients have the capacity to make decisions and must be given adequate information to assess the treatment options. This

information should be given in a way that they are able to understand. Patients must not be coerced, and some patients will decide not to undergo a particular treatment or surgical procedure.

> **Informed consent involves a continuing dialogue between the doctor and patient and is not simply a matter of obtaining the patient's signature on a consent form.**

Types of consent

Expressed consent is when a patient gives specific verbal or written permission for an investigation or treatment to be undertaken. It is essential if the proposed intervention has risks attached. Implied consent is verbal and occurs when a patient cooperates with a sim-

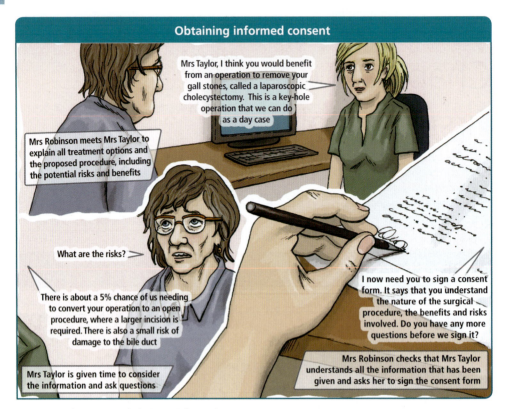

Figure 1.1 The process of obtaining informed consent.

ple action such as a physical examination or low-risk procedure (e.g. venesection). During the consent process, patients are informed of:

- The likely diagnosis and any uncertainty over this that exists
- The options available for treatment, including doing nothing
- The purpose of the proposed treatment
- The perceived benefits and risks

All questions posed by the patient or their relatives should be answered honestly, and information must not be intentionally withheld. It is good practice for the doctor performing the procedure to obtain consent. If obtaining consent is delegated, the individual must be appropriately trained. The patient can withdraw their consent and change their mind at any time.

Specific problems

Patients have autonomy, and the treatment of a competent adult cannot be decided by another individual. In an emergency situation, however, it sometimes may be impossible to obtain fully informed consent. Doctors must always act in the best interests of their patients so an emergency procedure (e.g. cardiopulmonary resuscitation) can be performed without consent. The action will be judged by the doctor's peers if its appropriateness is ever called in to question. Advanced care directives and living wills are legally binding and should be followed.

> **An advanced care directive is a written statement of the treatment a patient is willing to accept in the future,** should they ever 'lack capacity' to discuss treatment options. It sometimes includes an explicit desire not to undergo potentially life-saving treatment or surgery.

Consent in children

The cognitive ability of children to understand what medical treatment entails develops with age but is variable. By 16 years of age, a child is presumed to be able to understand and decide on their treatment. Below that age, children may still have the capacity to determine treatment. Based on a legal case, this is known as Gillick competence. If a Gillick-competent child refuses treatment, a person with parental responsibility (usually the mother, father or legal guardian) is able to authorise treatment that is in the child's best interests, thereby overruling the child.

Assessing patients for surgery

Surgery is inherently dangerous. The process of preoperative assessment aims to prepare patients for their proposed surgery and to inform them of what to expect and the likely recovery period. It also has benefits for the hospital by preventing unnecessary cancellations and reducing hospital stays.

> **Unexpected complications and postoperative deaths can occur in fit patients undergoing relatively minor elective surgery.** No surgery is risk free.

Evidence-based guidelines on the appropriateness of preoperative investigations reduce the time and cost associated with unnecessary investigations. An effective preoperative assessment process assesses the patient's fitness for anaesthesia and also gives them information on the proposed procedure. The issues to be addressed in a preoperative assessment are shown in **Table 1.1.**

Informed consent for the procedure may sometimes be obtained when assessing the patient.

American Society of Anesthesiologists grading system

A patient's fitness for anaesthesia depends on the presence or absence of pre-existing medical conditions. Important medical conditions that increase morbidity and mortality following surgery include cardiorespiratory

Preoperative assessment service	
Anaesthetic preassessment	Preassessment specific to the procedure
Past medical history	Specific prerequisites for the surgery planned
Current cardiorespiratory status	When to attend the hospital
Management of medication	Duration of and recovery from surgery
Duration of reduced oral intake prior to surgery	Postoperative care
Specific anaesthetic issues	Discharge date
	Follow-up arrangements
	Return to work or full activity

Table 1.1 Features of a preoperative assessment service

American Society of Anesthesiologists grading	
Grade	Definition
1	Normal healthy individual
2	Mild systemic disease that does not limit activity
3	Severe systemic disease that limits activity but is not incapacitating
4	Incapacitating systemic disease that is constantly life threatening
5	Patient moribund and not expected to survive 24 hours with or without surgery

Table 1.2 American Society of Anesthesiologists grading system

disease, diabetes, renal failure and obesity. The American Society of Anesthesiologists (ASA) grade is the system most commonly used to grade co-morbidity (**Table 1.2).** This accurately predicts morbidity and mortality after elective surgery. Over 80% of patients undergoing elective surgery are either ASA grade 1 or 2. The risk of death following anaesthesia in an ASA grade 1 patient is minimal but is never zero.

Preoperative investigations

The main purpose of preoperative investigations is to provide additional diagnostic and prognostic information with the aim of confirming the appropriateness of the clinical management. The information is used for risk assessment and to predict postoperative complications. Some of the results (e.g. haemoglobin levels prior to major abdominal surgery) provide a useful baseline measurement for later reference.

The choice of preoperative investigations is based on the findings of the clinical assessment and how likely it is that the patient has a clinical condition that is not producing symptoms. It also takes into consideration the severity of the surgery being considered.

The National Institute for Health and Care Excellence has produced guidelines on preoperative tests. These tests include:

- Chest radiograph
- ECG
- Echocardiography
- Full blood count
- Renal function
- Coagulation screen
- Glycated haemoglobin (HbA_{1c})
- Liver function
- Lung function

The tests recommended are based on the age of the patient, their ASA grade and the severity of the proposed surgery.

> Preoperative investigations rarely uncover unsuspected medical conditions and are not useful as a screening test for asymptomatic diseases. Only 5% of patients have abnormal results that have not been predicted from their clinical assessment. Only 0.1% of these investigations change the patient's management.

Cardiovascular disease

Of the cardiovascular diseases, hypertension and ischaemic heart disease in particular increase the risk associated with general anaesthesia. In patients with hypertension, an assessment is needed of both the severity of the hypertension and the presence of

end-organ damage, such as cardiac impairment or reduced renal function. The risk of postoperative cardiovascular morbidity is increased in poorly controlled hypertension. Elective surgery should be cancelled if the diastolic blood pressure is greater than 120 mmHg.

As postoperative mortality is significantly increased after a myocardial infarction, elective surgery is if possible be deferred for at least 6 months. The risk of postoperative reinfarction after a previous myocardial infarct is 35% between 0 and 3 months, 15% between 3 and 6 months and 4% at more than 6 months. The mortality following myocardial infarction is about 40%.

Cardiac function tests

Cardiac function can be assessed by simple non-invasive techniques or more complex and invasive investigations. Non-invasive tests include a chest radiograph, ECG and echocardiography.

> A routine preoperative chest radiograph is not required for all patients but needs to be considered if there are symptoms or signs of cardiorespiratory disease. Radiological signs associated with an increased morbidity from cardiac disease are cardiomegaly, pulmonary oedema and changes in cardiac outline that are specific to certain diseases.

An ECG taken when the patient is resting is normal in 25–50% of those with ischaemic heart disease. There may be characteristic features of ischaemia or previous infarction. Twenty-four-hour ECG monitoring is useful to detect and assess arrhythmias. Echocardiography is used to assess the cardiac muscle mass, the function of the ventricles, the ejection fraction, cardiac volumes and function of the heart valves. It can be performed percutaneously or via a probe placed in the oesophagus (the transoesophageal route). Doppler ultrasonography is used to measure blood flow and pressure gradients across the valves.

Respiratory disease

Lung disease leads to an increased risk of respiratory complications such as atelectasis (collapse of the bronchioles and alveoli) and hypoxaemia (a reduction in the partial pressure of oxygen in the arterial blood). Atelectasis predisposes to bronchopneumonia and respiratory failure.

> **Smoking doubles the risk of postoperative pulmonary complications.** This increased risk persists for 3–4 months after stopping smoking. Smoking increases blood carboxyhaemoglobin levels, interfering with the transport of oxygen. The increase in carboxyhaemoglobin persists for 12 hours after the last cigarette.

Respiratory function tests

The preoperative investigation of patients with respiratory disease either assesses lung function or images the thorax:

- Lung function tests predict the type (restrictive or obstructive) and severity of lung disease. They assess lung volumes, airway calibre and gas transfer.
- Potentially useful radiological investigations include a chest radiograph and high-resolution CT of the thorax.

Arterial blood gases provide additional helpful information in relation to the transport and transfer of oxygen and carbon dioxide.

> In obstructive lung disease (e.g. chronic obstructive pulmonary disease), the diameter of the airways is reduced, impeding the exhalation of air from the lungs. In restrictive lung disease (e.g. interstitial lung disease), expansion of the lungs is impaired due to a reduction in compliance of the lung tissue.

Lung volumes

Lung volumes are measured using spirometry (**Figure 1.2**). The total amount of air moved in and out of the lungs each minute depends upon the tidal volume (TV) and the respiratory rate (RR). Pulmonary ventilation equals RR × TV.

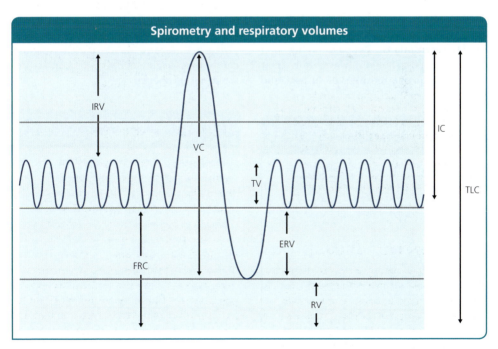

Spirometry and respiratory volumes

Figure 1.2 Spirometry and respiratory volumes. ERV, expiratory reserve volume; FRC, functional reserve capacity; IC, inspiratory capacity. IRV, inspiratory reserve volume; RV, residual volume; TLC, total lung capacity; TV, tidal volume; VC, vital capacity.

However, more than the TV can be inspired in any one breath, and the extra volume available is called the inspiratory reserve volume (IRV). Similarly, the extra volume that can be expired is called the expiratory reserve volume (ERV). Even after a maximum expiration, there is still some air in the lungs and this is known as the residual volume. The maximum volume available for breathing is called the vital capacity and is the sum of the IRV, TV and ERV.

Airway calibre

Airway calibre is assessed by peak flow measurements (**Figure 1.3**). Accurate assessment requires the patient's cooperation and maximum voluntary effort.

The flow rates measured include the forced vital capacity (FVC) and the forced expiratory volume in 1 second (FEV_1). The FEV_1/FVC ratio is a useful derived measurement. In restrictive lung disease, the FVC is reduced but the FEV_1/FVC is normal. In obstructive lung disease, the FVC is normal or reduced and the FEV_1/FVC is reduced.

Diabetes mellitus

The perioperative management of diabetic patients depends on the severity of their diabetes. Diet-controlled diabetes requires no specific precautions. Patients taking oral hypoglycaemics should always omit their medication on the morning of surgery and restart it when they are eating normally again. Patients with insulin-dependent diabetes should have an early position on the operating list. They should not have breakfast and their morning dose of insulin should be omitted.

The patient is given a glucose potassium insulin infusion or a sliding scale insulin regimen, administered at a rate dependent on the blood sugar level. An infusion of glucose potassium insulin is made up as 15 U of insulin, 10 mmol of potassium chloride and 500 mL of 10% dextrose. A sliding scale insulin is 50 U of insulin in 50 mL of normal saline. Either infusion is appropriate for non-insulin dependent diabetic patients undergoing major surgery.

> The perioperative management of a diabetic patient aims to keep the blood sugar level between 5 and 10 mmol/l until the patient is eating normally.

Obesity

Obesity leads to morbidity and mortality (**Table 1.3**) after any surgery, even in the absence of other diseases. The body mass index (BMI) is the best measure of the degree of obesity, where BMI = weight (kg)/height (m)^2. A normal BMI is 22–28 kg/m^2. A BMI >28 kg/m^2 indicates that the patient is significantly overweight. A BMI >35 kg/m^2 represents morbid obesity.

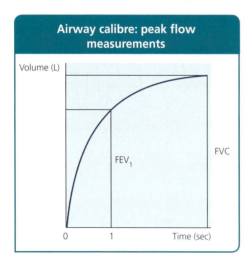

Airway calibre: peak flow measurements

Figure 1.3 Peak flow measurements. FVC, forced vital capacity; FEV$_1$, forced expiratory volume in 1 second.

Potential complications associated with obesity		
Cardiovascular	Respiratory	Other
Hypertension	Difficult airway	Gastro-oesophageal reflux
Ischaemic heart disease	Difficult mechanical ventilation	
Cerebrovascular disease	Chronic hypoxaemia	Abnormal liver function
Deep vein thrombosis	Obstructive sleep apnoea	Insulin resistance
Difficult vascular access	Pulmonary hypertension	Poor postoperative pain control
	Postoperative hypoxaemia	

Table 1.3 Potential complications associated with obesity

Stages of renal dysfunction		
Stage	Description	Creatinine clearance (mL/min/1.73 m²)
1	Normal	>90
2	Early renal insufficiency	60–89
3	Chronic renal failure	30–59
4	Pre-end stage failure	15–29
5	End-stage failure	<15

Table 1.4 Stages of renal dysfunction

Chronic renal failure

Chronic renal failure is defined as a glomerular filtration rate of <60 mL/min (**Table 1.4**). The metabolic consequences of this affect multiple organ systems (e.g. cardiac and respiratory system and coagulation).

Renal function tests

Serum urea and electrolytes measurements provide a basic assessment of renal function. If a more accurate measurement is required, the serum creatinine level is used to estimate the glomerular filtration rate. A formal assessment of creatinine clearance requires a 24-hour urine collection and serum creatinine level measurements during this time.

Prophylaxis of deep vein thrombosis

Venous thrombosis and its complications are a significant cause of morbidity and mortality in surgical patients. The formation and propagation of a venous thrombus depends on the presence of Virchow's triad (**Figure 1.4**). Immobility of the patient contributes to venous stasis. A hypercoagulable state can be caused by drugs or malignancy. Endothelial damage can result from external compression.

Risk factors for venous thrombosis are shown in **Table 1.5**. Most deep vein thromboses (DVTs) of the calf are clinically silent and about 80% of these lyse spontaneously without treatment. However, 20% of calf DVTs will spread to the thigh and this increases the risk of pulmonary embolism.

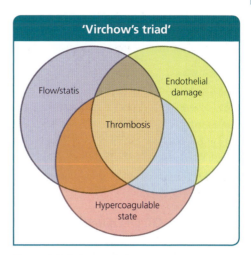

Figure 1.4 Virchow's triad.

Risk factors for venous thrombosis	
Patient factors	Disease or surgical procedure
Age	Trauma or surgery to pelvis, hip or lower limb
Obesity	
Varicose veins	Malignancy
Immobility	Heart failure
Pregnancy and puerperium	Recent myocardial infarction
High-dose oestrogen therapy	Lower limb paralysis
Previous deep vein thrombosis or pulmonary embolism	Infection
	Inflammatory bowel disease
Thrombophilia	Nephrotic syndrome
Deficiency of antithrombin III	Polycythaemia
Lupus anticoagulant	Paraproteinaemia

Table 1.5 Risk factors for venous thrombosis

> **Pulmonary emboli account for about 10% of all hospital deaths.** In many cases, they are preventable by performing a risk assessment and giving mechanical or pharmacological prophylaxis.

Risk assessment

The risk of venous thrombosis depends on the patient's age and co-morbidities, and the nature of the procedure. Surgical procedures can be divided into those with a low, moderate of high risk of venous thrombosis (**Table 1.6**).

Risk assessment of venous thrombosis		
Low risk	Moderate risk	High risk
Age <40 years	Age >40 years	Major orthopaedic surgery on the pelvis, hip or lower limb
Minor surgery	Major medical illness or malignancy	Major pelvis or abdominal surgery for cancer
Short duration	Major trauma or burns	Major trauma or pelvic surgery in patient with previous deep vein thrombosis or pulmonary embolism
No risk factors	Minor surgery in patients with previous deep vein thrombosis or pulmonary embolism	

Table 1.6 Risk assessment of venous thrombosis

Methods of prophylaxis

The risk of venous thromboembolic disease can reduced by patient education and physical and pharmacological mechanisms. Patient education is vital. Women should be advised to stop taking the contraceptive pill 4 weeks before elective surgery. Patients are also informed that immobility before or after surgery increases the risk of venous thrombosis. Before surgery, they should be given information on the risk of DVT and the effectiveness of prophylaxis.

Physical methods

Physical methods of prophylaxis include early mobilisation, graduated compression stockings and intermittent pneumatic compression (e.g. Flowtron boots). Graduated compression stockings reduce the incidence of DVT by 50%. It is recommended that patients wear compression stockings from admission until they resume normal mobility. Intermittent pneumatic compression devices are used during surgery, especially if it is high risk (**Table 1.6**).

Pharmacological methods

Pharmacological methods of prophylaxis invariably involve the use of daily subcutaneous injections of heparin, an acidic mucopolysaccharide (**Figure 1.5**). Unfractionated heparin has a molecular weight of 15 kDa. Low molecular weight heparin has a molecular weight of 5 kDa. Both potentiate antithrombin III activity by inactivating activated clotting factors. The side effects of unfractionated heparin include osteoporosis and thrombocytopenia.

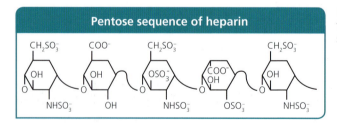

Pentose sequence of heparin

Figure 1.5 Pentose sequence forming part of the molecular structure of heparin.

Perioperative issues

The perioperative period begins when the patient is admitted for surgery and ends when they are stable and comfortable after their operation. Issues to consider in the perioperative period include pain management, fluid balance and the detection of early postoperative complications.

Preoperative fasting

General anaesthesia increases the risk of aspiration of the gastric contents. It is therefore necessary to limit the patient's intake of food and fluids prior to surgery. For elective surgery, patients can be allowed food and clear fluids until 6 hours and 2 hours before surgery, respectively. With emergency surgery, the oral intake should be limited for longer as many surgical emergencies are associated with delayed gastric emptying.

Safe Surgery Checklist

Surgery is inherently dangerous and errors during surgical procedures result in serious complications and even death. There are many contributory factors and these must be reduced to a minimum. Some complications are the result of human error.

In 2008, the World Health Organization proposed a Safe Surgery Checklist (**Table 1.7**). It has three parts – Sign In, Time Out and Sign Out – performed as the patient arrives in the anaesthetic room, before the start of surgery and at the end of the operation, respectively (**Figure 1.6**). Use of the checklist has been shown to reduce the risk of complications and death but errors still occur. These have been described as 'never events' (e.g. surgery on the wrong site or retained surgical instruments or swabs) as they should never occur.

Perioperative hypothermia

Due to the exposure of the skin and internal organs during surgical procedures, patients are at risk of hypothermia. This particularly occurs during operations that open body cavities or involve fluid loss. In addition, general anaesthesia impairs thermoregulatory heat-preserving mechanisms. Perioperative hypothermia (defined as a core temperature below 36.0°C) is a common but preventable complication of surgical procedures. It is prevented by keeping patients warm prior to surgery, the use of hot-air warming blankets and the administration of warmed intravenous fluids during the operation.

Fluid balance

A clear understanding of the size and composition of the body's different fluid compartments is needed to assess the changes that occur in surgical patients and manage them appropriately.

The 'average' 70 kg man has 42 L of total body water, which represents 60% of the body weight. This is made up of 28 L in the intracellular compartment and 14 L in the extracellular compartment. The plasma volume is 3 L and the extravascular volume is 11 L (**Table 1.8**).

There is 4200 mmol of total body sodium, of which 50% is in the extracellular fluid compartment. There is 3500 mmol of total body potassium, of which only 50 mmol is in the extracellular fluid compartment. The normal osmolality of extracellular fluid is 280–295 mosmol/kg.

Maintenance requirements

When calculating fluid replacement, it is necessary to consider:

WHO Safe Surgery Checklist		
Before induction of anaesthesia	**Before skin incision**	**Before patient leaves theatre**
Patient confirms identify and consent	Confirm patient's identity and consent	Confirm procedure performed
Surgical site marked	Confirm surgical site marked if required	Check instrument count is correct
Anaesthetic machine checked	Antibiotic prophylaxis required?	Label and sign any specimens
Any allergies?	Any surgical critical events?	Check any specific issues to be handed over to recovery team
Difficult airway?	Any anaesthetic critical events?	
Risk of >500 mL blood loss	Any imaging displayed?	
Adequate venous access?		

Table 1.7 World Health Organization Safe Surgery Checklist

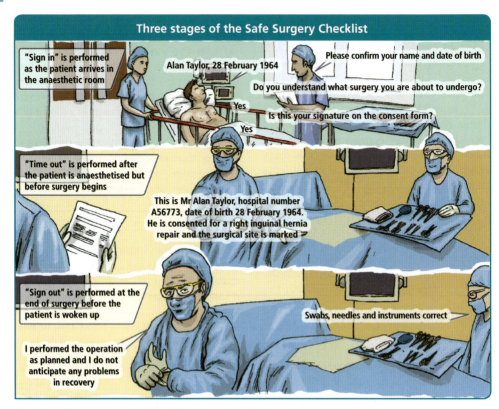

Figure 1.6 The three stages of the Safe Surgery Checklist.

Body fluid compartments		
Compartment	As a percentage of body weight	By volume
Total body water	60%	40 L
Intracellular fluid	40%	25 L
Extracellular fluid (ECF)	20%	15 L
Interstitial fluid	16%: 80% of ECF	12 L
Plasma volume	4%: 20% of ECF	3 L

Table 1.8 Body fluid compartments

- Maintenance requirements
- Pre-existing and ongoing losses
- Insensible losses

Daily maintenance fluid requirements depend on the individual's weight and renal function. For a 70 kg male, daily fluid and electrolyte requirements are about 3 L of water, 120 mmol of sodium and 70 mmol of potassium. For a 40 kg woman, the electrolyte requirements are 90 mmol of sodium and 40 mmol of potassium. The daily maintenance fluid requirements for children can be estimated as follows

- A child weighing 0–10 kg needs 100 mL/kg
- A child of 10–20 kg requires 1000 mL + 50 mL/kg for each kg over 10 kg
- A child of over 20 kg needs 1500 mL + 25 mL/kg for each kg over 20 kg

Pre-existing and other losses

Pre-existing and ongoing losses are rich in electrolytes. Most 'surgical' pre-existing and ongoing losses are rich in sodium and are replaced with 0.9% saline. These include:

- Vomit and diarrhoea
- Nasogastric aspirate
- Stomas, drains and fistula output

Insensible losses occur via the faeces (100 mL/day), the lungs (400 mL/day) and the skin (600 mL/day). Total insensible losses usually amount to about 1 L/day.

Fluid replacement therapy

Fluids can be replaced with crystalloid or colloid solutions. A crystalloid is an aqueous solution of salts, minerals or other water-soluble compounds. A colloid is a homogenous mixture dispersed within a liquid. Crystalloids are cheaper and are more widely used.

The composition of crystalloid solutions varies (**Figure 1.7**). Normal saline contains only sodium and chloride. Hartmann's solution has less chloride but also contains potassium, bicarbonate and calcium. Dextrose saline contains significantly less sodium and chloride in relation to its volume than normal saline. These are isotonic solutions – they have the same osmotic pressure as plasma.

Colloids include gelatins, albumin and starch. After intravenous administration, they disperse throughout the extracellular compartment. Colloids tend to remain in the intravascular space.

Assessment of fluid therapy

Clinical assessment and observations will provide a rough guide to the need for intravenous fluid resuscitation. Tachycardia, hypotension and reduced skin turgor are signs of dehydration. Urine output is a good estimate of the degree of hypovolaemia, with oliguria defined as a urine output of less than 0.5 mL/kg/h. If doubt remains over the extent of hypovolaemia, invasive monitoring and an assessment of central venous pressure should be considered. The response of the urine output or central venous pressure to a fluid challenge is one method to assess the adequacy of resuscitation.

A fluid challenge comprises a 200–250 mL bolus of crystalloid or colloid administered as quickly as possible. A response in the central pressure or urine output is usually seen in all patients within minutes. A rapid rise followed by a prompt fall suggests hypovolaemia. A rapid rise that is maintained indicates adequate intravascular volume replacement. The size and duration of the response is more important than the actual values recorded.

Prevention of infection

Infection is common in all surgical specialties and is one of the most common causes of postoperative morbidity and mortality. In addition, surgical disease often presents with infection (e.g. acute appendicitis and acute diverticulitis) and dictates the need for surgery. Although a surgeon cannot control pathologies that present with acute infection, surgical techniques can reduce the risk of postoperative infection and death. Aseptic surgical techniques, the sterilisation of surgical instruments and the appropriate use of antibiotics are used to do this.

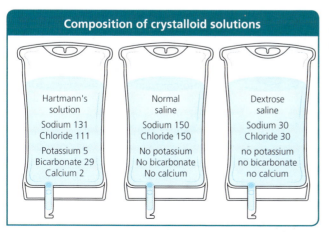

Composition of crystalloid solutions

Hartmann's solution	Normal saline	Dextrose saline
Sodium 131	Sodium 150	Sodium 30
Chloride 111	Chloride 150	Chloride 30
Potassium 5	No potassium	no potassium
Bicarbonate 29	No bicarbonate	no bicarbonate
Calcium 2	No calcium	no calcium

Figure 1.7 Composition of crystalloid solutions. The concentration of solutes is presented in mmol/L.

Asepsis and antisepsis

Antisepsis is the use of chemical solutions for disinfection. It involves removing microorganisms from the skin and reducing the number of skin flora. Asepsis is the complete absence of infectious organisms, usually by using sterile instruments and cloves. Aseptic techniques aim to minimise the risk of infection.

Sterilisation and disinfection

Sterilisation is the removal of all viable microorganisms including spores and viruses. Disinfection is a reduction in the number of viable organisms. These are achieved by different methods, as shown in **Table 1.9**.

> **Surgery must be performed using an aseptic technique.** All surgical instruments and sutures must be sterilised. The use of antiseptic techniques and disinfection is inadequate and subjects the patient to an increased risk of infections.

Antibiotics in surgery

Antibiotics are used to treat established infections or reduce the risk of postoperative sepsis.

Antibiotic prophylaxis is the use of antibiotics to prevent postoperative infections, particularly surgical site infections. The antibiotics are usually administered at the time of induction of anaesthesia via an intravenous route. Only one or a limited number of doses of antibiotics are required.

Methods of sterilisation and disinfection	
Sterilisation	Disinfection
Autoclaves	Low-temperature steam
Hot-air ovens	Boiling water
Ethylene oxide	Chemical disinfectants
Low-temperature steam and formaldehyde	
Irradiation	

Table 1.9 Methods of sterilisation and disinfection

> When planning antibiotic prophylaxis or treatment, consider the likely causative organisms and their antibiotic sensitivities.

Surgical nutrition

Malnutrition is common in surgical patients and results in:

- Delayed wound healing
- Reduced ventilatory capacity and increased risk of respiratory complications
- Reduced immunity
- An increased risk of infection

A nutritional assessment is recommended for all surgical patients. This simplest measure is the patient's BMI. Anthropometric measurements that provide additional information about nutritional status include the thickness of the triceps skin fold, the mid-arm circumference and the hand grip strength. Weight losses of 10% and 30% are regarded as mild and severe malnutrition, respectively.

Intestinal failure can be defined as a reduction in the functioning gut mass to below the minimum necessary for the adequate digestion and absorption of nutrients. It is a useful concept when assessing the need for nutritional support via either the enteral or parenteral route.

> Nutritional support can be given either via the gastrointestinal tract (enteral nutrition) or intravenously (parenteral nutrition).

Enteral nutrition

The gastrointestinal tract is used for nutritional support if it is available and able to absorb nutrients. Prolonged postoperative starvation is not required and feeding of patients in the early postoperative period, even after gastrointestinal surgery, is safe.

Enteral nutrition is cheaper than parenteral nutrition and has fewer complications. The polymeric liquid diet is made up of short peptides, medium-chain triglycerides, polysaccharides, vitamins and trace elements. Enteral feeding is often started at a low rate of infusion (e.g. 25 mL per hour) that is then increased.

Enteral feed can be taken orally or administered via a nasogastric tube. Long-term feeding can be via a surgical gastrostomy or jejunostomy, percutaneous endoscopic gastrostomy or needle-catheter jejunostomy, all of which involve placing a feeding tube directly into the gastrointestinal tract.

> **Early enteral nutrition is associated with reduced postoperative morbidity.** Enteral feeding prevents the intestinal mucosal from atrophy and supports the gut-associated immunological shield. It attenuates the hypermetabolic response to injury and surgery.

Complications of enteral feeding include malposition and blockage of the tube, gastro-oesophageal reflux and intolerance of the feed causing vomiting or diarrhoea.

Parenteral nutrition

Parenteral nutrition is a form of feeding that is given directly into either a peripheral or a central line. It is hyperosmolar and has a low pH. Parenteral nutrition is used for:

- Enterocutaneous fistula
- Moderate or severe malnutrition
- Acute pancreatitis
- Abdominal sepsis
- Prolonged ileus
- Major trauma and burns
- Severe inflammatory bowel disease

A typical parenteral feed contains amino acid, glucose, lipid emulsion, electrolytes, trace elements, water and fat-soluble vitamins. It is usually made up to a volume of 2.5 L and administered over a 24-hour period. The complications of parenteral nutrition are shown in **Table 1.10**.

Complications of parenteral nutrition	
Type	Examples
Metabolic	Fluid overload, hyperglycaemia, hyponatraemia, hyperkalaemia, hyperlipidaemia, vitamin and essential fatty acid deficiency
Infective	Bacteraemia, systemic fungal infection, line sepsis
Mechanical	Venous thrombosis, arrhythmias, air embolism
Other	Gallstone, bone demineralisation

Table 1.10 Complications of parenteral nutrition

Postoperative issues

The main issues that occur in the postoperative period relate to either pain control or the development of postoperative complications.

Pain management

Inadequate pain management is associate with an increased risk of complications and a poor patient experience during recovery from surgery.

Physiology of pain

Pain is defined as an unpleasant sensory and emotional experience associated with potential or actual tissue damage. The level of pain felt by two individuals with a similar degree of tissue damage varies as a result of a complex interaction of sensory, emotional and behavioural factors. Potentially damaging stimuli activate the pain or nociceptive system, which then conveys the information to the brain.

Somatic pain

There are two time courses of pain sensation: first or 'fast' pain, and secondary or 'slow' pain.

'Fast' pain First or 'fast' pain protects the individual by causing a rapid withdrawal from the painful stimulus.

Information on the pain is transmitted from skin receptors to the spinal cord by fast myelinated A fibres. These synapse in the dorsal horn of spinal cord with secondary fibres in the spinothalamic tract. The nerve impulse is transmitted along these to the posterior thalamic nuclei in the brain. From there, tertiary fibres transmit the stimuli to the somatosensory post-central gyrus of the cortex, which is the main area of the brain dealing with touch.

'Slow' pain This is a delayed sensation of pain that leads to behaviour to protect the damaged tissue. It is caused by the stimulation of high-threshold polymodal receptors (receptors that respond to mechanical, thermal and chemical stimuli). This leads to reflex responses such as tachycardia, hypertension and increased RR.

The information is transmitted from the receptors along slow unmyelinated C fibres, which enter the dorsal horn of the spinal cord. Here, they synapse with secondary fibres in the palaeo-spinothalamic tract, and these transmit the stimuli to the medial thalamic nuclei. From here, collateral fibres transmit the information to the midbrain, medullary reticular formation and hypothalamus, and on to the forebrain limbic system responsible for the emotional response to pain.

Gate control theory of pain

The gate control theory of pain (**Figure 1.8**) explains why the relationship between the severity of the injury and the patient's response is not linear. It suggests that pain is 'gated-out' in the dorsal horn by other stimuli or factors such as the person's emotional state.

Spinal level activation occurs in the dorsal horn of the spinal cord. It is a complex interaction between excitatory and inhibitory interneurones found between the afferent and efferent systems. It also involves tracts in the spinal cord that descend from the brain and inhibit the transmissions between neurones.

Visceral pain

There are fewer visceral nociceptors than somatic receptors and they are less densely represented in the cortex of the brain. Therefore visceral pain is poorly localised. It is also qualitatively different due to progressive

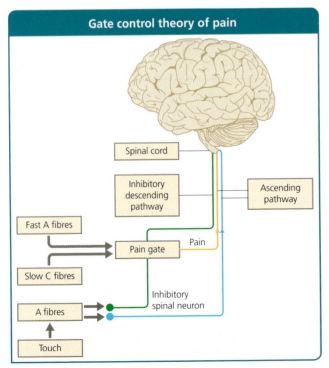

Gate control theory of pain

Spinal cord

Inhibitory descending pathway

Ascending pathway

Fast A fibres

Pain

Pain gate

Slow C fibres

Inhibitory spinal neuron

A fibres

Touch

Figure 1.8 The gate control theory of pain.

stimulation and summation. In addition, it may be referred to a site away from the source of stimulation.

Postoperative pain control

Postoperative pain tends to be inadequately managed by doctors. The adverse effects of postoperative pain are shown in **Table 1.11**.

Assessment of pain

Pain is a subjective experience. An observer's assessment of the patient's behaviour is not reliable enough to measure this. Therefore, pain is assessed and recorded using visual analogue scales, verbal numerical reporting scales and categorical rating scales.

Management of pain

The management of pain can be either pharmacological or non-pharmacological (**Table 1.12**).

Simple analgesia

Paracetamol is a weak anti-inflammatory agent. It is often combined with weak opiates such as dihydrocodeine. Paracetamol acts by reducing prostaglandin production in the central nervous system. It can be given orally, intravenously or rectally and is best taken regularly rather than 'as required'. Overdosing results in hepatic necrosis.

Adverse effects of inadequate pain control	
Respiratory	Reduced cough, atelectasis, sputum retention, hypoxaemia
Cardiovascular	Increased myocardial oxygen consumption, ischaemia
Gastrointestinal	Decreased gastric emptying, reduced gut motility, constipation
Genitourinary	Urinary retention
Musculoskeletal	Reduced mobility, pressure sores, increased risk of venous thrombosis
Neuroendocrine	Hyperglycaemia, protein catabolism, sodium retention
Psychological	Anxiety and fatigue

Table 1.11 Adverse effects of inadequate pain control

Pharmacological and non-pharmacological methods of pain control	
Pharmacological	Non-pharmacological
Simple analgesia	Preoperative explanation and education
Non-steroidal anti-inflammatory agents	Relaxation therapy and hypnosis
Opiates	Cold or heat
Local anaesthetic agents	Splinting of wounds
	Transcutaneous electrical nerve stimulation

Table 1.12 Pharmacological and non-pharmacological methods of pain control

Non-steroidal anti-inflammatory agents

Non-steroidal anti-inflammatory agents (e.g. ibuprofen) inhibit the enzyme cyclooxygenase. They decrease levels of prostaglandin, prostacyclin and thromboxane and also have a weak analgesic effect acting directly on the central nervous system. They are often used to prevent the need for opiates.

Their side effects include gastric irritation and peptic ulceration, bronchospasm in patients with asthma, impairment of renal function and platelet dysfunction and bleeding.

Opiates

The most commonly used opiate is morphine, which acts on mμ receptors in the brain and spinal cord.

Morphine can be administered via several routes. Intramuscular administration produces peaks and troughs in the plasma levels and variable pain relief. Subcutaneous infusion is useful for chronic pain relief, particularly in palliative care. Intravenous injection is reliable but can produce both sedation and respiratory depression. The side effects of morphine include sedation, nausea and vomiting, vasodilatation, myocardial depression, pruritus, delayed gastric emptying, constipation and urinary retention.

With patient-controlled analgesia, the morphine is administered intravenously but the patient determines their own analgesic requirement. A 'lock-out' period prevents accidental overdose. It is a safe means of administration as sedation occurs before respiratory depression.

Local and regional anaesthesia

Local anaesthetic agents act by reducing the permeability of the cell membranes to sodium. They act on the small unmyelinated C fibres before affecting the large A fibres. Therefore, they reduce pain and temperature sensation before touch and power.

Lignocaine has a rapid onset but a short duration of action. If adrenaline/epinephrine is added, the duration of action is increased to 2 hours. The main toxicity relates to the central nervous and cardiovascular systems.

Bupivacaine is chemically related to lignocaine but has a more prolonged onset and longer duration of action. It acts for 6–8 hours.

> **Plain lignocaine, without adrenaline/ epinephrine, is recommended for local anaesthesia of the digits and appendages** such as the ear or penis. The use of adrenaline/epinephrine containing a local anaesthetic solution reduces the blood supply and risks ischaemia.

Spinal and epidural anaesthesia

Spinal anaesthesia is the administration of local anaesthetic or opiate into the cerebrospinal fluid below the termination of the spinal cord at L1. Epidural anaesthesia is the administration of local anaesthetic or opiate into the fatty epidural space (**Figure 1.9**).

Both techniques requires an experienced anaesthetist as complications are common and can often be life-threatening (**Table 1.13**). The quality of the block is often better with a spinal anaesthetic. Contraindications to spinal or epidural anaesthesia are pre-existing neurological disease, known coagulopathy and sepsis.

Postoperative complications

Postoperative complications are common and can lead to significant morbidity and even death if not identified and adequately managed. Early recognition allows early intervention and favours a more positive outcome.

Postoperative pyrexia

Pyrexia (a core temperature >37.5°C) is a common problem after surgery and has both infective or non-infective causes. The underlying reason is often identified clinically from the time since the operation, the type of surgery undertaken and any associated clinical features (**Table 1.14**). Adequate assessment requires a full history and examination supplemented by appropriate investigations.

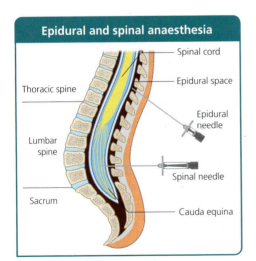

Figure 1.9 Epidural and spinal anaesthesia.

Complications of spinal and epidural anaesthesia			
	Characteristic	Spinal	Epidural
Immediate	Hypotension	Common	Less common
	Anaesthetic toxicity	Rare	Occasional
		Occasional	
	High blockade		Occasional
Early	Urinary retention	Common	Less common
		Rare	
	Headache	Almost never	Never unless dural puncture
	Local infection		
	Meningism	Uncommon	Uncommon
	Epidural haematoma	Rare	Very rare
		Common	Very rare
	Backache		Common

Table 1.13 Complications of spinal and epidural anesthesia

Causes of postoperative pyrexia		
Early (day 1–2)	**Intermediate (day 3–5)**	**Late (after day 5)**
Atelectasis	Pneumonia	Leak of an anastomosis
Aspiration pneumonitis	Superficial wound infection	Deep wound infection
Transfusion reaction	Deep vein thrombosis	Intra-abdominal abscess
Drug reaction		Infected prosthesis
Urinary tract infection		

Table 1.14 Causes of postoperative pyrexia

Respiratory complications often lead to breathlessness, cough and chest pain. Wound infections may cause erythema and purulent discharge. Abdominal pain, distension and ileus suggest an intra-abdominal abscess or a leaking anastomosis. Calf pain and tenderness suggest a DVT.

Potential causes of a postoperative pyrexia (the '6 Cs') are:

- Chest infection
- Catheter-related sepsis
- Cannula-related sepsis
- Cut – surgical site infection
- Collection – intra-abdominal abscess
- Calves – DVT

Investigations to assess a patient with a postoperative pyrexia include:

- Chest radiograph
- Arterial blood gases
- Midstream or catheter urine sampling
- Abdominal ultrasound or CT scan

Sepsis

Sepsis is a multiorgan clinical syndrome that complicates severe infection. It characterised by signs of inflammation occurring in organs away from the site of infection. The systemic inflammatory response syndrome (SIRS) has identical clinical features but is triggered by other conditions such as trauma, hypovolaemic shock, burns and pancreatitis. Both sepsis and SIRS can lead to multiple organ dysfunction. The definitions of sepsis, SIRS, bacteraemia and septic shock are shown in **Table 1.15**.

Definition of bacteraemia, SIRS, sepsis and septic shock	
Bacteraemia	The presence of viable bacteria in the blood stream
SIRS	A systemic inflammatory response with pyrexia (temperature > 38°C), hypothermia (temperature <36°C), tachycardia, tachypnoea and raised white cell count
Sepsis	SIRS with documented infection
Severe sepsis	Sepsis with hypotension and organ dysfunction
Septic shock	Sepsis with hypotension despite adequate fluid resuscitation

Table 1.15 Definition of bacteraemia, systemic inflammatory response syndrome (SIRS), sepsis and septic shock

Sepsis is a common cause of morbidity and death in surgical patients. Its early recognition is essential, in order to reduce complications and save lives. Treatment involves intravenous fluids, high-flow oxygen and the early administration of appropriate antibiotics.

The mnemonic for the immediate management and the investigation of sepsis is O₂ FLUID:

- Oxygen
- Fluids – intravenous
- Lactate measurement
- Urine output
- Infection screen
- Drugs – antibiotics

Wound complications

Wound and surgical site infections are one of the most common postoperative surgical complications.

Wound infections

A surgical wound can become contaminated by direct inoculation from the patient's skin flora or spread from the surgeon's hands or surgical instruments. Airborne contamination can also occur from the atmosphere in the operating theatre. Predisposing factors for wound infections are related to either the patient or the surgical technique (**Table 1.16**). Contaminated wounds are more likely to become infected than clean ones (**Table 1.17**).

Wound infections present with signs of inflammation – pain, redness, heat and sometimes a purulent discharge. The organisms involved usually depends on the type of surgery undertaken. *Staphylococcus aureus* is the organism most commonly involved in superficial skin wounds. Escherichia coli infections often occur after surgery on the gastrointestinal tract.

Prevention of infection is by either exogenous or endogenous methods (**Table 1.18**). Established infections are treated with appropriate antibiotics, based on antibiotic sensitivities, and the drainage of any purulent collections, usually by opening the wound.

Wound dehiscence

Wound dehiscence is a failure of wound closure that can be either superficial or deep, involving all the layers of a surgical wound. Even if the dehiscence seems to affect only part of the wound, it should be assumed that the underlying defect involves the whole wound. It affects about 2% of midline laparotomy wounds, resulting in exposure of the abdominal cavity.

Dehiscence is a serious complication with a mortality of up to 30%. It usually occurs between 7 and 10 days after surgery and is often heralded by a serosanguinous discharge from the wound.

Opiate analgesia should be given and a sterile dressing applied to the wound. Fluid resuscitation is necessary if the patient is hypovolaemic. A prompt return to theatre is necessary, where the wound is resutured under general anaesthesia.

Respiratory complications

Postoperative hypoxia (a reduced partial pressure of oxygen) can occur due to a lack of

Risk factors for wound infections	
Patient factors	Operative
Age	Duration of operation
Poor nutritional status	inadequate skin preparation
Diabetes mellitus	Poor instrument sterilisation
Smoker	Lack of antibiotic prophylaxis
Obesity	Foreign bodies (e.g. drains)
Malignant disease	Poor surgical technique
Immunosuppression	

Table 1.16 Risk factors for wound infections

Characteristics of a wound relative to its microbial content		
Type of wound	Characteristic	Example
Clean	Free from microorganisms	Breast surgery
Clean contaminated	Non-significant contamination	Biliary surgery
Contaminated	Contamination without infection	Colonic surgery
Infected	Infection and inflammation	Acute appendicitis

Table 1.17 Characteristics of a wound relative to its microbial content

Factors to prevent wound infections	
Exogenous factors	Endogenous factors
Sterilisation of instruments	Preoperative skin preparation
Surgical scrub procedures	
	Mechanical bowel preparation
Positive-pressure ventilation in theatre	Antibiotic prophylaxis
Exclusion of staff with infections	Good surgical technique

Table 1.18 Important factors to prevent wound infections

alveolar ventilation or perfusion. The causes are shown in **Table 1.19.**

Atelectasis

Hypoxaemia is a reduction in the arterial partial pressure of oxygen and is often seen during the first 48 hours after major surgery. It occurs as a result of a reduction in functional residual capacity.

Atelectasis is one cause of hypoxaemia and is collapse or closure of the lung resulting in reduced or absent gas exchange. Significant atelectasis is more common in patients with pre-existing lung disease and incisions in the upper rather than the lower abdomen. It also occurs more often in obese individuals and cigarette smokers. The mechanisms underlying atelectasis are:

- An increase in the volume of the bronchial secretions
- An increase in the viscosity of secretions
- A reduction in TV and in the ability to cough

Atelectasis usually presents as a postoperative pyrexia starting about 48 hours after surgery. It is often accompanied by tachycardia and tachypnoea. On examination, there is reduced air entering the lungs, dullness on percussion of the lungs and reduced breath sounds. A chest radiograph may show consolidation (lung tissue filled with fluid) and collapse (reduction in lung volume). The management of atelectasis involves intensive chest physiotherapy, nebulised bronchodilators and appropriate antibiotics for any associated infection.

There is no evidence that prophylactic antibiotics reduce the risk of pneumonia.

Aspiration pneumonitis

Aspiration of the gastric contents results in a chemical pneumonitis (inflammation of the lung tissue) **(Figure 1.10)**. Due to the anatomy of the main bronchi, it most commonly occurs in the apical segments of the right lower lobe. If it is not identified or is inadequately treated, a secondary bacterial infection can result. Secondary infection is usually with Gram-negative and anaerobic organisms.

Immediate treatment involves tilting the head of the operating table down and sucking out the patient's pharynx. Intubation and endotracheal suction should be considered if simple measures fail to result in improvement of the clinical condition. Prophylactic antibiotics are given. There is no evidence that steroids reduce the inflammatory response.

Cardiovascular complications

Postoperative cardiovascular complications include:

- Hypotension
- Hypovolaemia
- Ventricular failure
- Cardiogenic shock
- Arrhythmias

Causes of postoperative hypoxaemia	
Poor alveolar ventilation	Poor alveolar perfusion
Hypoventilation (airway obstruction, opiates)	Ventilation–perfusion mismatch (e.g pulmonary embolism)
Bronchospasm	
Pneumothorax	Impaired cardiac output
Arteriovenous shunting (collapse, atelectasis)	Decreased alveolar diffusion
	Pneumonia
	Pulmonary oedema

Table 1.19 Causes of postoperative hypoxaemia

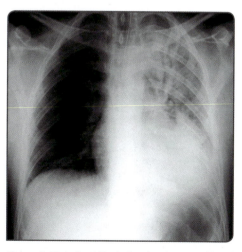

Figure 1.10 A chest X-ray showing pneumonitis affecting the left lung

- Conduction defects
- Hypertension

Perioperative arrhythmias can occur as result of physiological or pathological disturbances. Physiological causes include acidosis, hypercapnoea and hypoxaemia, electrolyte imbalance, and hypovolaemia. Pathological causes include myocardial ischaemia, pulmonary embolus and drugs (medications the patient has been given).

Renal complications

Both acute renal failure and urinary tract infections are common in the postoperative period, particularly in those with underlying comorbidity and patients with a urinary catheter.

Acute renal failure

Acute renal failure is commonly seen in the perioperative period. As it is associated with high morbidity and mortality, it must be either prevented it or recognised and treated early. The causes of postoperative renal failure are classified into prerenal, renal and postrenal (**Table 1.20**):

- Renal hypoperfusion from any cause leads to concentration of urine by the kidney and a decreased urinary output. Therefore, prerenal dysfunction is a normal response to inadequate renal perfusion. Prompt treatment of the precipitating cause may reverse the renal dysfunction. Established renal injury may occur if there is a

superimposed insult such as exposure to a nephrotoxic agent
- Postrenal renal failure occurs when there is obstruction of the urine flow anywhere distal to the renal pelvis. Obstruction is always the most likely diagnosis when there is anuria (a total absence of urine)

> If a patient is anuric (has no urine output), first make sure that the patient does not have a blocked urinary catheter and then look for a post-renal cause or acute renal failure.

Urinary tract infections

Approximately 10% of all surgical patients admitted to hospital have a urinary catheter inserted during their admission. The risk of catheter-related infection depends on the patient's age and sex, how long the catheter has been in place and why it was needed.

Catheters are commonly colonised with bacteria increasing the risk of urinary tract infections: 90% of patients whose catheter has been in situ for more than 2 weeks will develop bacteriuria (bacteria in the urine). The organisms most commonly identified are *Enterobacter* and enterococci. Colonisation does not require treatment unless the patient is systemically unwell. Colonisation can be reduced and infection can be prevented by maintaining a closed drainage system and good infection control standards. Backflow of urine from the catheter bag must also be prevented.

> Consider whether it is essential to insert a catheter. If a catheter is required, it must inserted using an aseptic technique. The catheter must be managed carefully and removed at the earliest opportunity to avoid the risk of catheter-related urinary tract infections.

Postoperative confusion

Postoperative confusion occurs in 10% of postoperative patients. It is associated with increased morbidity and mortality and

Causes of postoperative renal failure		
Prerenal	Renal	Postrenal
Shock	Acute tubular necrosis	Bladder outflow obstruction
Renal artery disease	Glomerulonephritis	Single ureter (calculus, tumour)
	Interstitial nephritis	Both ureters (bladder malignancy)

Table 1.20 Causes of postoperative renal failure

leads to longer stays in hospital. The clinical features include a reduced level of consciousness, impaired thinking and memory, abnormalities of perception (e.g. hallucinations) and disturbances of emotion (e.g. acute anxiety). The causes of postoperative confusion are shown in **Table 1.21**. As hypoxia and hypovolaemia are important factors in the aetiology of postoperative confusion, Patients are given oxygen and intravenous fluids and the underlying cause is identified.

Causes of postoperative confusion	
Cause	Examples
Respiratory	Hypoxia, bronchopneumonia, respiratory failure
Cardiac	Cardiac failure, arrhythmia
Infective	Bacteraemia, cannula or catheter sepsis
Metabolic	Hyponatraemia, hyperkalaemia, hypercalcaemia, vitamin deficiency
Endocrine	Hypothyroidism, hyperthyroidism, Addison's disease
Neoplastic	Primary and secondary cerebral tumours
Drug	Opiate analgesia
Trauma	Head injury

Table 1.21 Causes of postoperative confusion

Answers to starter questions

1. Even simple operations are multistep procedures with risks at each stage: preoperative, intraoperative and postoperative. Patients submit themselves to either a local or general anaesthetic. Surgery is then performed with either local or systemic risks of complication. Surgery involves numerous steps performed by several individuals all of which have the potential for human error. Risk management strategies need to be in place to ensure that the correct operation is performed on the right patient, at the right time, by an appropriately trained practitioner trying to ensure the best possible outcome.

2. Informed consent is the process of getting the patient's permission to undertake the procedure. In order to achieve this the patient must have the capacity to understand what the procedure involves and what are the benefits and risks. They must also be informed of the likely outcome if no treatment is undertaken. Obtaining informed consent takes time and information must be conveyed in a fashion that the patient understands. Patients must not be coerced and their autonomy should be respected at all times

3. As children grow their understanding of the risks and benefits of surgery increases and they become better able to process information presented to them to determine their own treatment. Gillick competence is used to decide whether a child (≤16 years) is able to consent to their own treatment without the need for parental permission.

4. Infective organisms, usually bacteria, occur on patients' and surgeons' skin, and in the surgical environment. They have the potential to cause infective postoperative complications ranging from minor wound infections to potentially life-threatening sepsis. To reduce the threat of postoperative infection, sterilisation of surgical instruments and sutures and surgical skin preparation are used to create asepsis, i.e. the complete absence of infective organisms from the environment.

Answers *continued*

5. Antibiotics are used in surgery to either prevent or treat infection. Antibiotic prophylaxis is the use of antibiotics to prevent postoperative infections, particularly surgical-site infections. Antibiotics should be administered before surgery, usually at the time of induction of anaesthesia and via an intravenous route. Only one or a limited number of doses of antibiotics are required. In the treatment of established infection it is important to take appropriate microbiological cultures before starting antibiotic treatment. Initial choice of antibiotics should be based on the likely organisms involved. This may need to be adapted once cultures and sensitivities are available. Treatment of established infection usually requires administration of antibiotics for several days or weeks.

6. Pain is defined as an unpleasant sensory and emotional experience associated with potential or actual tissue damage. It is often dependent on the presenting pathology or the extent of surgery performed. However, the amount of pain and the response felt by two individuals with a similar degree of tissue damage is variable. This is a result of complex interactions between sensory, emotional and behavioural factors. As a Therefore, the analgesic requirements and the management of pain should be tailored to the individual.

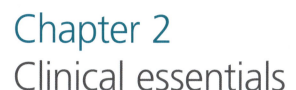

Chapter 2
Clinical essentials

Introduction. 23
Common symptoms of
surgical diagnoses 23
Common signs of surgical
diagnoses 26

Investigations 35
Screening programmes 38
Surgical techniques 39

Starter questions

Answers to the following questions are on page 44.

1. What imaging modalities are used to assess patients with surgical diseases and what are the pros and cons of each?
2. How do you recognise a surgical emergency?
3. How do surgical assessments differ from the assessment of a medical patient?
4. How do patients presenting through screening programmes differ from those presenting with symptoms?
5. Why is a tourniquet useful during surgery and how can it be dangerous?

Introduction

With increasing knowledge and technological advances, general surgery is evolving and surgeons are becoming increasingly specialised. As a result, they work in specific subspecialties during their elective surgical practice. However, many surgical patients still present as emergencies and general surgeons need a broad knowledge and skills in assessing them. They also need core generic surgical skills in order perform safe surgery in both their elective and emergency practice.

Common symptoms of surgical diagnoses

Surgical pathology, in both the elective and the emergency setting, often presents with a lump or pain, either alone or combined. A thorough history and clinical examination often allow a clinical diagnosis to be reached without extensive investigation. In the modern era of increasing technological advancements, the value an accurate clinical assessment and acumen acquired through experience must not be underestimated.

This chapter presents an over view of the common clinical features of both elective and emergency surgical diseases. The general assessment of the patient will be considered. Specific clinical features that indicate potential pathology in various bodily systems or anatomical sites will be discussed in more detail in subsequent chapters.

Pain

Pain is a symptom complained about by a patient. Tenderness is a sign elicited by a clinician.

Everyone experiences pain at some stage in their life. It is an unpleasant sensation of varying intensity. Although many diseases present with pain, it has several features that allow it to be accurately described. Pain is also a common symptom of surgical disease.

> The essential features of pain can be described using the mnemonic SOCRATES:
>
> Site
> Onset
> Character
> Radiation
> Associations
> Timing
> Exacerbating and relieving factors
> Severity

Abdominal pain

Acute abdominal pain is one of the most common presentations of surgical pathology. Many patients undergo emergency admission to hospital with abdominal pain but only about 10% of them proceed to surgery.

Site of pain

The site of abdominal pain can be described by approximately dividing the abdomen into regions. The simplest description is to divide the abdomen into right, left, upper and lower quadrants. Alternatively, the abdomen can be divided into nine regions (**Figure 2.1**).

Due to the embryology of the gastrointestinal tract, pain from the foregut (stomach, duodenum, liver and gallbladder) midgut (small bowel and proximal colon) and hindgut (distal colon) is often felt at different sites (**Figure 2.2**). The site of pain sometimes changes as the disease progresses and some disease processes (e.g. biliary diseases) have characteristic regional sites for pain (**Table 2.1**).

Onset of pain

The onset of pain is either gradual or sudden. A gradual onset with increasing severity is seen in several inflammatory conditions (e.g. acute diverticulitis). A sudden onset, with the exact time recalled by the patient, is seen with a perforated viscus (e.g. perforated peptic ulcer).

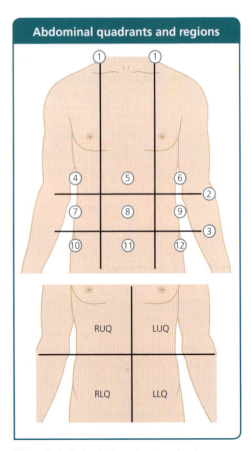

Abdominal quadrants and regions

RUQ   LUQ

RLQ   LLQ

Figure 2.1 Abdominal quadrants and regions. ① Midclavicular lines ② Subcostal plane ③ Transtubercular plane ④ Right hypochondrium ⑤ Epigastric ⑥ Left hypochondrium ⑦ Right lumbar ⑧ Central/umbilical ⑨ Left lumbar ⑩ Right iliac fossa ⑪ Suprapubic/hypogastrium ⑫ Left iliac fossa

Sites of foregut, midgut and hindgut pain

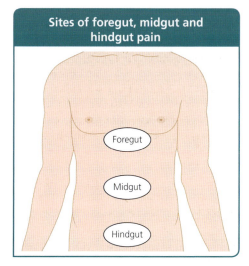

Foregut

Midgut

Hindgut

Figure 2.2 Sites of foregut, midgut and hindgut pain.

Cardinal features of acute inflammation

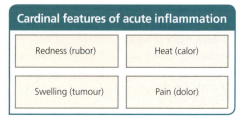

Redness (rubor)	Heat (calor)
Swelling (tumour)	Pain (dolor)

Figure 2.3 Cardinal features of acute inflammation.

improvement or worsening of the pain. For example, the pain associated with peritonitis is relieved by remaining still. On other occasions, the pain improves when the patient moves around. Sometimes the same behaviour produces a different result. For example, taking food sometimes relieves or exacerbates the symptoms.

Abdominal pain often spreads or radiates to other areas within or outside the abdomen. Typical areas of radiation that occur with surgical pathology include the back, shoulder tip, scapula and groin. Abdominal pain is often associated with other symptoms. These include anorexia, nausea, vomiting and a change in bowel habit.

> **Medical conditions that can mimic acute surgical abdominal conditions** include lower lobe pneumonia, myocardial infarction, hypercalcaemia and diabetic ketoacidosis.

Sites of abdominal pain

Site of pain	Examples of possible pathology
Right hypochondrium	Gallbladder disease
Epigastrium	Peptic ulcer disease, abdominal aortic aneurysm, pancreatitis
Central abdomen	Small bowel obstruction, early appendicitis, gastroenteritis
Right iliac fossa	Acute appendicitis, Crohn's disease, pelvic inflammatory disease, ovarian cyst
Left iliac fossa	Diverticulitis, large bowel obstruction, ulcerative colitis, constipation
Suprapubic region	Cystitis, urinary retention, ectopic pregnancy
Loin	Ureteric colic, pyelonephritis

Table 2.1 Characteristic sites of abdominal pain

Nature of pain

The nature of the abdominal pain sometimes indicates its underlying cause. Pain is often described as aching, burning, stabbing or colicky. The character of pain may often change over time. For example, pain that is initially colicky sometimes becomes constant. Pain can also increase or decrease in intensity over time.

Symptomatic improvement is often a reassuring symptom for both the patient and doctor. The patient's behaviour can lead to an

Inflammation

Inflammation is the body's response to tissue injury and is a common cause of surgical pathology. The many causes of inflammation include:

- Physical injury
- Chemical injury
- Infection
- Immunological disorders

The cardinal features of acute inflammation are shown in **Figure 2.3**. Pain is often the main symptom. There is often also a loss of function of the tissue or organ involved.

The clinical features can be explained by hyperaemia (an increase in blood flow), exudation (an increase in capillary permeability)

Outcomes of acute inflammation	
Outcome	Effect
Resolution	Restoration of normal function
Suppuration	Accumulation of pus and abscess formation
Repair and organisation	Replacement of dead tissue with fibrous tissue
Chronic inflammation	Persistent inflammation

Table 2.2 Possible outcomes of acute inflammation

Differential diagnosis of a leg ulcer	
Cause	Examples of possible pathology
Venous	Chronic venous hypertension, varicose veins
Arterial	Chronic limb ischaemia
Neuropathic	Diabetes mellitus, neurological disorder
Traumatic	Trauma, pressure sores
Neoplastic	Squamous cell carcinoma, basal cell carcinoma
Infective	Syphilis, tuberculosis
Other	Pyoderma gangrenosum

Table 2.3 Differential diagnosis of a leg ulcer

and the migration of white cells. The inflammatory process is influenced by the body's physical and immunological response to the initial insult resulting in four possible outcomes of acute inflammation (**Table 2.2**), which also affect the clinical features.

Ulceration

An ulcer is defined as a break in the continuity of an epithelial surface. Ulcers occur on any surface that has an epithelial covering and have numerous causes. Various disease processes causes ulcers at specific sites.

The leg is one of the most common sites of ulceration. The differential diagnosis of a leg ulcer is shown in **Table 2.3**. Venous ulcers are usually found on the lower medial third of the lower limb. Arterial ulcers are usually found on the toes and the heal. Neoplastic ulcers often occur on sun-exposed skin.

Common signs of surgical diagnoses

The physical examination begins with the measurement of vital signs and a general assessment of the patient. This is followed by a clinical examination that focuses on the underlying organ system.

General appearance

Looking at the patient's general appearance usually suggests whether they have a significant illness and hence indicates the urgency of investigation and treatment. This is often referred to as the 'end-of-the-bed-o-gram' (**Figure 2.4**).

An initial rapid assessment identifies significant physiological derangement, particularly if the patient appears pale or sweaty, is confused, is hyperventilating or is restless. Some diseases (e.g. thyrotoxicosis or Cushing's syndrome) have almost pathognomic signs that are instantly recognised by an experienced clinician. The inability to give a coherent history is a worrying sign.

The examination sometimes reveals cachexia and loss of weight. In patients with abdominal pathology, it is important to assess the degree of dehydration. The physical signs of dehydration are showed in **Table 2.4**.

The vital signs of temperature, pulse, blood pressure and respiratory rate are recorded for all patients presenting as an emergency. These provide objective evidence of physiological normality or derangement.

Body temperature

The body/s normal temperature is between 36.5°C and 37.5°C. It is tightly controlled by the hypothalamus and thermoregulatory mechanisms. However, in many medical conditions it is raised or lowered.

An increase in core temperature is known as a pyrexia and is often a sign of inflammation or infection. Both the extent and pattern of the

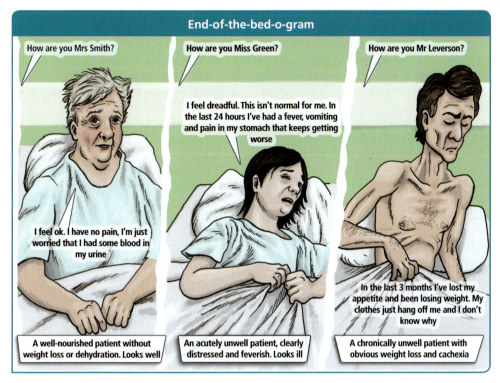

Figure 2.4 'End-of-the-bed-o-gram'.

Signs of dehydration	
Mild (<5%)	Moderate (5–8%)
Mild thirst	Moderate thirst
Dry mucous membranes	Reduced skin turgor
Concentrated urine	Increased heart rate
Severe (9–12%)	Severe (>12%)
Significant thirst	Comatose
Collapsed veins	Moribund
Sunken eyes	Signs of shock
Postural hypotension	
Reduced urine output	
Percentage is of total body water	

Table 2.4 Signs of dehydration

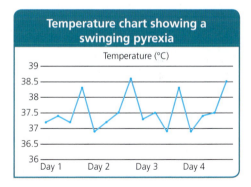

Figure 2.5 Temperature chart showing a swinging pyrexia.

pyrexia give an indication of the underlying cause. Some diseases (e.g. acute appendicitis) show a minimal elevation in temperature while others (e.g. acute pyelonephritis) often cause a high fever. A swinging pyrexia (**Figure 2.5**) fluctuates with time and often occurs with intra-abdominal abscesses.

Pulse and blood pressure

The normal resting pulse rate in adults is between 60 and 90 beats per minute. Tachycardia (an increase in resting pulse rate) is general regarded as being more than 100 beats per minute. Bradycardia (a decrease in resting pulse rate) is a pulse rate of less than 60 beats per minute. Tachycardia is a common observation in patients undergoing emergency surgery and often is an appropriate response to a pyrexia or a sign of hypovolaemia.

The normal blood pressure varies with sex and age. Blood pressure is higher in men and increases with age. As a general rule, a systolic blood pressure of less than 100 mmHg is called hypotension.

Cardiovascular observations are more useful when combined with measurements of vital signs than when used in isolation. For example, a combination of increasing hypotension and tachycardia in a surgical patient indicates an increasing level of hypovolaemic shock (**Table 2.5**).

Respiratory rate

A normal respiratory rate is less than 15 breaths per minute. An increase in respiratory rate in a surgical patient often indicates pulmonary pathology (e.g. atelectasis or an aspiration pneumonia) or hypovolaemia and a metabolic acidosis.

The summation of vital scores provides an early warning score. The higher the score, the greater the degree of physiological derangement. An example of a early warning score is shown in **Table 2.6**. This can be supplemented by simple invasive measurements such as recording urinary output.

> If the initial assessment and measurement of vital signs indicate that patient is in extremis, resuscitation and life-saving interventions are required before a detailed history and examination is performed.

Description of a lump

Certain principles are used to describe a lump in any part of the body. Following a consistent approach allows an accurate assessment to be performed, recorded and conveyed to others.

Vital signs in hypovolaemic shock				
Vital sign	Class 1	Class 2	Class 3	Class 4
% Blood loss	<15%	15–30%	30–40%	>40%
Pulse rate (beats per minute)	<100	>100	>120	>140
Systolic blood pressure	Normal	Normal	Decreased	Decreased
Respiratory rate (breaths per minute)	14–20	20–30	30–40	>40
Urine output (mL per hour)	>30	20–30	<30	Negligible

Table 2.5 Vital signs in different classes of hypovolaemic shock

Variables and scores of an early warning system							
Variable	3	2	1	0	1	2	3
Heart rate (beats per minute)		≤40	41–50	51–100	101–110	111–130	≥130
Mean blood pressure (mmHg)	≤70	71–80	81–100	101–199		≥200	
Respiration (breaths per minute)		≤8		9–14	15–20	21–29	≥30
Temperature		≤35	35.1--36.5		36.6–37.4	≥37.5	
Level of consciousness				Awake	Responds to voice	Responds to pain	No response

Table 2.6 Physiological variables and scores of an early warning system

A lump can be described in relation to its:

- Site
- Shape
- Size
- Surface
- Edge
- Colour
- Composition
- Temperature
- Tenderness
- Reducibility
- Relation to surrounding structures

The site of the lump is recorded in exact anatomical terms in relation to fixed landmarks. Lumps are three-dimensional structures and are also described in relation to their shape, size and surface appearance. The size is measured in several dimensions, particularly if the lesion is asymmetrical. The measurement is more accurate if performed with a tape measure or calipers.

The edge of the lesion is eithe clearly defined or indistinct. Measuring the temperature indicates whether the lesion is hot or at body temperature. The lump is also recorded as tender or non-tender.

The different composition of lumps often results in a characteristic feel. The consistency of a lump varies from soft to very hard depending on both the structure from which it arises and the tension within the lump. Other features assessed in relation to consistency are:

- **Fluctuation** – pressure on the lump causing it to protrude at the side
- **Fluid thrill** – a percussion wave that is conducted across the lump
- **Translucency** – the appearance when a light is held against the lump
- **Resonance** – whether the lump sounds hollow when tapped
- **Pulsatility** – which suggests a connection to the arterial system
- **Compressibility and reducibility** – whether it reduces in size or disappears with pressure

Finally, the regional lymph nodes are examined, and the lump is auscultated to determine whether it has a bruit.

Abdominal examination

Abdominal examination follows the sequence of inspection, palpation, percussion and auscultation.

The patient lies flat with their head comfortably supported on a pillow. The abdomen is exposed from 'the nipples to the knees' while respecting the patient's modesty as much as possible. It is acceptable to cover the groin and genitalia for most of the examination, but they must be examined at the appropriate points.

Inspection

On inspection, the abdomen may appear normal or distended. There are often scars from previous surgical procedures. The position of these is noted and an explanation sought for surgical incisions that have not previously been declared. The movement of the abdomen with respiration is assessed. Large abdominal masses are sometimes seen and, depending on the underlying pathology, may be pulsatile. The groins are inspected for hernias.

Palpation

The flat of the hand is used to palpate the abdomen. The examiner kneels on the floor so that their shoulder is positioned at a similar height to their hand.

The abdomen is first gently palpated to elicit any obvious tenderness. Deep palpation allows obvious masses to be identified (**Figure 2.6**). The presence of hepatomegaly (an enlarged liver) or splenomegaly (an enlarged spleen) is also sought (**Figure 2.7**).

Signs of peritoneal inflammation include:

- Rigid abdomen – involuntary contraction of all the abdominal muscles
- Guarding – involuntary localised contraction of the abdominal muscles
- Rebound tenderness – pain and involuntary contraction on release of pressure
- Percussion tenderness – pain and involuntary contraction on percussion

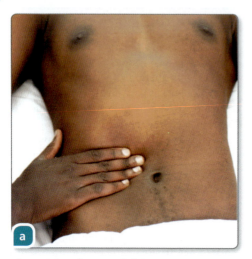

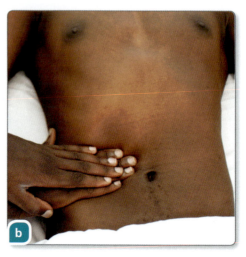

Figure 2.6 Techniques of abdominal palpation

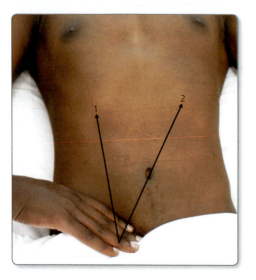

Figure 2.7 Technique for eliciting hepatomegaly (1) and splenomegaly (2).

Percussion

Percussion is performed by placing the spread, flattened fingers of the left hand on the abdomen and gently tapping this hand with the middle finger of the right hand. The sound that is produced will vary according to whether there is a solid or a fluid-filled cavity below the fingers. Solids organs (e.g the liver or spleen) and lesions are dull to percussion (**Figure 2.8**). Gas-filled organs (e.g the stomach) and cavities are tympanic.

Shifting dullness is elicited by first percussing the abdomen with the patient supine and then asking them to roll onto their side (**Figure 2.9**). Ascites is present if the flanks are initially dull to percussion but become tympanic as the patient rolls to the side.

The presence of a fluid thrill transmitted across the abdomen is also a sign of ascites (**Figure 2.10**).

Auscultation

Auscultation of the abdomen is the use of a stethoscope to listen to the bowel sounds. The diaphragm of the stethoscope is placed in the centre of the abdomen.

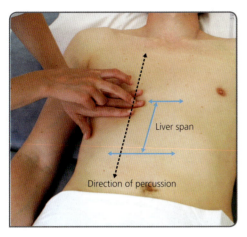

Figure 2.8 Technique of abdominal percussion.

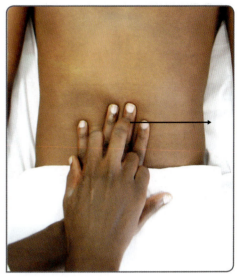

Figure 2.9 Technique for eliciting shifting dullness.

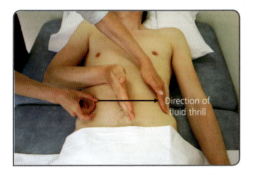

Figure 2.10 Technique for eliciting fluid thrill.

The bowel sounds are either normal or high-pitched. High-pitched, 'tinkling' bowel sounds are present in intestinal obstruction. If bowel sounds are absent, an ileus is present.

Auscultation also allows a bruit, a noise created by turbulent blood flow, to be detected.

Rectal examination

A rectal examination is an important part of all abdominal examinations (**Figure 2.11**). The patient must be informed about the examination to be performed. They then adopt the left lateral position, with the knees flexed to 90°. The anal skin is first inspected for lumps, ulceration and scars.

A gloved finger is then inserted into the anal canal and the tone of the anal sphincter is observed. Tenderness and lumps within the

anal canal are also noted. The presence, absence and firmness of any stool are recorded. The lower rectal mucosa is then felt by gently moving the finger around the circumference of the rectum. If a lump is felt, an assessment is made of whether it is within or outside the rectum.

In men, the prostate gland is palpated and a note is made of its size, its shape, the presence of any nodules and whether the medial groove is maintained. In women, the cervix can be felt and any tenderness or irregularity recognised.

Finally, when the gloved finger is removed, the presence or absence of blood, fresh or dark is sought.

> During any intimate examination such as a rectal examination, the patient's dignity must be maintained at all times. Implied consent must be obtained. A chaperone should be offered to all patients.

Abdominal distension

In women, pregnancy is the most common cause of abdominal distension, with the

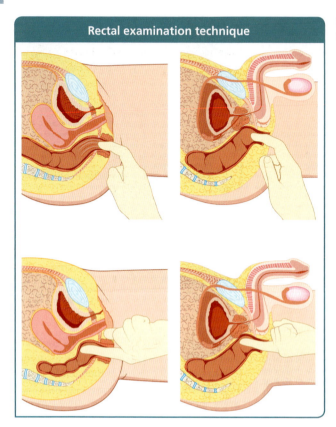

Rectal examination technique

Figure 2.11 Technique of rectal examination in a woman and man.

gravid uterus reaching the umbilicus by 22 weeks of gestation. However, abdominal distension is a common sign of surgical disease and determining its cause can be challenging. The presence of specific physical signs often allows the underlying pathology to be determined.

Gas within any part of the intestine can cause considerable distension, and visible peristalsis of the small intestine is sometime seen seen in patients with small bowel obstruction. Gently shaking the patient may cause a splashing sound or succussion splash in those with gastric distension due to gastric outlet obstruction. Faecal impaction presents with abdominal distension or a palpable abdominal mass. Faecal masses usually lie in the periphery of the abdomen and are indentable.

With obesity becoming more common in the developed world, abdominal adiposity is increasingly seen as a cause of an enlarged abdominal girth.

The causes of abdominal distension can be remembered by the six 'F's:

- Fetus
- Faeces
- Flatus
- Fat
- Fluid
- Fibroids

Abdominal masses

There are numerous causes of abdominal masses (**Table 2.7**).

When an abdominal mass is identified, it is described as for any other lump. Its site is recorded in relation to either the quadrants or regions (Figure 2.1) of the abdomen. Its site, shape and surface contour are assessed. Tenderness often indicates the presence of infection or ischaemia. Pulsation usually indicates the presence of an aneurysm. An at-

Causes of abdominal masses	
Right iliac fossa	Left iliac fossa
Appendix abscess	Faeces
Carcinoma of the caecum	Carcinoma of the
Crohn's disease	sigmoid colon
Ovarian cyst or tumour	Diverticular abscess
Psoas abscess	Ovarian cyst or tumour
Hernia	Psoas abscess
Transplanted kidney	Hernia
	Transplanted kidney
Upper abdomen	Pelvis
Abdominal aortic aneurysm	Distended bladder
Retroperitoneal lymphadenopathy	Ovarian cyst or tumour
Pancreatic pseudocyst	Uterus – pregnancy or fibroids
Carcinoma of the stomach	
Carcinoma of the transverse colon	
Omental mass	

Table 2.7 Causes of abdominal masses

Differential diagnosis of a groin lump	
Above inguinal ligament	Below inguinal ligament
Inguinal hernia	Femoral hernia
Undescended testis	Lymph node
Hydrocele of the cord	Saphena varix
Lipoma of the cord	Femoral artery aneurysm

Table 2.8 Differential diagnosis of a groin lump

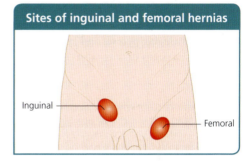

Sites of inguinal and femoral hernias

Figure 2.12 Anatomical sites of inguinal and femoral hernias. An inguinal hernia occurs above and medial to the pubic tubercle. A femoral hernia occurs below and lateral to pubic tubercle.

tempt should be made to assess whether the lump moves with respiration and whether it is reducible, suggesting the presence of a hernia.

> **When examining the abdomen, remember also to examine the supraclavicular lymph nodes, hernial orifices, genitalia and rectum.** An incomplete examination means that important clinical signs are occasionally missed.

Hernias

A hernia is a protrusion of an organ through the wall that contains it. Although hernias occur at many different sites of the body, the abdomen is the most common.

Inguinal and femoral hernias are the most frequent presentation. On examination, a lump is often obvious in the groin. In the absence of complications, this is non-tender and reducible. It may be possible to demonstrate a cough impulse.

The position of the lump in the groin usually allows inguinal and femoral hernias to be

differentiated (**Table 2.8**). Firstly, it is important to determine whether the lump is above or below the inguinal ligament. The inguinal ligament runs between the pubic tubercle and the anterior superior iliac spine. If the lump lies above and medial to the pubic tubercle, it is likely to be an inguinal hernia. If it is below and lateral to the pubic tubercle, it is likely to be a femoral hernia (**Figure 2.12**).

The level of clinical concern is greater if the lump is red, tender and irreducible. These are signs of strangulation.

> **If a patient provides a history of a groin lump but no hernia is apparent,** ask the patient to stand up as hernias are easier to identify in the erect position.

Abscesses

An abscess is a localised collection of pus that usually occurs within the soft tissues. It is a response to acute inflammation and is often seen when the patient's response to the infection is inadequate. Predisposing factors include a foreign body (e.g. a suture or drain) in a wound, haematoma formation or the presence of ischaemic or necrotic tissue.

Abscesses that occur in the superficial tissues (e.g. infected sebaceous cysts) may be clinically obvious. They often appear as a red and tender lump. An untreated abscess may fluctuate and 'point'. If it remains untreated, the abscess will often eventually discharge spontaneously.

Deep abscesses (e.g. an appendix abscess) usually present with systemic signs of infection (e.g. a swinging pyrexia and tachycardia). Local physical signs of deep abscesses are often difficult to demonstrate.

> **Fluctuation occurs when a lump is full of fluid.** It is elicited by applying pressure on one surface (usually the top) of the lump and feeling expansion in two other directions (usually the sides).

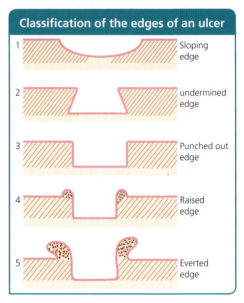

Classification of the edges of an ulcer

1 — Sloping edge
2 — undermined edge
3 — Punched out edge
4 — Raised edge
5 — Everted edge

Figure 2.13 Classification of the edges of an ulcer

Ulcers

The examination of an ulcer follows the same principles as that of a lump and a number of features need to be recorded. The site, shape and dimensions of the ulcer help to identify the likely underlying pathology and assess whether treatment is leading to an improvement in the ulcer over time. Caliper measurements or clinical photographs are often useful for recording purposes.

The edge

The edge of an ulcer is the most important part to assess as this is the junction between the healthy and diseased tissue. Benign and malignant underlying disease processes often display characteristic forms. The edges of an ulcer are described as sloping, punched out, undermined, rolled or everted (**Figure 2.13**).

The base

The base of the ulcer must be carefully examined. Overlying necrotic tissue is removed if necessary so the ulcer's base is seen.

The base of the ulcer may comprise granulation tissue, dead tissue or tumour. Granulation tissue is made up fine capillaries and fibroblasts and has a red velvety appearance. A thin rim of pink epithelium at the edge indicates that the ulcer is healing. Dead tissue is called slough and often has a green or black colour. Tumour tissue is often very vascular but does not have the same healthy appearance as granulation tissue.

Recognisable structures such as bone or tendons are occasionally visible.

Depth and discharge

The discharge from an ulcer can be described as serous, sanguinous or purulent. The quantity of the discharge is assessed by direct observation or from the state of the dressings. The condition of the local tissue and regional lymph nodes is also assessed.

> **The clinical appearance of an ulcer can be described using the mnemonic BEDS:**
>
> - **Base** – colour and appearance
> - **Edge** – flat, punched out, rolled, everted
> - **Depth and discharge** – serous or purulent discharge
> - **Surroundings** – skin changes, colour

Surgical sieve

Having taken a detailed history and performed an appropriate clinical examination, it is then necessary to formulate a differential diagnosis. The 'surgical sieve' is a useful aid for structuring thoughts on the possible cause. This ensures that all aetiological factors are considered and a potentially important diagnosis is not omitted.

> **The mnemonic MIDNITE is the best to use for remembering the surgical sieve:**
> - Metabolic
> - Inflammatory
> - Degenerative
> - Neoplastic
> - Infective
> - Traumatic
> - Endocrine

Investigations

Investigations are used to confirm or refute the differential diagnosis. If a thorough history and examination have not been completed, it is likely that inappropriate investigations will be requested. This is costly and subjects the patient to inappropriate risk.

> **The overuse of investigations is no substitute for an adequate clinical assessment.** When requesting an investigation, consider what information will be obtained and how that will influence the patient's management.

Common blood tests in surgical patients	
Test	Relevance
Full blood count	Blood loss, presence of infection
Urea and electrolytes	Dehydration, hypovolaemia, adequacy of resuscitation
Liver function tests	Jaundice
Amylase	Pancreatitis
Clotting screen	Jaundice, clotting disorders, major haemorrhage
Group and save	Prior to anticipated blood loss or transfusion

Table 2.9 Common blood tests in surgical patients

Blood tests

Blood tests are often the initial investigations when assessing a surgical patient. Investigations may be diagnostic, allow an assessment of disease severity or provide an indication of the patient's fitness for a surgical procedure. Blood tests commonly performed for surgical patients are shown in **Table 2.9**.

No blood tests are regarded as diagnostic as all have some degree of limitation of either sensitivity or specificity. For example, the measurement of serum amylase is useful in the diagnosis of acute pancreatitis, but sometimes it may be only minimally increased. It is also often raised in other conditions such as a perforated peptic ulcer or intestinal ischaemia.

Arterial blood gases

Arterial blood gases are measured on blood drawn from an accessible artery. This is commonly the radial artery. The sample is used to measure both the partial pressures of oxygen and carbon dioxide and the arterial pH. Other variables are derived using the Henderson–Hasselbach equation and are summarised in **Table 2.10**. Arterial blood gas analysers also measure arterial lactate levels and are useful in the assessment of a patient's acid-base status.

Derangements of acid–base status are common in emergency surgical patients, and a metabolic acidosis often occurs. Assessment of the acid–base balance is a useful measure

Variables reported by a blood gas analyser	
Variable	Normal values
Temperature	37°C
pH	7.36–7.44
Partial pressure of carbon dioxide	4.6–5.6 kPa
Partial pressure of oxygen	10.0–13.3 kPa
Bicarbonate	22–26 mmol/L
Total carbon dioxide	24–28 mmol/L
Standard bicarbonate	22–26 mmol/L
Base excess	−2 to +2 mmol/L
Standard base excess	−3 to +3 mmol/L
Oxygen saturation	More than 95%
Haemoglobin	11.5–16.5 g/dL

Table 2.10 Variable reported by a blood gas analyser

of the severity of physiological disturbances. It also has a role in monitoring the response to resuscitation.

Plain radiography

Plain radiographs are simple and cheap to acquire and are universally available. They have limited sensitivity and specificity and their limitations need to be understood. However, some plain radiographs have uses in the assessment of surgical patients, including plain abdominal radiographs, erect chest radiographs and kidney–ureter–bladder radiographs. The indications for these are discussed in later chapters.

When interpreting radiographs, it is important to have a mental schema to ensure that they are the correct radiographs of the correct patient and that an appropriate assessment is made of them. A good outline for performing the initial assessment of a radiograph is as follows:

- Check the name of the patient and the date of the investigation
- Check the projection or view of the film and confirm that an adequate area has been covered
- Check the exposure and consider under- or overexposure

- Comment on any obvious artefacts
- Follow a routine to look at the bone and the hollow and solid organs
- Make sure the whole film is viewed and compared with any previous films that are available

Ultrasound

Ultrasound is non-invasive imaging technique that has several well recognised uses in the assessment of surgical patients, for example imaging solid organs such as the liver and gallbladder and assessing vascular disease.

Ultrasound is cheap and easily available, but the quality and interpretation of the images obtained depend on the user. Many different types of image are produced. The most well known is B-mode ultrasound, which displays a two-dimensional cross-section of the tissue being imaged. Doppler ultrasound is used to measure blood flow.

CT scanning

CT scanning is based on the ability to differentiate between different anatomical structures depending on the variation in how X-rays are absorbed by different tissues. Modern spiral scanners can rapidly acquire data in thin slices. The information is then manipulated by computer to convert two-dimensional data into high-resolution three-dimensional tomographic (sliced) images in different planes. Images are acquired relatively quickly but the radiation dose is high.

In surgical patients, CT scanning is used to image the thorax, abdomen and pelvis. It allows pathology to be confirmed and cancers to be staged.

Radiation exposure from different investigations varies significantly. The radiation dose from an abdominal CT scan is about 500 times more than that from a chest radiograph. Excessive radiation exposure has the potential to induce tissue damage.

Magnetic resonance imaging

MRIs uses magnetic fields that are rapidly switched on and off around the patient. Hydrogen atoms are energized by these oscillating magnetic fields at various resonant frequencies. The images are acquired by detecting the radiofrequency signals that are emitted. Different frequencies are emitted by different tissues as the excited hydrogen ions return to their state of equilibrium.

As MRI does not involve the use of radiation, the scanners are generally safe. However, some patients find them claustrophobic. Implanted metal objects can potentially be moved by the strong magnetic fields. Therefore, caution is required in patients with cochlear implants, cardiac pacemakers and metallic foreign bodies in their orbits. However, modern surgical implants are often made of titanium and are not affected by magnetic fields. MRI scans are relatively expensive and acquiring the images is a slow process sometimes taking up to an hour.

MRI scanning has increasing utility in the assessment of surgical patients. It is used to assess the biliary tree without the need for endoscopy. It is also be used to assess the arterial tree without the risk associated with vascular puncture and angiography.

Interventional radiology

Interventional radiology uses minimally invasive, image-guided procedures to diagnose and treat diseases. In many specialties, (e.g vascular surgery) it has been proved to be a useful adjunct to surgery, and in some areas it has replaced surgical intervention. Using percutaneous or endoluminal techniques, ultrasound and CT scanning can be used to enter body cavities or organs and perform procedures. However, this is not always successful, has associated risks and needs surgical support if complications occur.

> **Interventional radiology is expensive and time-consuming.** However, it often spares patients from more extensive surgery associated with higher risks and longer recovery periods.

Many patients with arterial disease who would previously have been treated with surgical bypass procedures can now be managed by radiologists using angiography, balloon angioplasty and stenting. Intra-abdominal abscesses resulting from primary pathology (e.g. an appendix or diverticular abscess) can be managed by percutaneous drainage.

Microbiology

Sepsis is a common cause of surgical pathology and one of the most common complications of surgical procedures. It can vary from minor wound infections to life-threatening septic shock.

Management requires the appropriate collection and processing of microbiological specimens. Common specimens include blood, urine and tissue fluids or pus, which should be transported directly to the laboratory.

When possible, the samples are taken before the patient starts taking antibiotics. The choice of antibiotic therapy is based on the likely infecting organism known to cause specific diseases or complications. However, it may need to be adjusted once antibiotic sensitivities are available.

> **When possible, microbiological samples are taken before the patient is started on antibiotics.** This will increase the chances of identifying the causative organism so that an appropriate treatment can be instigated.

Screening programmes

Most patients with surgical disease present to either their general practitioner or the emergency department with symptoms or signs that require further investigation. However, some diseases (e.g. breast or colorectal cancer) are present for a period of time before they cause symptoms. For these, it is possible to test individuals to detect the disease before it becomes symptomatic. Asymptomatic healthy individuals are contacted and invited to attend for the investigation. This process allows early intervention and improves the outcome, measured in terms of population mortality.

To justify the establishment of a screening programme, various criteria must be met in relation to the disease, test and treatment (**Table 2.11**). A mnemonic to remember the criteria is IATROGENIC:

- Important – the condition should be common
- Acceptable treatment is available for the disease
- Treatment and diagnostic facilities are available
- Recognisable at an early stage of symptoms
- Opinions on who to treat as patients must be agreed
- Guaranteed safety of the test
- Examination must be acceptable to the patient
- Natural history of the disease must be known
- Inexpensive test

- Continuous or repeated screening is available

> **The success of screening programme** is judged by whether there is a reduction in population mortality from the disease once the programme has been implemented.

Cancer screening programmes have been established, for example, in the UK's National Health Service (**Table 2.12**). Various biases within screening programmes can sometimes skew the apparent success of screening programmes (**Table 2.13**).

Sensitivity and specificity

A screening test, like any other investigation, can give either a positive or negative result.

UK cancer screening programmes			
Disease	Test	Age range (years)	Frequency (years)
Breast	Mammograms	47–70	3
Cervix	Cervical smear	25–49 and 50–64	3 and 5 (respectively)
Bowel	Faecal occult blood	60–69	2

Table 2.12 UK National Health Service cancer screening programmes

Criteria for an effective screening programme		
Disease	Test	Treatment
Common and important problem	A specific and sensitive test exists	Appropriate treatment options exist
Natural history of the disease is established	The test is acceptable with a high uptake	Treatment for asymptomatic disease reduces the population mortality
	Facilities must exist to implement the test	Benefits of screening outweigh any adverse effects
		Financial costs are acceptable

Table 2.11 Criteria for an effective screening programme

Potential biases in a screening programme	
Bias	Definition
Selection bias	Patients select themselves into a treatment group by attending for screening
Lead time bias	Early detection appears to improve survival by increasing the time from diagnosis to death but mortality remains unchanged. The patient is simply aware that they have the disease for longer
Length bias	Slower growing tumours with a better prognosis are more likely to be detected by screening

Table 2.13 Potential biases within a screening programme

Possible outcomes of an investigation	
Outcome	Definition
True positive	A positive test result in the presence of the disease
True negative	A negative test result in the absence of the disease
False positive	A positive test result in the absence of the disease
False negative	A negative test result in the presence of the disease

Table 2.14 Possible outcomes of an investigation

The does not, however, imply that the patient does or does not have the disease.

There are four possible outcomes of a test (**Table 2.14**). The sensitivity of a test is the ability of the test to detect the presence of the disease. The specificity of a test is the ability to exclude the disease in the absence of the disease. Tests are ideally both 100% specific and 100% sensitive. However, this is not seen in practice.

Surgical techniques

A limited number of surgical principles and techniques are fundamental to all types of surgery. Before surgeons undertake complex surgery, they need to understand these basic principles. They also need to master the surgical techniques, such as making an incision and suturing a wound closure, that are fundamental to all types of surgery.

Surgical incisions

Incisions need to allow access to the surgical site and also:

- Allow adequate access to perform safe surgery
- Be capable of being extended to improve access to the operative field
- Be able to be closed with a low risk of complications
- Be associated with minimal pain
- Have a good cosmetic result when healed

Commonly used abdominal incision are shown in **Figure 2.14.**

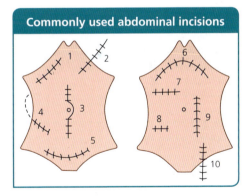

Commonly used abdominal incisions

Figure 2.14 Commonly used abdominal incisions. ① Kocher. ② Thoracoabdominal. ③ Midline. ④ Muscle splitting loin. ⑤ Pfannenstiel. ⑥ Gable. ⑦ Transverse muscle splitting. ⑧ Lanz. ⑨ Paramedian. ⑩ McEvedy.

Open versus laparoscopic surgery

Minimal access surgery reduces the trauma associated with access to body cavities without compromising the ability to perform the operation adequately. The most common forms of minimal access surgery are use laparoscopy and thoracoscopy to access the abdomen and thorax, respectively. The advantages and disadvantages of minimal access surgery are shown in **Table 2.15.**

Robotic surgery has recently been developed. This uses three-dimensional technology and even smaller instrumentation to extend the scope and range of minimally invasive surgery.

Diathermy

Diathermy is the use of a high-frequency electrical current to produce heat. The technique is used to cut tissue or produce coagulation. The electrical frequency used in diathermy is in the range of 300 kHz to 3 MHz, compared with 50 Hz for mains electricity. In diathermy, the patient's body forms part of the electrical circuit but the current has little effect on the muscles and myocardium. As a result of its lower frequency, mains electricity leads to intense activation of the muscles and nerves.

Monopolar diathermy

With monopolar diathermy (**Figure 2.15**), an electrical plate placed on the patient acts as a neutral or indifferent electrode. The current flows between the instrument and this electrode. As the surface area of the instrument is an order of magnitude less than that of the area of the plate, localised heating is produced at the tip of instrument and a minimal heating effect is at the indifferent electrode.

The effects of diathermy depend on the intensity and waveform of the current. Coagulation is produced by interrupted pulses of current (at 50–100 pulses per second) and a square waveform. Cutting is achieved using a continuous current with a sinus waveform.

Diathermy does, however, carry risks. Metal instruments and implants occasionally produce arcing. Superficial burns can occur due to ignition of spirit-based skin preparations. Burns are also seen under the indifferent electrode if the plate is not properly applied. In addition, channelling effects and tissue damage will occur if diathermy is used on a viscus with a narrow pedicle (e.g. the penis or testis).

Minimally invasive surgery	
Advantages	Disadvantages
Less tissue trauma	Lack of tactile feedback
Less postoperative pain	Increased technical expertise required
Faster recovery	Possible longer duration of surgery
Fewer postoperative complications	Increased risk of iatrogenic injuries
Better cosmesis	Difficult removal of bulky organs
	More expensive

Table 2.15 Advantages and disadvantages of minimally invasive surgery

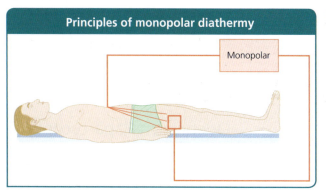

Principles of monopolar diathermy

Monopolar

Figure 2.15 Monopolar diathermy.

Bipolar diathermy

With bipolar diathermy (**Figure 2.16**), the two electrodes are combined in the instrument (e.g. forceps) and the current passes between the tips and not through the patient. The advantage of bipolar diathermy is that the electrical current does not pass through parts of the body that are not being treated. Thus, the quantity of tissue being coagulated is more precisely controlled.

Tourniquets

A tourniquet is a device used to control both the venous and arterial circulation to an extremity for a period of time by compressing both the arteries and veins. Tourniquets are commonly used in surgical practice to reduce blood loss in the operative field.

A tourniquet requires correct placement and connection to the inflation source. Adequate padding must be placed under the cuff and the limb exsanguinated before the tourniquet is inflated. The least pressure (usually 100 mmHg above the systolic blood pressure) is applied for the shortest possible time (no longer than 90 minutes). Relative contraindications to the use of tourniquets include:

- Previous deep vein thrombosis or pulmonary embolus
- Arterial disease
- Vasculitic disorders
- Sickle cell anaemia

When a tourniquet is properly applied, it provides excellent haemostasis. When it is incorrectly used, it can be dangerous by causing damage to the underlying skin and tissues.

Complications of tourniquet use include:

- Nerve injury
- Vascular injury
- Postoperative embolic events
- Increased blood viscosity
- Increased postoperative pain
- Tourniquet burns

Rubber tubing and surgical gloves must not be used as tourniquets on fingers as they can inadvertently be left on the digit at the end of the procedure. Specific brightly coloured digital tourniquets are available.

The excessive use of diathermy and prolonged tourniquet times can cause tissue damage, resulting in long-term morbidity and a risk of litigation.

Drains

Surgical drains are often used to evacuate established collections of pus, blood or other fluids (e.g. lymph) and to drain a space where potential fluid collections may form. Their use is, however, controversial and some surgeons consider that they cause more harm

Figure 2.16 Bipolar diathermy.

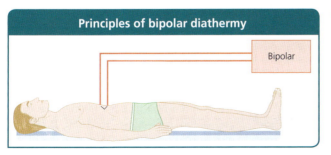

Principles of bipolar diathermy

Bipolar

than good. Most modern drains are made from an inert silastic material that produces only minimal tissue reactions. However, older red rubber drains induce severe tissue reactions that allow tracts to form that will allow continued drainage after the drain is removed. They are therefore now only used for specific purposes (e.g. biliary T-tubes).

Drains are open or closed and active or passive. Open drains include corrugated rubber or plastic sheets that collect the fluid into a gauze pad or stoma bag. They carry an increased risk of infection. Closed drains consists of a tube draining into a bag or bottle, for example in a chest and abdominal drain. These have a lower risk of infection.

Active drains are maintained under low- or high-pressure suction. They can drain more fluid but the pressure may cause tissue damage. Passive drains do not involve suction. These function as a result of the different pressures of the body cavities and the exterior.

Nasogastric tubes

After abdominal surgery, gastrointestinal motility is reduced for a variable period, ranging from hours to days. As a result, gastrointestinal secretions accumulate in the stomach and proximal small bowel. This

leads to postoperative distension and vomiting and a risk of aspiration pneumonia.

Nasogastric tubes are often used to remove fluid and secretions. They are of proven value for gastrointestinal decompression in intestinal obstruction and after emergency abdominal surgery. Nasogastric tubes are usually left on free drainage and intermittently aspirated. They are removed when the volume of nasogastric aspirate has reduced and gastrointestinal motility has returned.

There is little clinical evidence to support the routine use of nasogastric tubes after elective gastrointestinal surgery. They may in fact increase the risk of pulmonary complications.

Urinary catheters

A urinary catheter is a form of drain that is placed in the bladder (**Figure 2.17**). It is commonly used to either transurethrally or suprapubically. Catheters vary in terms of:

- The material from which they are made (latex, plastic or silastic or with a Teflon coating)
- The length of the catheter (38 cm for men or 22 cm for women)
- The diameter of the catheter (10 Fr to 24 Fr)
- The number of channels (two or three)
- The size of the balloon (from 5 mL to 30 mL)
- The shape of the tip

The catheter must be of an appropriate size, inserted using an aseptic technique and never placed using force. The residual volume of urine needs to be recorded. To avoid urethral damage, a catheter introducer (a metal guide) is best avoided unless the operator has been trained in its use. If difficulty is encountered inserting a urethral catheter, consider the suprapubic route. The catheter is removed as early as possible.

> **Never inflate the balloon of a urinary catheter until urine is seen coming from the catheter.** Inflation before urine is seen can result in trauma to the urethra.

The common indications for urinary catheterisation are shown in **Table 2.16**. The only absolute contraindication to the place-

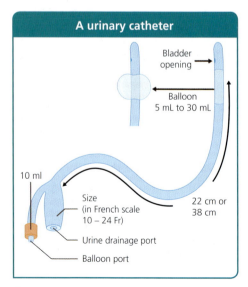

A urinary catheter

Bladder opening

Balloon 5 mL to 30 mL

10 ml

Size (in French scale 10 – 24 Fr)

22 cm or 38 cm

Urine drainage port

Balloon port

Figure 2.17 A urinary catheter.

Indications for urinary catheterisation

Intermittent	Management of patients with neurogenic bladder
	Intravesical chemotherapy
Short term	Management of acute urinary retention
	Assessment of fluid status during surgery
	Measurement of urinary output in critically ill patients
	Management of haematuria with clots
	Improved patient comfort during end-of-life care
	After surgery on the genitourinary tract
Long term	Management of patients with neurogenic bladder
	Management of urinary incontinence
	Management of immobile patients

Table 2.16 Indications for urinary catheterisation

ment of a urethral catheter is the presence of urethral injury. Relative contraindications include a urethral stricture and recent urinary tract surgery. Complications of urethral catheterisation include:

- Paraphimosis (the inability to pull the foreskin forward)
- Blockage
- By-passing of urine
- Infection
- Failure of the balloon to deflate
- Urethral stricture

Suprapubic catheterisation

In suprapubic catheterisation, the catheter is inserted directly into the bladder through the abdominal wall. This approach is used when urethral catheterisation is inappropriate. It can be used for patient comfort, dignity or convenience. Insertion requires a palpable bladder. Complications include misplacement, bleeding and bowel perforation.

Wound closure

The technique for wound closure is a matter of personal preference influenced by the surgeon's experience. The aim is to achieve secure healing with minimal pain and a favourable cosmetic outcome. If there is concern about possible wound infection, due to the presence of an established infection, the skin wound can be left open.

Sutures

Sutures hold a wound together until the natural healing process has been established and makes the support of the suture material unnecessary. The ideal suture material:

- Has good handling characteristics
- Does not induce a significant tissue reaction
- Allows secure knots to be tied
- Has adequate tensile strength
- Does not cut through the tissue
- Is sterile
- Is non-allergenic
- Is cheap

The choice of suture for a particular purpose will depend on the properties of the suture material as well as its absorption rate and handling and knotting properties. Sutures are connected to needles that also vary in size and shape.

The physical characteristics of suture materials differ. Monofilament sutures (e.g. polypropylene) are smooth. They slide well in tissues but can break if handled inappropriately. Multifilament sutures (e.g. polyglactin) are braided. They are easier to handle and knot well. Some suture materials have a 'memory' and return to their former shape when the tension on them is removed.

A number of suture materials are non-absorbable and remain within the body for ever. Absorbable sutures are broken down by proteolysis or hydrolysis. The rate of breakdown varies between individual suture materials.

Sutures must be removed as soon as possible. Skin incisions in different parts of the body heal at different rates. Sutures on the head and face, limbs and abdomen can be removed at 5, 7 and 10 days, respectively.

Answers to starter questions

1. The common imaging modalities used in the assessment of surgical diseases are ultrasound, CT scanning and MRI. Ultrasound is a non-invasive technique that is cheap and readily available. However, its successful use is very user dependent. CT scanning is able to rapidly produce high resolution images and is very useful for producing images of the thorax, abdomen and pelvis that can be reconstructed and manipulated in different planes. It does however require the patient to be exposed to a high radiation dose. MRI scanning does not involve radiation exposure and produces high resolution images but it is an expensive technique and the images do take a period of time to be acquired. Each imaging technique has its strengths and weaknesses that often complement each other.

2. Rapid recognition of surgical emergences is essential in order to start appropriate investigation and timely intervention. The presenting complaint and associated features should alert the clinician to the potential pathology. The measurement of vital signs, often interpreted as part of an Early Warning System, highlight the degree of physiological derangement. A focused clinical examination should complement the history and confirm a specific diagnosis. The overall clinical picture, supplemented by test results, will determine both the need for and timing of surgery

3. The assessment of any patient, medical or surgical, should include a full history and examination, allowing the formulation of a differential diagnosis and investigation plan. However, in surgical patients one also needs to consider whether an operation is required, what operation should be performed and when. When dealing with surgical pathology, there are often several different approaches that can be adopted. The outcome needs to be that the correct operation is performed on the correct patient, at the right time with the most favourable clinical outcome.

4. Most patients who present with surgical disease present to either their general practitioners or as emergencies with symptoms or signs of the underlying disease. Appropriate investigations will define the underlying cause and extent of the disease. Patients who present through screening programmes are invariably asymptomatic. They access the health care system by being invited to undergo a screening test. Most of these investigations are normal and no further intervention is required. However, some patients are shown to have an abnormal test that requires further investigation. Diseases detected through screening programmes are often at an early stage and intervention produces a better outcome; this is the main rationale for establishing the screening programme.

5. A tourniquet is a device used to control both the venous and arterial circulation to an extremity by compressing both the arteries and veins. They are commonly used in surgical practice to reduce blood loss in the operative field. When properly applied they provide excellent haemostasis. When incorrectly used, they are dangerous. Safe use requires adequate padding with inflation to the minimum pressure for the shortest duration. Complications of tourniquet use include nerve injury and vascular injury, postoperative embolic events, myoglobinuria and tourniquet burns.

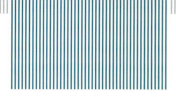

Chapter 3
Breast disease

Introduction. 45
Case 1 Breast lump 46
Core sciences 47
Triple assessment 50
Disorders of breast development . 54

Benign breast disease 54
Breast pain 57
Breast cancer 57
Gynaecomastia 62

Starter questions

Answers to the following questions are on page 63.

1. Why is oestrogen important in the development of breast cancer?
2. How should women presenting with breast symptoms be evaluated?
3. What factors determine the surgical approach in a woman shown to have breast cancer?
4. Why does the United Kingdom have one the highest breast cancer mortality rates in the world?
5. How should the assessment of breast lumps differ between women and men?

Introduction

Concerns related to the breast, such as lumps, nipple discharge and pain, are one of the most common reasons why women consult their general practitioners. Most symptoms are due to benign disease and many patients, particularly those with breast pain, can be managed in primary care. However, as breast cancer is one of the most common malignant diseases in women, patients presenting with a breast lump require prompt evaluation in a breast clinic.

Case 1 Breast lump

Presentation

A 58-year-old woman, Elizabeth Green, presents to her general practitioner with a 1-week history of a painless lump in her right breast.

Initial interpretation

In a postmenopausal woman, the most likely cause of a painless breast lump is either a breast cancer or a breast cyst. Other less common causes include fat necrosis, fibroadenomas and phyllodes tumours. Further clinical assessment and investigation aims to confirm or refute the diagnosis of breast cancer.

History

Elizabeth has noticed a lump associated with some indrawing of her nipple and distortion of the breast tissue and overlying skin. She has not noticed any nipple discharge. Her general health is good.

Interpretation of history

A painless breast lump in a postmenopausal woman that is associated with indrawing of the nipple and skin dimpling is highly suspicious of a breast cancer. In most cases, the patient's general health is good, unless the tumour is advanced and/or metastasis has occurred. Other diagnoses to consider include a breast cyst and fat necrosis.

Further history

Elizabeth has a past history of breast cysts but no history of breast trauma and no family history of breast cancer. She had

Breast disease: investigation

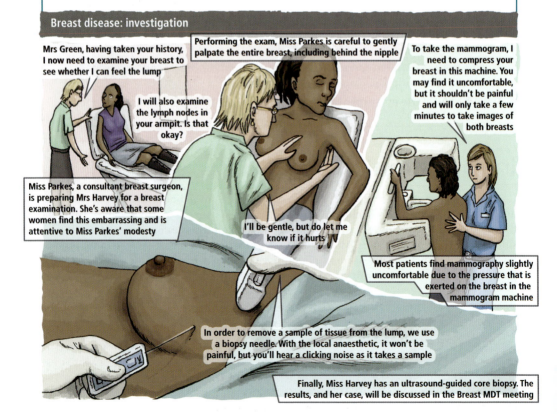

Case 1 *continued*

normal screening mammograms under the UK National Health Service Breast Screening Programme 2 years ago.

Examination

On examination, there is a 3 cm irregular lump in the upper outer quadrant of Elizabeth's right breast. There is indrawing of the nipple and dimpling of the skin over the lump. The lump is not fixed to either the skin or the chest wall. Several lymph nodes are palpable in the axilla. The left breast is normal on palpation.

Interpretation of findings

Women with a history of breast cysts do not have an increased risk of breast cancer. A woman with a first-degree relative with breast cancer has double the risk of developing the disease. Having two first-degree relatives with breast cancer increases the risk by approximately five times.

Breast cancers invariably have an irregular shape. The presence of skin dimpling or indrawing of the nipple is suggestive of tumour infiltration along the suspensory ligaments. The palpable lymph nodes represent axillary lymphadenopathy, supporting a diagnosis of breast cancer.

Investigations

Mammography shows a 3 cm 'spiculate' (i.e. irregular) mass, which is also seen on ultrasound. The axillary ultrasound shows several enlarged lymph nodes with an irregular outline. These are highly suspicious of nodal metastases. A core biopsy of the breast lump and fine-needle aspirate of the axillary lymph nodes are obtained under ultrasound guidance. Histological analysis of the breast biopsy shows an invasive ductal carcinoma. Cytological analysis of the fine-needle aspirate shows malignant cells in the lymph nodes.

Diagnosis

The biopsy and aspirate confirm a diagnosis of an invasive ductal carcinoma with axillary lymph node involvement. Breast imaging suggests that the tumour is only 2.5 cm in diameter, i.e. it is a small tumour in a relatively large breast and is therefore suitable for breast-conserving surgery with removal of the lump only.

A wide local excision (lumpectomy) and axillary node clearance are performed and the specimens are submitted for histopathological assessment. The tumour is excised with clear resection margins (i.e. no tumour at the edge of what was excised). Overall, 15 lymph nodes are removed from the axilla, five of which are shown to contain metastases. The tumour is shown to be oestrogen receptor positive and human epidermal growth factor receptor 2 (HER2) receptor negative.

Core sciences

Breast embryology

During the 4th and 6th weeks of gestation, an ectodermal 'mammary ridge' of 15–20 breast buds develops that extends from the axilla to the groin (**Figure 3.1**). In the embryo, these buds coalesce so that usually only one breast bud remains on each side. This is situated in the fourth or fifth intercostal space. The buds grow into the underlying mesoderm with branching lactiferous ducts. The mesenchyme develops into the supporting connective tissue and the fat of the breast.

Breast embryology

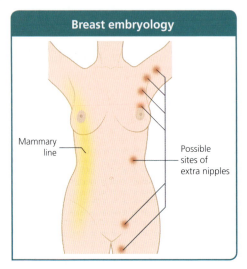

Figure 3.1 Breast embryology.

Neonatal, or 'witch's', milk is secreted in many newborns, both male and female. It is a result of stimulation of the neonatal pituitary gland, which secretes prolactin, and of the effect of maternal oestrogens. These oestrogens cross the placenta to cause either unilateral or bilateral neonatal breast enlargement or sometimes secretion.

Breast development

From birth until puberty, the breast consists of lactiferous (mammary) ducts that have no milk-producing alveolar epithelial cells. At puberty, oestrogen causes the breast ducts to grow and the breast bud to develop. Following the onset of ovulation, progesterone causes the formation of lobular elements and side branches on the ducts.

Oestrogens are responsible for proliferation of the lactiferous ducts, the branching network of tubes that transports milk from the lobules to the nipple. Both oestrogen and progesterone are responsible for the development of the breast lobules. During pregnancy, the levels of oestrogen and progesterone increase significantly, and full lobular alveolar growth occurs.

Breast anatomy

The adult breast is made up of both fatty and glandular tissue (**Figure 3.2**). The ratio

Breast anatomy

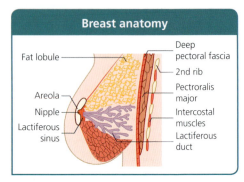

Figure 3.2 Breast anatomy.

of fat to glandular tissue varies between individuals and changes with age. After the menopause, the relative amount of fatty tissue increases as the glandular tissue diminishes.

Approximately 25 breast lobes drain into about 10 major ducts. The lobes contain numerous lobules that produce and secrete milk. They are connected by ducts and lactiferous sinuses that collect the milk and deliver it to the nipple. The distal end of the ductal system is the terminal ductal lobular unit. Each lobe has thousands of these, each with an inner layer of secretory cells and an outer layer of myoepithelial cells. The myoepithelial cells contain contractile fibres that eject the milk into the ducts during lactation.

The nipple is surrounded by the areola, which contains large sebaceous glands that are often visible to the naked eye – the glands of Montgomery. The base of the breast overlies the pectoralis major muscle between the second and sixth ribs. A tongue of tissue extends towards the axilla and is known as the axillary tail. The breast is fixed to the pectoralis major fascia by the suspensory ligaments that run throughout the breast tissue parenchyma from the deep fascia beneath the breast to the dermis of the skin.

Blood supply and lymphatics

The blood supply to the breast skin is via the plexus of blood vessels that lie underneath the skin. These communicate with deeper vessels supplying the breast tissue. The blood supply to the breast (**Figure 3.3**) is derived from the:

Arterial blood supply of the breast

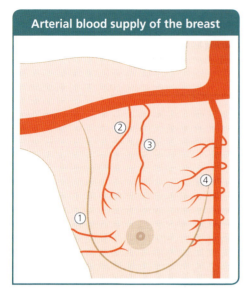

Figure 3.3 Arterial blood supply of the breast. ① Intercostal perforators. ② Lateral thoracic artery. ③ Thoracromial artery. ④ Internal mammary artery.

- Internal mammary artery
- Thoracoacromial artery
- Lateral thoracic artery
- Perforating vessels arising from the intercostal perforators

The lymphatic drainage of the breast is into the axilla, although the lower inner quadrants can drain to the internal mammary nodes (**Figure 3.4**).

Innervation

The sensory innervation of the breast skin is dermatomal, i.e. supplied by a single spinal nerve. The nerve supply is via the anterolateral and anteromedial branches of the thoracic intercostal nerves. Supraclavicular nerves from the lower fibres of the cervical plexus also innervate the upper and lateral portions of the breast. The sensation to the nipple is derived from the lateral cutaneous branch of T4.

> **The premenopausal breast contains a large proportion of glandular tissue,** making it radiologically dense and limiting the sensitivity of mammograms. Therefore mammography is of limited use in women under the age of 40 years.

Lymphatic drainage of the breast

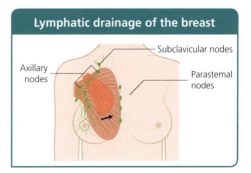

Figure 3.4 Lymphatic drainage of the breast.

Breast physiology

All women experience changes in their breasts throughout their life. For example, fluctuating hormone levels during the menstrual cycle cause changes in the appearance and feel of the breasts.

During pregnancy, the ducts grow and branch, and the breasts enlarge to twice their normal weight. There is an increase in mammary blood flow and in areolar pigmentation. During lactation, the acini (the terminal parts of the lobules) are dilated and engorged with first colostrum (a fluid rich in proteins and antibodies) and then milk, rich in nutrients. After the menopause, the breast lobules begin to involute, leaving mostly ducts, adipose tissue and fibrous tissue.

Lactation

After oestrogen and progesterone have caused the initial development of the mammary secretory tissue, lactogenic hormones initiate the production of milk. There are two lactogenic hormones:

- Prolactin is secreted by the anterior pituitary gland
- Human placental lactogen is produced by the maternal placenta

The secretion of human placental lactogen reaches a peak during the final weeks of gestation to prepare the breast for milk production. After birth, this hormone disappears from the maternal circulation, and prolactin functions as the sole lactogenic hormone.

Oxytocin plays an important role in lactation. It is produced in the hypothalamus and stored in the posterior pituitary. Breastfeeding stimulates its release, which in turn causes contraction of the myoepithelial cells around the ducts to propel more milk to the ducts. During lactation, about 1 L of milk is produced each day.

Triple asssessment

In any woman presenting with a concern regarding her breasts, first consider her age as certain diseases present in specific age groups (**Figure 3.5**). The most common symptoms and signs of breast disease are shown in **Table 3.1**.

History

The most common symptoms with which women present to a breast clinic are breast lumps and breast pain. These are assessed in the same fashion as a lump or pain elsewhere in the body.

The patient's menstrual history and menopausal status must also be elicited. Correlate the patient's symptoms to her menstrual cycle as many benign conditions (e.g. benign nodularity) fluctuate with the period. A nipple discharge is another symptom of breast disease and is often described as watery, purulent or blood-stained.

Any family history of breast or ovarian cancer should be established, in particular which relatives were affected.

Examination

First ensure a female chaperone is present. Ask the patient to undress from the waist up, including her bra. Then she is asked to sit on the couch facing towards the examiner with her arms by her sides.

Inspection

Inspect the breasts from the front and the sides. Ask the patient to place her hands on her hips and press down. This contracts the pectoral muscles and tightens the suspensory ligaments, making it easier to see any abnormalities in the contour or shape of the breast. Finally, ask her to raise her arms above her head. This allows the axilla to be inspected.

During inspection it is important to assess:

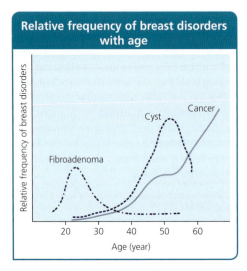

Relative frequency of breast disorders with age

Relative frequency of breast disorders

Cancer
Cyst
Fibroadenoma

20   30   40   50   60
Age (year)

Figure 3.5 Relative frequency of breast disorders with age.

Symptoms and signs of breast disease	
Symptoms	Signs
Breast pain	Breast lump
Breast lump	Nipple discharge
Skin distortion	Axillary lymphadenopathy
Nipple discharge	Peau d'orange
Indrawn nipple	

Table 3.1 Common symptoms and signs of breast disease

- Breast size
- Breast symmetry
- Contour – any obvious lumps or dimpling
- Scars – any previous breast surgery
- Dimpling or tethering of the skin
- Ulceration
- Peau d'orange – skin resembling orange peel that overlies a carcinoma
- The appearance of the nipples

A breast examination is embarrassing for some women. Explain the purpose and method of the examination and respect the patient's dignity throughout. A female chaperone must be present.

Palpation

Ask the patient to lie supine on the couch with her hands by her sides. Assess the contralateral breast first to assess what is normal for that patient. Examine the breast with the palm flat, the fingers palpating the breast in small circular motions. Use the right hand to examine the left breast and axilla, and the left hand to examine the right breast and axilla.

Clinically, the breast is divided into four quadrants: upper outer, upper inner, lower outer and lower inner (**Figure 3.6**). If a lesion is identified within the breast, it is described in terms of its:

- Site
- Size
- Shape
- Surface and overlying skin
- Tenderness
- Consistency
- Mobility and attachment of any lump

If the lump cannot be moved, this implies that it is fixed to the underlying muscle and likely to be malignant. The features of benign and malignant breast lumps are shown in **Table 3.2**.

When assessing a breast lump, consider the patient's age. Fibroadenomas occur during breast development. Cysts occur around the time of the menopause, and breast cancer is uncommon below the age of 30 years.

If the patient mentions a nipple discharge, she is asked to squeeze her nipple to show the discharge. A nipple discharge is described:

- As unilateral or bilateral
- As single or multiduct
- By its colour and volume

Finally, the regional lymph nodes are examined. Lift the patient's arm up and palpate for any nodes. Axillary lymph nodes are described as lower, posterior, lateral and apical (**Figure 3.7**).

This full history and examination form the initial step of the assessment and often lead to a clinical diagnosis that should be confirmed by further investigations. The 'triple assessment' allows women with benign conditions to be rapidly reassured and an appropriate management plan to be formulated.

The triple assessment is a full clinical, radiological and pathological examination of a lump in any woman presenting with breast symptoms.

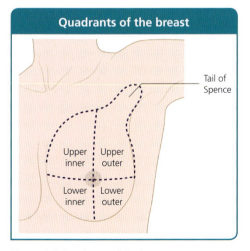

Figure 3.6 Quadrants of the breast.

Quadrants of the breast

Tail of Spence

Upper inner | Upper outer

Lower inner | Lower outer

Features of benign and malignant breast lumps

Benign lumps	Malignant lumps
Smooth	Hard
May be painful	Painless
Well defined	Irregular edge
Mobile	Fixed or tethered to skin or muscle
No skin dimpling	Skin dimpling
No nipple retraction	Nipple retraction

Table 3.2 Features of benign and malignant breast lumps

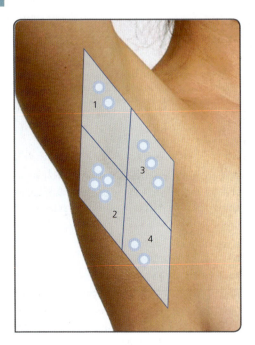

Figure 3.7 Position of axillary nodes. ① Apical nodes. ② Lateral nodes. ③ Pectoral nodes. ④ Low axillary nodes.

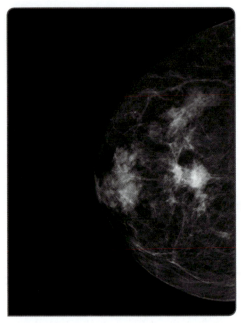

Figure 3.8 Spiculate mass on mammography due to a breast cancer.

Investigation

Breast imaging forms the second strand of the triple assessment.

The breast can be imaged using mammography (low-energy X-rays), ultrasound scanning or MRI. Mammography is the most sensitive modality but its sensitivity is reduced in young women due to the increased presence of glandular tissue. In women under the age of 40 years, ultrasound is the modality of choice.

Mammography

Abnormalities detected on mammography can be classified in to one of four categories:

Spiculate masses are soft tissue mass with spicules ('spikes') extending into the surrounding tissue (**Figure 3.8**). About 95% of spiculate masses are due to invasive cancer. Other causes include a radial scar or complex sclerosing lesion and fat necrosis.

Stellate lesions are localised distortions of the breast tissue with no perceptible mass lesion. They are caused by invasive cancers, radial scars and surgical scars.

Circumscribed masses are well defined and have a uniform density and clear outlines. They are caused by fibroadenomas, cysts, mucinous carcinoma and lipomas.

Microcalcification is due to debris within the duct wall or lumen. Malignant microcalcification has a characteristic appearance and is usually linear or branching. Benign microcalcification is usually rounded and punctuate. Causes of microcalcification include ductal carcinoma in situ (DCIS), invasive cancer, papillomas, fibroadenomas and fat necrosis.

> Radial scars appear malignant on mammograms but are pathologically benign.

Breast ultrasound

Ultrasound scanning is useful in the assessment of breast lumps irrespective of the patient's age. It complements mammography by enabling solid and cystic lesions to be differentiated. It is also used to guide fine-needle aspiration and core biopsies.

On an ultrasound scan, cysts have smooth walls, sharp anterior and posterior borders and

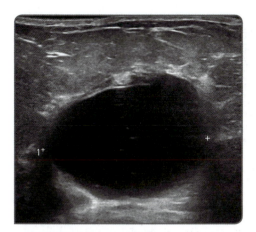

Figure 3.9 Ultrasound appearance of a cyst.

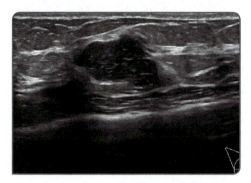

Figure 3.10 Ultrasound appearance of a fibroadenoma.

hypoechoic centres (Figure 3.9). Solid lesions have internal echoes. Benign tumours (e.g. a fibroadenoma) have isoechoic or hypoechoic patterns, smooth walls and well-defined borders, and cast no shadows (Figure 3.10). Malignant tumours have hypoechoic areas and irregular edges, and cast hypoechoic shadows.

Breast MRI

This is a recently developed technique that is very sensitive but not very specific in imaging breast tumours. Its uses include:

- Assessing the size of breast cancers

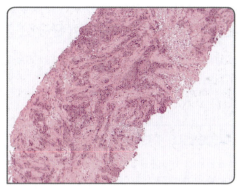

Figure 3.11 Breast core biopsy showing an invasive carcinoma.

- Determining whether lobular cancers are unifocal or multifocal
- Imaging the breast for occult disease in the presence of axillary metastases
- Differentiating between scar tissue and recurrences of cancer
- Assessing the integrity of breast implants.

Fine-needle aspiration

Fine-needle aspiration is used to remove a sample of cells from a lesion. It is performed without anaesthesia using an 18 Fr needle and a 10 mL syringe. Gentle suction is applied while the needle is advanced and withdrawn through the lesion. The sample is then washed into a fixative, before being centrifuged and smeared onto a microscope slide. It allows tissue to be obtained from solid lesions for cytological assessment. It is also used to drain cysts.

Core biopsy

A core biopsy obtains more pathological information about a lesion (Figure 3.11) than fine-needle aspiration. However, there are greater risks associated with the procedure as it can result in extensive bruising and rarely in complications such as a pneumothorax.

Disorders of breast development

Aberrations of breast development are common, and their clinical features are best understood from an embryological perspective.

Accessory nipples

Accessory nipples are seen in about 2% of the population, with an equal incidence in the two sexes. The nipples develop along the mammary line (Figure 3.1), and almost all are seen in the inframammary region, below the nipple. They can be unilateral or bilateral and sometimes have a relatively well-developed areola.

No treatment is required unless the nipple causes irritation or the patient wishes it to be excised for cosmetic reasons.

Accessory breast tissue

Accessory breast tissue or supernumerary breasts are seen in approximately 1–2% of the population. The most common site is in the axilla, where the tissue sometimes has its own nipple–areola complex. Accessory breast tissue is susceptible to all the changes that normally occur in a breast, such as pregnancy-related increases in size, and to all breast diseases, including malignancy. The tissue can be excised if bulky and embarrassing.

Benign breast disease

Benign breast conditions are an almost universal phenomenon that affect almost all women at some time in their lives. There was previously a tendency to include all benign breast disorders under the designation of 'fibrocystic disease', which implies an underlying pathological process.

However, the term 'aberrations of normal development and involution' is now preferred to describe most benign breast disorders (Table 3.3). The classification is based on the fact that most benign breast disorders are relatively

minor aberrations of normal processes of development, cyclical hormonal response and involution.

Fibroadenomas

These are benign breast lumps derived from the breast lobule and are classified as simple or giant. They have both epithelial and connective tissue elements, but their pathogenesis is unclear. They are not true neoplasms as they are polyclonal (i.e. produced from

Classification of benign breast disease			
Condition	Normal	Benign disorder	Benign disease
Development	Duct, lobular and stromal development	Nipple inversion Fibroadenoma Breast hypertrophy	Giant fibroadenoma
Cyclical change	Hormonal activity	Mastalgia and nodularity	
Pregnancy and lactation	Epithelial hyperplasia	Blood-stained nipple discharge	Galactocele
Involution	Duct involution	Duct ectasia Nipple retraction	Periductal mastitis
Lobular involution	Cysts Sclerosing adenosis	Epithelial hyperplasia	Lobular and ductal hyperplasia with atypia

Table 3.3 Classification of benign breast disease

several different cell types) rather than monoclonal (i.e. produced from one cell).

Simple fibroadenoma

Most simple fibroadenomas are smooth or slightly lobulated in appearance. They usually present soon after breast development. The incidence decreases in the years approaching the menopause. They may present as a hard-calcified mass in the elderly. Approximately 10% of fibroadenomas are multiple.

Over a 5-year period, 50% increase in size, 25% remain stable and 25% decrease in size. Most fibroadenomas do not require surgical excision.

Giant fibroadenoma

Giant fibroadenomas have a bimodal age presentation, with a peak incidence in teenagers and a second smaller peak around the menopause. They are more common in women of Afro-Caribbean or Far-East Asian descent. They grow rapidly and typically present with pain, breast enlargement, nipple displacement and characteristic skin changes with erythema and dilated veins.

Treatment is by excision, choosing an area that will leave a cosmetically acceptable scar. Any resulting breast distortion is usually self-correcting.

Phyllodes tumour

Phyllodes tumours are fibroepithelial lesions composed of an epithelial and a cellular stromal component. They invariably occur in premenopausal women. They show a wide spectrum of activity varying from entirely benign to locally aggressive. They are classified as benign, borderline and malignant.

Phyllodes tumours should be excised with a 1 cm margin of normal tissue. Even those classified as 'malignant' rarely spread and do not usually require adjuvant chemotherapy or radiotherapy.

Breast cysts

Breast cysts are fluid-filled sacs lined with epithelium that lie within the breast tissue. Approximately 10% of women develop a clinically palpable cyst at some stage of their lives. They usually occur in perimenopausal women. Cysts are often multiple, sometimes appear suddenly and are frequently painful.

The initial treatment is simple aspiration. Surgical excision is rarely required but is considered if a cyst recurs repeatedly or there is a residual lump after aspiration.

Breast papillomas

Breast papillomas are hyperplastic epithelial growths with a fibrovascular core. They occur in large or small ducts and can be solitary or multiple. When multiple and small, the term 'papillomatosis' is used. Papillomas often present with a blood-stained nipple discharge from a single duct. Treatment is by surgical excision.

Breast infections

Breast infections occur either during lactation or in non-lactating young or middle-aged women. The pathological process and organisms involved are different in the two groups.

Lactational breast abscess

Lactational breast sepsis is most commonly due to *Staphylococcus aureus* infection. The resulting abscess is usually peripherally situated. The need for surgical drainage may be pre-empted by early diagnosis.

If the diagnosis is suspected, aspiration is attempted, ideally under ultrasound guidance. Repeated aspiration may be required if the abscess refills and formal incision and drainage can often be avoided. Antibiotics, dependent on the likely organisms involved, are given and continued until confirmed by sensitivities from culture of the pus.

Advise patients to express milk from the affected side and to continue breastfeeding from the opposite breast. There is no need to suppress lactation.

Non-lactational breast abscess

Non-lactational breast sepsis often occurs in the periareolar tissue (**Figure 3.12**). Bacterial

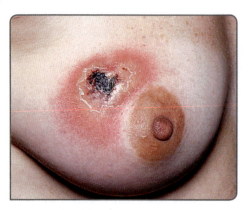

Figure 3.12 Non-lactational breast abscess.

culture often yields *Bacteroides* species, anaerobic streptococci or enterococci. It is usually a manifestation of duct ectasia or periductal mastitis. It most commonly occurs in women aged between 30 and 60 years. It is more common in smokers, and patients often give a history of recurrent breast sepsis.

Repeated aspiration is the treatment of choice. Formal incision and drainage through a small incision should be considered if the abscess does not resolve with conservative management. If definitive treatment is necessary, it should be carried out when the sepsis is quiescent. It usually involves a major duct excision. Spontaneous discharge or surgical excision can result in a mammary duct fistula.

> **A mammary-duct fistula is an abnormal connection between a subareolar breast duct and the overlying skin.** It usually occurs in the periareolar region following the spontaneous discharge of a non-lactational breast abscess associated with periductal mastitis.

Galactorrhoea

Galactorrhoea is milk secretion that is unrelated to childbirth or breastfeeding. It is common and usually benign, although it sometimes has a pathological cause (**Table 3.4**). It is usually a bilateral, multiduct, milky discharge. Copious volumes are produced, and the discharge sometimes occurs spontaneously.

Fat necrosis

Fat necrosis is the enzymatic destruction (by lipases) of fat tissue that sometimes follows a trivial or unnoticed injury. Fat released from damaged adipocytes induces an inflammatory response leading to subsequent fibrosis and calcification.

The patient usually presents with a painless breast lump. There is sometimes a history of trauma and a suggestion that the lump is reducing in size over time. Examination usually reveals a hard, irregular lump, which may be tethered to the skin. Clinically, it may be difficult to differentiate it from a carcinoma so a full triple assessment is indicated. Mammography may show a spiculate mass identical to that seen in breast cancer, but a core biopsy will confirm the diagnosis. No specific treatment is required.

Causes of galactorrhoea			
Physiological	**Drugs**	**Pathological**	**Others**
Mechanical stimulation	Dopamine-receptor blocking agents	Hypothalamic and pituitary lesions	Oestrogens
Post-lactational		Pituitary tumours	Opiates
Stress	Dopamine-depleting agents	Ectopic prolactin secretion	
		Hypothyroidism	
		Chronic renal failure	

Table 3.4 Causes of galactorrhoea

Breast pain

Breast pain (mastalgia) is one of the most common reasons women why consult their general practitioners. It is also the most common reason for referral to a breast clinic. It is classified as cyclical or non-cyclical mastalgia, depending on its variation in intensity during the menstrual cycle.

> **Breast pain is an uncommon symptom of breast cancer,** with fewer than 5% of patients reporting pain at their initial presentation.

Cyclical mastalgia

Cyclical mastalgia is breast pain that varies with the menstrual period.

Clinical features

Cyclical mastalgia is usually bilateral, localised in the upper outer quadrant of the breast, and worsens prior to the menstrual period. It is usually mild and accepted as a 'part of normal life'. No consistent hormonal abnormality has been identified. However, prolactin levels may be increased and essential fatty acid profiles are occasionally abnormal. No imaging is required unless there is a palpable mass.

Management

Most women require only reassurance that breast pain is an unfortunate aspect of 'normal' physiology. However, if it is present for 6 months, or for more than 7 days during each menstrual cycle, treatment options include the following:

Evening primrose oil is often recommended but there is little evidence to support its use. It needs to be used for at least 4 months and has a 50% response rate. Side effects are rare, but about 1% of patients develop nausea.

Danazol is a derivative of the synthetic steroid ethisterone, a modified testosterone, and has an 80% response rate. Unfortunately, 25% of patients develop complications, including acne, weight gain and hirsutism.

Bromocriptine is a dopamine agonist. It has a 50% response rate with 20% of patients developing complications, including postural hypotension.

Non-cyclical mastalgia

Non-cyclical mastalgia usually affects older women, with an average age of onset of 45 years. It is usually unilateral and often localised. True non-cyclical mastalgia often has a musculoskeletal cause. Treatment involves a supportive bra and anti-inflammatory analgesia.

Breast cancer

Breast cancer is the most common cause of cancer death in women. Its most frequent presentation is with a painless breast lump, which is the most common reason for women being referred to a breast clinic. The assessment and investigation of breast lumps should be tailored to rapidly identify women with breast cancer and to reassure women whose lumps are benign.

Types

The World Health Organization classifies breast cancer as non-invasive or invasive. Non-invasive disease is confined to the ducts or lobules, and classified as either DCIS or lobular neoplasia. Invasive breast cancer is further categorised by histological type:

- Ductal (85%)
- Lobular (10%)

- Mucinous
- Papillary
- Medullary

Mucinous, papillary and medullary carcinomas are uncommon, their treatment is as other forms of breast cancer and their prognosis is good.

Ductal carcinoma in situ

DCIS is a premalignant condition in which the malignant cells remain within the basement membrane of the breast lobules. It does not have the ability to metastasise. Not all cases progress to invasive cancer. It is usually asymptomatic and was rarely seen prior to the establishment of breast screening services.

DCIS usually presents as malignant microcalcification on screening mammography. Its management depends on the extent and grade of the lesion. Surgery by either wide local excision or mastectomy alone is often adequate. However, postoperative radiotherapy is considered for those undergoing breast-conserving surgery for high-grade DCIS. The role of tamoxifen in the management of DCIS is controversial.

Invasive breast cancer

The histological assessment of invasive breast cancer shows malignant cells invading the basement membrane. In addition, the myoepithelial layer around the breast lobules is no longer intact. Malignant cells are found within the surrounding parenchymal tissue and have the potential to metastasise.

Epidemiology

Breast cancer affects one out of nine women worldwide. In the UK, there are 48,000 new cases and 15,000 deaths each year, accounting for 6% of all deaths in females. Despite its breast cancer treatment being some of the most advanced in the world, the UK has one of the highest rates of mortality from breast cancer worldwide. This is almost certainly the result of delayed presentation of the disease.

Aetiology

Most breast cancers arise sporadically, with no obvious aetiology. Identified risk factors include those relating to total oestrogen exposure:

- Early menarche
- Late menopause
- Oral contraceptive use or hormonal replacement therapy

About 5% of breast cancers have a genetic basis, most commonly a *BRCA1* or *BRCA2* gene mutation. Women with an abnormal *BRCA1* or *BRCA2* gene have a 60% lifetime risk of developing breast cancer.

> **BRCA1** and **BRCA2** are tumour **suppressor genes.** Their inactivation by a mutation therefore leads to an increased probability of cancer.

Screening

The UK's National Health Service Breast Screening Programme was introduced in 1988. All women between 47 and 70 years are invited every 3 years for two-view mammography. If an abnormality is seen on a mammogram, the woman is recalled for clinical examination, further imaging and fine-needle aspiration cytology or core biopsy as required.

> About 70% of screen-detected abnormalities are shown to be of no clinical significance, and about 25% of all breast cancers are screen-detected.

Pathogenesis

Malignant change occurs in the epithelium of the terminal ductal lobular unit. When invasion of the basement membrane occurs, invasive breast cancer has developed. This then has the potential to spread to the axillary or internal mammary lymph nodes. If distal metastases occur, they are often seen in the bones, liver and lungs.

Clinical features

Symptomatic breast cancer usually presents with a painless breast lump, most commonly in the upper outer quadrant or subareolar region of the breast. This may be associated with skin dimpling or nipple retraction due to involvement of the suspensory ligaments of the breast. Clinical evaluation includes an assessment of tethering or fixation to the skin or pectoral muscle, and an examination of the axillary and supraclavicular lymph nodes.

Uncommon clinical presentations of breast cancer include inflammatory breast cancer and Paget's disease of the nipple. In patients with inflammatory breast cancer, obstruction of the lymphatic system in the dermis can give the skin an appearance like orange peel that is called peau d'orange. Paget's disease presents with nipple ulceration.

A quarter of breast cancers are asymptomatic and are picked up through breast screening programmes.

Investigations

All women presenting with a breast lump need to undergo breast imaging and a core biopsy. If the lump has radiological features of malignancy, an axillary ultrasound scan is performed and a core biopsy or fine-needle aspiration sample taken from any abnormal lymph nodes. Breast imaging should measure the size of the lesion. If a diagnosis is confirmed on a biopsy, an assessment should be made of the tumour type, histological grade and oestrogen receptor and HER2 receptor status as these will influence management.

Management

In patients who are fit enough, the management of breast cancer invariably involves surgery and adjuvant therapy. Adjuvant therapy incorporates chemotherapy, radiotherapy, hormonal treatment and biological therapies depending on the age of the patient and the pathological features of the tumour.

Surgery

This is either breast-conserving surgery or mastectomy (**Figure 3.13**). Breast-conserving surgery involves excision of the tumour with a cuff of surrounding normal breast tissue. Mastectomy involves removal of the whole breast, preserving the underlying pectoral muscles.

Tumours considered suitable for breast conservation are usually small single lesions in a large breast, often in a peripheral location with no evidence of skin or extensive nodal involvement. There is no difference in survival between breast-conserving surgery with radiotherapy and mastectomy.

> **Mastectomy often has a huge emotional impact on the patient.** In women undergoing mastectomy, breast reconstruction should be considered either at the time of the mastectomy or as a delayed procedure.

Axillary surgery

Overall, 30–40% of patients with early breast cancer have nodal involvement at first presentation. The aims of axillary surgery in breast cancer are to eradicate local disease and to determine the prognosis to guide adjuvant therapy. Surgical evaluation of the axilla is important and is considered for all patients with invasive cancer. The status of the axilla can be staged by:

- Axillary node clearance
- Axillary four-node sampling
- Sentinel lymph node biopsy

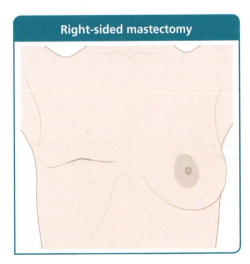

Right-sided mastectomy

Figure 3.13 A right-sided mastectomy

Axillary node clearance involves removing the lymph nodes in levels 1–3 of the axilla. The levels of the axilla are shown in **Table 3.5**. Axillary node clearance is an extensive surgical procedure. Its complications include seroma formation (i.e. a postoperative fluid collection), paraesthesia and lymphoedema. The risk of complications depends on the extent of the surgery.

Sentinel lymph node biopsy is less invasive and is regarded as the optimal method of staging in those with a clinically and radiologically disease-negative axilla. Sentinel node biopsy aims to stage disease in the axilla accurately without the morbidity of axillary clearance. The technique attempts to identify the first nodes that the tumour drains to by mapping the axilla after injecting of a combination of an isotope and a blue dye.

Prognosis

About 40% of women with operable breast cancer who receive surgery as the only treatment will die from metastatic disease. Prognostic factors (**Table 3.6**) are therefore important in order to:

- Select the appropriate adjuvant therapy
- Allow a comparison of treatment between similar groups of patients
- Improve understanding of the disease

Levels of the axilla in relation to pectoralis minor	
Level	Relation to pectoralis minor
Level 1	Below pectoralis minor
Level 2	Up to the upper border of pectoralis minor
Level 3	To the outer border of the first rib

Table 3.5 Levels of the axilla in relation to pectoralis minor

Prognostic factors in breast cancer	
Chronological factors	Biological factors
Age	Histological type
Tumour size	Histological grade
Lymph node status	Lymphatic or vascular invasion
Metastases	Hormone and growth factor receptors

Table 3.6 Prognostic factors in breast cancer

Although individual prognostic factors are useful, combining independent prognostic variables in the form of an index allows the identification of patients with different prognoses. This can then be used to predict survival and select adjuvant therapies.

> **The Nottingham Prognostic Index gives a quantifiable measure of post-surgical prognosis.** It incorporates tumour size, nodal status and histological grade:
>
> Nottingham Prognostic Index score = 0.2 × size (cm) + node stage + tumour grade

Chemotherapy

This is given either before or after surgery for breast cancer.

Primary (neoadjuvant) chemotherapy

Chemotherapy can be given prior to surgery to a patient with a large or locally advanced tumour. About 70% of tumours respond by decreasing in size, and in 30% of patients the lesion becomes impalpable. Primary chemotherapy has not been shown to improve survival when compared with chemotherapy given after surgery, but it can make breast-conservation surgery possible where a mastectomy would otherwise be required.

Adjuvant chemotherapy

The use of adjuvant chemotherapy depends primarily on the risk of recurrence. Factors to consider when planning possible chemotherapy include the age of the patient, the menopausal status, nodal status, tumour grade and receptor status. The greatest effect of chemotherapy is seen in premenopausal women.

Hormonal treatment

Tamoxifen is an oestrogen receptor antagonist that blocks the effects of endogenous oestrogens. It is only effective in those with oestrogen-receptor-positive disease. The optimum duration of treatment is unclear but current recommendations cite 5 years. A benefit is seen in both premenopausal and postmenopausal women.

Several new endocrine therapies are available. Aromatase inhibitors (e.g. letrozole) reduce the peripheral conversion of androgens to oestrogens. They are only effective in postmenopausal women and may be superior to tamoxifen in women at high risk of recurrence.

Biological therapy

Epidermal growth factor receptors are proteins embedded in the cell membrane that regulate cell growth, adhesion and migration. HER2 is overamplified in 20% of breast cancers. Therefore, HER2 positivity is an independent factor indicating a poor prognosis.

Trastuzumab (Herceptin) is a monoclonal antibody that binds selectively to the HER2 receptor, negating the effect of growth factors (**Figure 3.14**). It only works in patients whose cancers are HER2-positive as detected by immunocytochemistry and fluorescent in situ hybridisation testing. Around 5% of patients receiving it develop cardiac dysfunction as a side effect. Trastuzumab has been shown to improve survival in both the adjuvant and the metastatic setting.

Radiotherapy

Treatment with radiotherapy is indicated after breast-conserving surgery for all breast cancers, and after mastectomy in patients with large, high-grade, node-positive tumours. It has been shown to reduce the risk of local recurrence following breast-conserving surgery and to improve survival.

Paget's disease of the nipple

Paget's disease of the nipple is an uncommon condition characterised by eczematous-like changes of the nipple (**Figure 3.15**). It usually occurs in women over 50 years of age.

The early symptoms are redness and scaling of the nipple. Late features are nipple ulceration or erosion, bleeding and pain. Clinical features that allow the differentiation between Paget's disease and eczema of the nipple are shown in **Table 3.7**. The diagnosis can be confirmed by a nipple biopsy that shows Paget cells in the deep layers of the epidermis. The treatment is the same as for the underlying breast cancer.

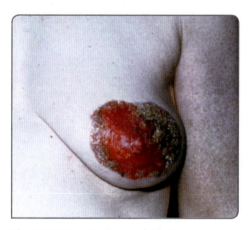

Figure 3.15 Paget's disease of the nipple.

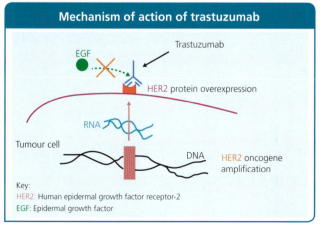

Figure 3.14 Mechanism of action of trastuzumab (Herceptin).

Paget's disease versus nipple eczema	
Paget's disease	Nipple eczema
Unilateral	Bilateral
Minimal itching	Significant itching
Nipple destroyed	Nipple architecture maintained
Possible lump	
Nipple discharge or bleeding	No lump
	Other features of atopic disease

Table 3.7 Differential diagnosis of Paget's disease and nipple eczema

Paget's disease is strongly associated with an underlying breast cancer. About 50% of patients presenting with Paget's disease have a palpable breast lump, usually an invasive ductal carcinoma.

Male breast cancer

About 1% of all breast cancers occur in men. Pathologically, the disease is similar to that in women. The principles of treatment are the same although the proportion of men undergoing mastectomy is obviously higher as men have smaller volumes of breast tissue and breast conserving surgery is often impossible. Adjuvant therapy is the same as for women.

Gynaecomastia

Gynaecomastia is benign enlargement of the male breast. It is the most common breast condition affecting men. It represents enlargement of both ductal and stromal tissue (**Figure 3.16**). 'True' gynaecomastia is enlargement of the breast glandular tissue, whereas 'pseudo' gynaecomastia is due to excess adipose tissue.

Gynaecomastia is benign and often reversible. Most cases are idiopathic (**Table 3.8**). The physiological effects are due to a relative excess of oestrogen, which occur in the neonatal period, during puberty and in old age.

Clinical features

Gynaecomastia usually presents as unilateral or bilateral non-tender breast enlargement.

The history or examination should give an indication of an underlying cause. A detailed drug history is taken and assessment includes

Pathological causes of gynaecomastia	
Causes	Examples
Primary testicular failure	Anorchia
	Klinefelter's syndrome
	Bilateral cryptorchidism
Acquired testicular failure	Mumps
	Irradiation
Secondary testicular failure	Generalised hypopituitarism
	Isolated gonadotrophin deficiency
Endocrine tumours	Testicular
	Adrenal
	Pituitary
Non-endocrine tumours	Bronchial carcinoma
	Lymphoma
	Hypernephroma
Hepatic disease	Cirrhosis
	Haemochromatosis
Drugs	Oestrogens and oestrogen agonists
	Gonadotrophins
	Testosterone target cell inhibitors

Table 3.8 Pathological causes of gynaecomastia

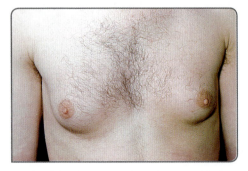

Figure 3.16 Bilateral gynaecomastia.

abdominal and testicular examinations. The diagnosis is essentially clinical so extensive investigation is not usually required.

> **Gynaecomastia is a very common cause of male breast lumps at all ages.** Male breast cancer is extremely uncommon and rarely presents in patients below 50 years of age.

Treatment

Most patients simply need reassurance that gynaecomastia is a benign and self-limiting condition without any underlying cause. Drug treatment is rarely required but danazol reduces the breast size in 80% of patients.

Surgery

The results of cosmetic surgery can be disappointing, and patients are often unhappy with the cosmetic appearance both before and after surgery. An operation is considered if gynaecomastia is painful or cosmetically embarrassing. Small areas of gynaecomastia can be excised through periareolar incision, whereas more extensive areas require either liposuction or a breast reduction via a circumareolar incision.

Answers to starter questions

1. Most of the risk factors that predispose a woman to breast cancer are related to prolonged oestrogen exposure. They include an early menarche, late menopause and consuming medications that contain oestrogen, such as the oral contraceptive pill and hormone replacement therapy. The World Health Organisation (WHO) classifies oestrogens as carcinogenic, and there are two main theories why. Firstly, by its direct action on cell membrane receptors, oestrogen increases breast cell division, increasing the risk of DNA mutations as cells divide and DNA is copied. It is also known to have metabolites that interfere directly with DNA to increase the chance of mutations.

2. Women presenting with any breast symptom should be evaluated by Triple Assessment. This involves a full clinical, radiological and pathological evaluation. This will allow the vast majority of patients with benign breast disease to be rapidly reassured and discharged. In those shown to have breast cancer an appropriate treatment plan is formulated.

3. Surgery for breast cancer usually involves an operation on the breast and an axillary staging procedure. The type of breast surgery depends on the size of the tumour in relation to the size of the breast and involves either breast conserving surgery or a mastectomy. If the axillary lymph nodes are likely to show no evidence of metastases, then a sentinel node biopsy is the axillary staging procedure of choice. If the lymph nodes are known or are likely to have metastatic disease then an axillary node clearance is required.

4. Whilst the mortality from breast cancer in the UK is improving, it remains significantly higher than in other countries in Europe. The standard of treatment in this country is comparable to other developed counties and the higher mortality is almost certainly related to lack of population awareness and late presentation of the disease.

5. Breast lumps in both women and men should be assessed by Triple Assessment. However, the causes of breast lumps significantly differ between the sexes. Only 1% of breast cancers occur in men and it is very uncommon below the age of 50 years. The majority of men with a breast lump have gynaecomastia. Assessment in women should be aimed at identifying those with breast cancer. In men, assessment should be aimed at confirming gynaecomastia and reassuring the majority that it is simply physiological.

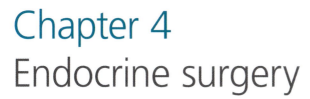

Chapter 4
Endocrine surgery

Introduction. 65
Case 2 Neck lump 66
Core sciences 68
History, examination and
investigation 73
Altered thyroid states 76
Thyroglossal cysts 78
Solitary thyroid nodules 79
Thyroid neoplasms 80
Thyroiditis 82
Parathyroid conditions 83
Adrenal conditions 85
Carcinoid tumours 89

Starter questions

Answers to the following questions are on page 90.

1. What are hormones and how are their levels controlled?
2. Can a benign endocrine tumour be dangerous?
3. How do you know if a thyroid lump is 'sinister'?
4. Why is knowledge of the anatomy of the recurrent laryngeal nerve important in thyroid surgery?
5. How do primary and secondary hyperparathyroidism differ?

Introduction

The endocrine system consists of a series of glands (**Figure 4.1**) that produce chemicals called hormones. These have diverse actions that regulate the function of many other physiological systems. Endocrine diseases result from either a local change to an endocrine gland (e.g. goitre) or from systemic metabolic effects as a result of an under- or overproduction of hormones.

Endocrine disorders can be managed with drugs but some patients need surgical intervention to control the disease or manage its complications.

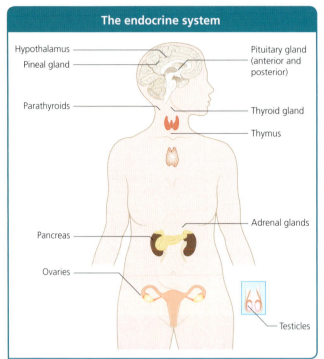

The endocrine system

Hypothalamus

Pineal gland

Pituitary gland
(anterior and
posterior)

Parathyroids

Thyroid gland

Thymus

Adrenal glands

Pancreas

Ovaries

Testicles

Figure 4.1 The endocrine system.

Case 2 Neck lump

Presentation

A 64-year-old man, William Penfield, presents to his general practitioner with a 4-month history of a painless neck lump.

Initial interpretation

Neck lumps are a common presentation of surgical disease. A thorough history and examination guides subsequent investigations to determine both the site and the cause of the lump. There are many, mostly benign, causes of neck lumps. However, a small proportion are malignant.

History

William first noticed the lump 4 months ago. It is situated in the left side of his neck. It is painless and has slowly increased in size.

Interpretation of history

A painless, slow-growing neck lump to one side of the midline in an elderly man suggests that the lump is either a thyroid nodule or a cervical lymph node. Both thyroid nodules and cervical lymphadenopathy arise from benign or malignant pathological processes.

Further history

William is otherwise fit and well. His weight is steady. He has noticed no change in his voice. He has had no palpitations.

Examination

On examination, William looks well. His pulse rate is normal. Examination of his outstretched hands shows no evidence of a tremor. His eyes appear normal.

Case 2 *continued*

Inspection of his neck shows a 2 cm lump in the left lobe of his thyroid gland. The lump moves up when William is asked to swallow a mouth full of water. Palpation confirms a smooth, non-tender lump in the thyroid gland. Auscultation shows no bruit. There is no cervical lymphadenopathy.

Interpretation of findings

General examination shows no physical signs to suggest thyroid disease. Examination of the neck shows a benign nodule in the left lobe of the thyroid gland.

Investigations

William is referred to an ENT surgeon in the local hospital who arranges an ultrasound scan (**Figure 4.2**). This confirms a 2 cm solitary nodule in the left lobe of the thyroid gland. A fine-needle aspiration cytology specimen is taken under ultrasound guidance (**Figure 4.3**). This shows follicular cells. A radioiodine scan shows the lump to be cold (i.e. to not take up the

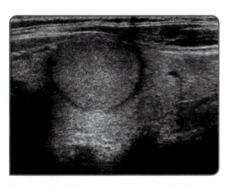

Figure 4.2 Ultrasound appearance of a benign thyroid nodule.

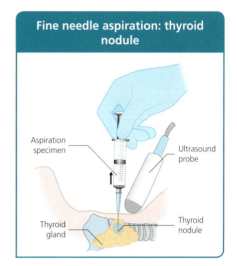

Fine needle aspiration: thyroid nodule

Aspiration specimen

Ultrasound probe

Thyroid gland

Thyroid nodule

Figure 4.3 Fine-needle aspiration of a thyroid nodule.

radioisotope). Serum total thyroxine (T_4) and thyroid stimulating hormone (TSH) levels are normal.

Diagnosis

The clinical picture, confirmed by ultrasonography, shows the lump to be a solitary thyroid nodule. The patient has normal results on thyroid function tests.

Fine-needle aspiration shows cells from either a follicular adenoma or a carcinoma. As it is impossible to differentiate between follicular adenomas or carcinoma on fine-needle aspiration cytology, a thyroid lobectomy is undertaken. This shows no evidence of invasion of the capsule around the lesion, confirming the lesion to be a follicular adenoma. William makes an uncomplicated recovery from his surgery.

Core sciences

Endocrine physiology

Hormones are blood-borne messengers that are produced by one organ, secreted into the circulation and carried to other parts of the body where they have an effect on other organ systems. Only those organs that have specific receptors for a particular hormone are able to respond to it. Hormones have a key role in both homeostasis and adaptation.

Many hormones are amines, proteins or steroids (**Table 4.1**). Some are transported bound to proteins. Only hormones unbound within the plasma are biologically active. Hormones have a short half-life and are rapidly removed from the circulation.

Control of salt, water and osmotic pressure

Homeostasis is the maintenance of a constant internal environment. It requires a close regulation of body salt and water.

Antidiuretic hormone (ADH) is produced in the posterior pituitary and increases water resorption in the collecting ducts of the kidney. Aldosterone is produced in the adrenal cortex and increases sodium reabsorption. If the osmotic pressure of the blood increases or the blood volume falls, increases occur in the secretion of ADH and aldosterone, respectively.

A number of hormones (e.g. parathyroid hormone) are involved in the control of serum calcium.

Categories of hormones		
Amine	**Protein**	**Steroids**
Thyroxine	Insulin	Oestrogens
Adrenaline/ epinephrine	Parathyroid hormone	Testosterone
Melatonin	Growth hormone	Aldosterone
	Prolactin	Cortisol

Table 4.1 Categories of hormones

Reproductive function

Follicle stimulating hormone (FSH) and luteinising hormone (LH) control both the growth of the ovaries and testes and the secretion of the sex hormones oestrogen, progesterone and testosterone. Oxytocin, produced by the posterior pituitary, causes contraction of the uterine muscles particularly during childbirth. Milk production involves many hormones, including prolactin. Milk ejection during lactation is controlled by oxytocin.

Growth and metabolism

Thyroxine increases the metabolic rate of many tissues including the heart and skeletal muscles. Glucagon, adrenaline, cortisol and growth hormone aid metabolism by raising the blood glucose level increasing its availability. Conversely, insulin lowers the blood glucose. Erythropoietin supports metabolism by regulating the number of red cells in the blood. Thyroxine is important in the regulation of growth; excesses or deficiencies of either result in specific growth disorders (e.g. acromegaly).

Thyroid anatomy and physiology

The thyroid gland is found close to the trachea in the front of the neck and has a central role in the control of metabolism.

Thyroid embryology

In the embryo, the thyroid gland develops from the floor of the pharynx. It arises at a site between the tuberculum impar and copula linguae at the junction between the anterior two-thirds and the posterior one-third of the tongue. This point is known as the foramen caecum.

A diverticulum called the thyroglossal duct invaginates and descends in close relation to the hyoid bone (**Figure 4.4**). The gland develops into a bilobed structure to form the thyroid lobes.

Embryology of the thyroid gland

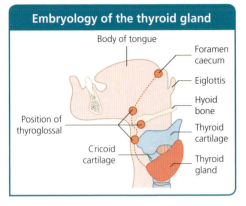

Figure 4.4 Embryology of the thyroid gland. Dotted line shows path of descent of the thyroid gland.

Anatomy of thyroid gland

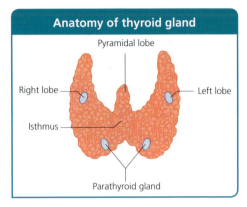

Figure 4.6 Thyroid and parathyroid: gross anatomy.

Thyroid gland: relationship to the trachea

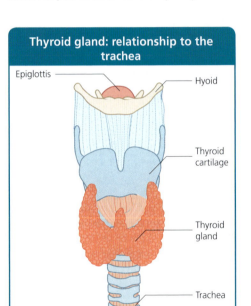

Figure 4.5 Relationship of the thyroid gland to the trachea

Recurrent laryngeal nerve relationship to thyroid gland, trachea and oesophagus

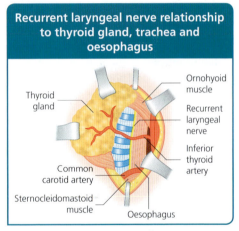

Figure 4.7 Relationship of the recurrent laryngeal nerve to the thyroid gland, trachea and oesophagus: anterior oblique view.

Blood and lymph supply of the thyroid

The thyroid gland is supplied by the superior and inferior thyroid arteries (Figure 4.8). The superior thyroid artery is a branch of the external carotid artery. The inferior thyroid artery is a branch of the thyrocervical trunk. In turn, the thyrocervical trunk is a branch of the subclavian artery.

The venous drainage of the thyroid gland is to the superior, middle and inferior thyroid veins. The superior thyroid vein drains into the internal jugular vein. The middle thyroid vein drains into the internal jugular vein. The inferior thyroid vein drains into the brachiocephalic vein.

Thyroid anatomy

The thyroid gland lies in the front of the neck below the thyroid cartilage (Figure 4.5). The carotid sheath lies posteriorly and laterally. The parathyroid glands lie posterior to the gland (Figure 4.6). The recurrent laryngeal nerves (Figure 4.7) and external laryngeal nerves lie medially. The recurrent laryngeal nerve is closely related to the inferior thyroid artery.

The two lobes of the thyroid gland are connected at the thyroid isthmus (Figure 4.6).

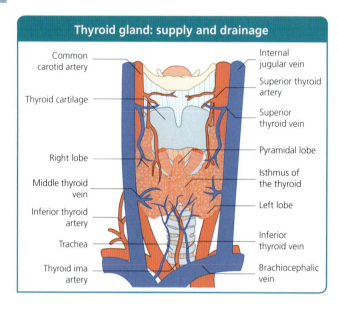

Thyroid gland: supply and drainage

Common carotid artery

Thyroid cartilage

Right lobe

Middle thyroid vein

Inferior thyroid artery

Trachea

Thyroid ima artery

Internal jugular vein

Superior thyroid artery

Superior thyroid vein

Pyramidal lobe

Isthmus of the thyroid

Left lobe

Inferior thyroid vein

Brachiocephalic vein

Figure 4.8 Arterial supply to and venous drainage of the thyroid gland.

The lymphatics of the thyroid gland drain into the deep cervical nodes.

Thyroid histology

The thyroid gland is composed of follicles that selectively absorb iodine and concentrate it in the production of thyroid hormones. As a result, 25% of the body's iodine is found in the thyroid gland.

The follicles are made up of a single layer of cuboidal epithelial cells. These contain a colloid that is rich in a thyroglobulin. This serves as a reservoir of materials for thyroid hormone production.

The spaces between the thyroid follicles contain the second type of thyroid cell – the parafollicular cells or C cells.

Thyroid physiology

Thyroxine and triiodothyronine

The thyroid gland produces T_4 and triiodothyronine (T_3). These are contained within the follicles and are stored bound to thyroglobulin. In the circulation, 99% of the T_4 and T_3 is bound to albumin, thyroxine binding pre-albumin and thyroxine binding globulin. Only the 1% of the hormones that remains unbound is physiologically active. T_3 is quick acting (hours) and T_4 is slow acting (days).

Both thyroid hormones act on most cells of the body except those of the brain. They promote carbohydrate, protein and lipid metabolism. In addition, they increase the basal metabolic rate and oxygen consumption, and regulate tissue growth and development.

Calcitonin

The parafollicular C cells produce calcitonin, which and acts on skeletal tissue and bone. Its main action is to lower serum calcium. Calcitonin inhibits osteoclast activity and bone resorption. It also stimulates osteoblast activity and inhibits the release of ionic calcium from bone.

Parathyroid anatomy and physiology

The parathyroid glands are found in close relation to the thyroid gland and have a role in calcium homeostasis.

Parathyroid embryology

The parathyroid glands are derived from the pharyngeal pouches (**Figure 4.9**). The third pharyngeal pouch gives rise to the two inferior parathyroid glands, and the fourth pharyngeal pouches give rise to the two superior parathyroid glands.

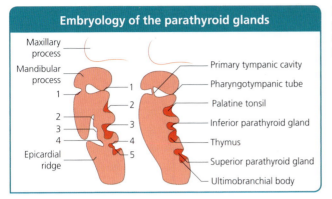

Embryology of the parathyroid glands

- Maxillary process
- Mandibular process
- 1
- 2
- 3
- 4
- Epicardial ridge
- 1
- 2
- 3
- 4
- 5
- Primary tympanic cavity
- Pharyngotympanic tube
- Palatine tonsil
- Inferior parathyroid gland
- Thymus
- Superior parathyroid gland
- Ultimobranchial body

Figure 4.9 Embryology of the parathyroid glands. Numbered structures are the pharyngeal pouches and sinuses.

Abnormalities of the position and number of the parathyroid glands are common. About 5% of the population have fewer than four glands and 25% have supernumerary glands, often in aberrant positions.

Parathyroid anatomy

The four parathyroid glands are usually found near the posterior aspect of the thyroid gland. They have a distinct, encapsulated, smooth surface that differs from the adjacent thyroid tissue. They are typically light brown in colour because of their fat content and vascularity.

The superior parathyroid glands are commonly located close to the superior pole of the thyroid gland near the cricothyroid cartilage. They lie close to the intersection of the inferior thyroid artery and the recurrent laryngeal nerve. The inferior parathyroid glands are more variable in location and are found near the lower pole of the thyroid.

Parathyroid physiology

Parathyroid hormone is made up of 84 amino acids. Its half-life is measured in minutes. In bone, it increases bone turnover and calcium release. In the kidney, it increases the production of 1,25 dihydroxy-vitamin D_3. In the gut, parathyroid hormone increases calcium absorption. The overall effect is to increase serum calcium levels.

Pituitary anatomy and physiology

The pituitary gland has two lobes. It has a pivotal role in homeostasis as it controls several other endocrine systems.

Anatomy of the pituitary gland

The pituitary gland is situated below the third ventricle of the brain. It lies in the pituitary fossa of the sella turcica in the sphenoid bone and is covered by a fold of dura mater known as the diaphragma sellae. It is connected to the brain by the infundibulum and has anterior and posterior lobes.

The anterior lobe of the pituitary is formed in the embryo from Rathke's pouch and consists of the pars anterior and pars intermedia. The hormones it produces are transported to the hypothalamus in the blood supply. The posterior lobe is a downgrowth of the floor of the third ventricle. Nerve fibres extend from hypothalamus to the posterior pituitary.

The gland is overhung by the anterior and posterior clinoid processes, dorsum sellae and diaphragma sellae. The infundibulum of the pituitary passes posteriorly to the optic chiasma. Superior to the optic chiasma is the anterior communicating artery. A cavernous sinus lies on each side of the pituitary gland. In the lateral wall of each cavernous sinus lie several

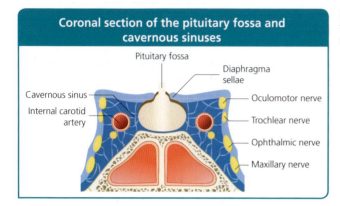

Coronal section of the pituitary fossa and cavernous sinuses

Pituitary fossa
Diaphragma sellae
Cavernous sinus
Internal carotid artery
Oculomotor nerve
Trochlear nerve
Ophthalmic nerve
Maxillary nerve

Figure 4.10 Coronal section of the pituitary fossa and cavernous sinuses.

cranial nerves as well as the internal carotid arteries (**Figure 4.10**).

Anterior pituitary physiology

The hypothalamus is a major control centre in homeostasis. It constantly monitors the status of body and regulates several bodily functions via both nerves and hormones. It is responsible for the control of emotional responses, temperature regulation, appetite and water balance.

The hypothalamus controls the anterior pituitary through a series of releasing hormones, which travel in a portal system (i.e. a blood system that joins directly to organs) to the pituitary gland. These either stimulate or inhibit the release of anterior pituitary hormones. The anterior pituitary is in turn controlled by negative feedback loops (**Figure 4.11**).

Adrenocorticotrophic hormones

Corticotrophin releasing hormone is produced by the hypothalamus. It stimulates the release of adrenocorticotrophic hormone (ACTH) from the anterior pituitary. ACTH in turn stimulates the adrenal cortex to release hormones including glucocorticoids, androgens and mineralocorticoids. Increased levels of glucocorticoids reduce ACTH release via a negative feedback loop. Levels of ACTH are increased in fever, stress and hypoglycaemia.

Thyroid stimulating hormone

Thyrotropin releasing hormone is produced in the hypothalamus. It stimulates the release of TSH from the anterior pituitary.

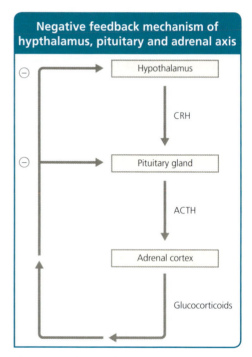

Negative feedback mechanism of hypthalamus, pituitary and adrenal axis

Hypothalamus
CRH
Pituitary gland
ACTH
Adrenal cortex
Glucocorticoids

Figure 4.11 Negative feedback mechanism of the hypothalamus, pituitary and adrenal axis. ACTH, adrenocortotrophic hormone; CRH, corticotrophin releasing hormone.

TSH stimulates thyroid hormone production. Raised levels of thyroid hormones inhibit the release of both thyrotropin releasing hormone and TSH. Levels of thyrotropin releasing hormone are increased during exercise and as part of the stress response.

Gonadotrophins

Gonadotrophin releasing hormone is produced by the hypothalamus. It stimulates the release of LH and FSH from the anterior pituitary. FSH stimulates sperm and egg production. LH causes maturation of the ovarian follicle and ovulation. LH also causes the release of the gonadal hormones testosterone and oestrogen. Rising levels of gonadal hormones inhibits the release of gonadotrophin releasing hormones, LH and FSH.

Growth hormone

The hypothalamus produces growth hormone releasing hormone. This stimulates the release of growth hormone by the anterior pituitary.

Growth hormone has a direct action on non-endocrine cells. It is an important anabolic hormone, stimulating many cells to grow and divide. It also promotes the growth of bones and skeletal muscles. It increases protein production by the liver and muscle, and stimulates gluconeogenesis. In addition, it converts glucose to glycogen.

Posterior pituitary physiology

Nerves pass directly from the supraoptic and paraventricular nuclei in the hypothalamus to the posterior pituitary. The cell bodies of these nerves produce the posterior pituitary hormones. These hormones are then transported down the axons by axoplasmic transport to the posterior pituitary gland. Finally, they are released from the pituitary by neurosecretion.

The posterior pituitary releases two hormones. ADH acts on the collecting ducts of the kidney to increase water retention. Oxytocin stimulates the uterus to contract during childbirth. It also causes vasoconstriction and raises blood pressure.

Adrenal anatomy and physiology

There are two adrenal glands, situated in close relation to the superior borders of the two kidneys. Each adrenal gland is divided into the cortex and medulla (**Figure 4.12**), both of which have endocrine functions. The adrenal medulla is part of the sympathetic nervous system and releases adrenaline/epinephrine and noradrenaline/norepinephrine into the circulation. The adrenal cortex produces both mineralocorticoids and glucocorticoids.

Aldosterone is produced by the zona glomerulosa of the adrenal cortex. It acts on the

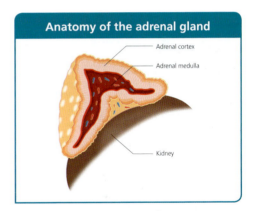

Anatomy of the adrenal gland

- Adrenal cortex
- Adrenal medulla
- Kidney

Figure 4.12 Anatomy of the adrenal gland. The adrenal cortex is divided into the zona glomerulosa, zona fasciculata and zona reticularis.

distal convoluted tubule of the kidney to increase sodium reabsorption. Sodium reabsorption occurs at the expense of potassium and hydrogen ion loss. Cortisol is produced by the zona fasciculata of the adrenal cortex and has widespread effects on carbohydrate metabolism increasing blood glucose levels.

History, examination and investigation

The clinical features that result from disorders of an endocrine gland have two underlying causes: the local effects of the physical changes in the gland, and systemic changes resulting from the levels of the hormones that the gland produces.

Common symptoms of endocrine disease	
System	Features
General	Weight gain or loss
	Heat intolerance or sweating
	Skin and hair changes
	Menstrual irregularity
	Erectile dysfunction
Cardiovascular	Palpitations
Gastrointestinal	Changes in bowel habit
Urinary	Polyuria and polydipsia
Neurological	Anxiety or nervousness
	Irritability or mood changes

Table 4.2 Common symptoms of endocrine disease

Differential diagnosis of neck lumps	
Midline	Lateral
Thyroglossal cyst	Solitary thyroid nodule
Submental lymph node	Goitre
	Salivary gland
	Cystic hygroma
	Branchial cyst
	Pharyngeal pouch
	Carotid artery tumour or aneurysm

Table 4.3 Differential diagnosis of neck lumps

History

When taking a history from a patient with a suspected endocrine disorder, it is important to identify both the local and the systemic features. Common systemic symptoms of endocrine disorders are shown in **Table 4.2**.

Thyroid gland

Disorders of the thyroid gland are the most common endocrine disorders presenting to surgeons. Diseases of the thyroid cause local symptoms related to a lump or swelling in the neck or to systemic effects resulting from changes in the endocrine activity of the gland.

Comparison of hypothyroidism and hyperthyroidism	
Hypothyroidism	Hyperthyroidism
Increased weight	Weight loss
Slow thoughts	Nervousness
Slow speech	Hyperactivity and irritability
Hair loss	Insomnia
Muscle fatigue	Tremor
Preference for warm weather	Tachycardia and palpitations
	Dyspnoea
	Increased appetite
	Sweating
	Diarrhoea
	Eye signs e.g ophthalmoplegia
	Preference for cold weather

Table 4.4 Comparison of clinical features of hypothyroidism and hyperthyroidism

Common signs of endocrine disease	
System	Features
General	Change in mental state
	Change in energy levels
Skin	Sweating
	Skin thinning
	Bruising
	Moon face
	Hirsutism
	Hair loss
Eyes	Exophthalmos
	Cranial nerve palsy
	Visual field defects
Breast	Gynaecomastia
	Galactorrhoea
Musculoskeletal	Muscle weakness

Table 4.5 Common signs of endocrine disease

Local symptoms

The majority of thyroid swellings present with a lump in the neck, either in the midline or more lateral. The differential diagnosis of neck lumps is shown in **Table 4.3**.

Most thyroid swellings remain static or slowly increase in size over an extended period. Some thyroid swellings are painful and appear suddenly. Large thyroid swellings can obstruct the oesophagus and cause discomfort on swallowing (dysphagia) or compress the trachea, causing difficulty in breathing (dyspnoea). A change in the quality of the voice or hoarseness suggests a recurrent laryngeal nerve palsy due to direct tumour invasion and is a symptom that should raise suspicion of a malignant disease.

General symptoms

A comparison of the general symptoms of hypothyroidism and hyperthyroidism is shown in **Table 4.4**.

Examination

The physical signs of endocrine disease are also local or systemic. The most common systemic features of endocrine disease are shown in **Table 4.5**. The examination of patients with potential thyroid disease first elicits signs of an altered thyroid state. This is followed by an examination of the thyroid gland looking for either a goitre or a discrete thyroid lump.

Thyroid gland

General examination

Look first for the presence or absence of signs of hypothyroidism or hyperthyroidism. Examine the hands for sweating, tremor or tachycardia. Examine the eyes for:

- **Lid retraction** – upward displacement of the upper eye lid margin
- **Lid lag** – delayed movement of the upper lid
- **Exophthalmos** – protrusion of the eyes
- **Ophthalmoplegia** – weakness of the eye muscles
- **Chemosis** – swelling of the conjunctiva

There can also be stridor, a high-pitched sound resulting from turbulent airflow through the upper airway.

Inspection

This aims to ascertain whether the lump is in the anatomical site of the thyroid gland.

The patient is given a glass of water and asked to hold a mouthful before swallowing it. The lump is observed for elevation on swallowing. Ask the patient to protrude their tongue to see whether the lump moves up.

> **All thyroid swellings ascend on swallowing.** If the lump rises on tongue protrusion, it must be connected to the hyoid bone which ascends during this movement.

Palpation

The thyroid gland is palpated with the doctor standing behind the patient. The patient's neck is slightly flexed (**Figure 4.13**). The size, shape, surface and consistency of the thyroid gland are assessed, and tenderness is noted.

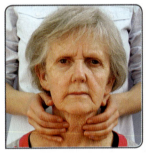

Figure 4.13 Palpation of the thyroid gland

Functional assessment of a goitre or solitary thyroid nodule		
Thyroid examination	Thyroid function	Causes
Diffuse goitre	Euthyroid	Physiological goitre
		Autoimmune thyroiditis
Diffuse goitre	Hyperthyroid	Primary hyperthyroidism
Multinodular goitre	Euthyroid	Multinodular goitre
Multinodular goitre	Hyperthyroid	Toxic nodular goitre
Solitary nodule	Euthyroid	Thyroid cyst
		Thyroid adenoma
		Thyroid carcinoma
Solitary nodule	Hyperthyroid	Functioning adenoma

Table 4.6 Functional assessment of a goitre or solitary thyroid nodule

A normal thyroid gland is impalpable. If a lump is palpated, it is important to determine whether it is solitary, multiple or part of a diffuse enlargement of the gland. The position of the trachea is checked by placing the tip of the finger in the suprasternal notch. The trachea may be deviated laterally by a goitre. The cervical and supraclavicular lymph nodes are palpated and the gland is auscultated for a possible bruit.

Goitre

'Goitre' is a non-specific term describing enlargement of the thyroid gland. This does not imply the presence of any specific pathology. Goitres are either diffuse or multinodular (**Table 4.6**).

Investigation

The investigation of potential endocrine disease aims to confirm the underlying clinical impression, formulated following the taking of history and examining the patient, to assess the functional endocrine status and identify the underlying cause. For all endocrine disorders this requires a combination of biochemical assays and radiological imaging.

Thyroid function tests

Thyroid function tests are a series of blood tests used to assess the overall function of the thyroid gland. They include measurement of TSH, T_4 and T_3.

> In hyperthyroidism, T_4 and/or T_3 are raised and TSH is immeasurable. In hypothyroidism, TSH is elevated.

Thyroid ultrasound

Thyroid ultrasound is a safe and effective method of determining the number, size and presence of any solid or cystic components within the thyroid gland. Unfortunately, malignant thyroid nodules cannot be differentiated from benign nodules by this technique alone.

Fine-needle aspiration cytology

Fine-needle aspiration cytology is the diagnostic tool of choice for pathological evaluation of the thyroid nodules. It involves using a needle and syringe to aspirate a sample from the gland and can be performed under ultrasound guidance (see **Figure 4.3**).

Specimens are classified as benign, malignant, indeterminate or insufficient. The accuracy of fine-needle aspiration cytology in assessing thyroid lesions is closely related to the histological type of the lesion under investigation.

Radioisotope scanning

Radioisotope scanning, also known as scintigraphy, allows thyroid nodules to be classified according to their ability or lack of ability to accumulate the radioactive isotope. The most commonly used isotopes are ^{131}iodine, ^{123}iodine and ^{99}technetium, which provide a functional assessment of the thyroid. Nodules are classified as:

- **Cold**, which are hypofunctional
- **Warm**, which are normal
- **Hot,** which are hyperfunctional

Thyroid radioisotope scanning cannot distinguish between benign and malignant thyroid nodules. A cold nodule can be malignant, but most cold nodules are still benign.

Altered thyroid states

An alteration in the thyroid state results in in either an underproduction or an overproduction of thyroid hormones. The clinical features will reflect the physiological and metabolic properties of thyroid hormones.

Thyrotoxicosis

Thyrotoxicosis is due to an overproduction of T_4 or T_3. It affects 2% women and 0.2% of men. The most common causes are Graves' disease, toxic nodular goitre, a toxic solitary nodule and thyroiditis.

Clinical features

The many clinical features of thyrotoxicosis are shown in **Table 4.4**.

Pretibial myxoedema occurs in 1–2% patients with Graves' disease. It presents with painless thickening of the skin in nodules or plaques. These usually occurs on the shins or on the dorsum of foot.

Thyroid acropachy occurs in fewer than 1% patients with thyrotoxicosis. It closely resembles finger clubbing.

> **Graves' disease is an autoimmune disorder resulting from the production of antibodies against the TSH receptor.** The antibodies cause thyrotoxicosis by binding to the TSH receptor, causing chronic stimulation.

Diagnostic approach

The diagnostic approach to a patient with clinical features of thyrotoxicosis is first to establish the diagnosis and then to elucidated the underlying cause.

Investigations

The diagnosis of thyrotoxicosis is confirmed by measuring the serum TSH level which will be low and suppressed. The serum free T_4 level is normally increased. The serum total T_4 level varies due to changes in the amount of thyroid binding globulin. Free T_3 is occasionally increased in isolation in patients with T_3 toxicosis. A normal TSH level excludes a diagnosis of thyrotoxicosis.

Anti-TSH antibodies are increased in patients with Graves' disease. Thyroid scintigraphy will show a hot nodule (with suppression of the normal gland) in patients with a toxic solitary nodule.

Management

In patients with severe thyrotoxicosis, rapid symptomatic relief is achieved using beta-blockers. Thyroid function can be reduced by anti-thyroid drugs, radioactive iodine or surgery.

Medication

Anti-thyroid drugs

These inhibit the synthesis of T_4 by reducing the incorporation of iodine into tyrosine residues. The most commonly used drug is carbimazole. Treatment with this should be used in the short term (3–4 months) prior to definitive treatment (radioiodine or surgery) or in the long term (12–24 months) to induce remission in patients with Graves' disease. Overall, 40% of patients with Graves' disease respond to carbimazole.

The advantage of anti-thyroid drugs is that surgery and the use of radioactive materials are avoided. The disadvantages are that treatment is prolonged and the failure rate is high at approximately 50%. It is impossible to predict which patients will remain in remission.

> **The side effects of carbimazole include agranulocytosis, aplastic anaemia and hepatitis.** Patients should be warned to seek medical attention if they develop a sore throat or other signs of infection. as these can be life threatening in the presence of agranulocytosis.

Radioactive iodine

[131]Iodine is the isotope most commonly used to treat thyrotoxicosis. A single oral dose of 400 MBq renders 50% of patients hypothyroid but about 20% remain hyperthyroid - the remainder are euthyroid. It is contraindicated in children, pregnancy and breastfeeding. Pregnancy should be avoided for 4 months after treatment.

The advantage of radioiodine treatment is that surgery and prolonged drug therapy are not required. The disadvantage is that 80% of patients will be hypothyroid at 10 years.

Surgery

This is indicated in patients with Graves' disease if there is relapse after an adequate course of anti-thyroid drugs or a large goitre at diagnosis. Subtotal thyroidectomy is the operation of choice. This preserves about 10% of the thyroid tissue. To reduce the risk of cardiovascular complications and thyroid storm, patients must have normal thyroid function prior to surgery.

The advantages of surgery are that the goitre is removed and the cure rate is high. The disadvantages are that 5% of patients develop recurrent thyrotoxicosis, 20% develop postoperative hypothyroidism and 0.5% develop parathyroid insufficiency.

> **A thyroid storm is an uncommon, life-threatening exacerbation of thyrotoxicosis.** It has a mortality of up to 50%. Precipitating factors include thyroid surgery, radioiodine and the withdrawal of antithyroid drugs. Clinical features include severe thyrotoxicosis, fever, delirium, seizure and jaundice. Treatment is with propylthiouracil, Lugol's iodine, beta-blockers and supportive measures.

Hypothyroidism

Hypothyroidism is due to an underproduction of T_4. Worldwide, iodine deficiency is the most common cause. In the developed world, hypothyroidsm is most commonly due to Hashimoto's thyroiditis, thyroid surgery or radioiodine therapy. It affects about 5% of the adult population.

Early disease can be asymptomatic or associated with minimal symptoms. Common presenting clinical features are:

- Tiredness
- Lethargy
- Muscle weakness
- Weight gain
- Depression
- Skin thinning
- Bradycardia

An examination may show a goitre. The diagnosis is confirmed by showing a raised TSH level, and treatment is with T_4 replacement.

Thyroglossal cysts

Thyroglossal cysts arise from remnants of thyroid tissue that are found in the line of descent of the thyroglossal duct. They are cystic lesions with thyroid tissue in the wall. The cysts are present in about 5% of the population, with an approximately equal male to female distribution. About 40% of cases present in children less than 10 years of age.

Clinical features

A thyroglossal cyst presents as a painless midline neck swelling, almost always below the hyoid bone (**Figure 4.14**). The remainder are found in the base of the tongue or as far laterally as the tip of the hyoid bone. As the cyst is attached to the foramen caecum, the classical clinical sign is that the lump moves up when the patient protrudes their tongue.

Cysts occasionally present with a painful lump as a result of infection, or as a discharging wound if an infected cyst ruptures.

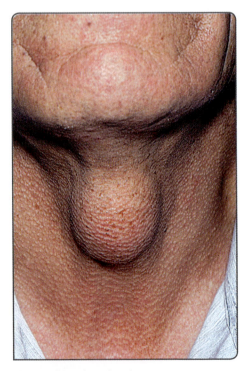

Figure 4.14 A thyroglossal cyst.

Management

Treatment is by surgical excision. A Sistrunk operation is the surgery of choice. First, a transverse skin crease incision is made. The platysma muscle is elevated and the cyst dissected. It is important to remove the middle third of the hyoid bone and any remnants of the thyroglossal duct that extend above the hyoid bone. This reduces the risk of recurrence.

Solitary thyroid nodules

A solitary thyroid nodule is an isolated lump occurring in an otherwise normal thyroid gland. It should be differentiated from a goitre, in which the thyroid gland is diffusely enlarged or there are multiple nodules – a multinodular goitre.

Epidemiology

About 5% of population have a palpable solitary thyroid nodule, with over 80% occurring in women. Malignant thyroid nodules are more common in children, men and those over the age of 60 years.

Aetiology

Solitary thyroid nodules are caused by thyroid cysts, colloid nodules and benign and malignant thyroid tumours. Fewer than 10% of solitary thyroid nodules are malignant.

Clinical features

A solitary thyroid nodule usually presents with a slow-growing, painless neck lump. Rapid growth or the presence of pain suggests either malignancy or haemorrhage into a nodule. The report of a family history of thyroid cancer is important as about 20% of medullary carcinomas are familial. A history of radiation exposure should also be sought as radiation exposure increases the risk of thyroid malignancy.

Most patients will be clinically euthyroid, and examination of the neck will show a mobile solitary nodule within the thyroid gland. Evidence of fixation or cervical lymphadenopathy suggests malignancy. Obstructive signs include stridor, tracheal deviation and engorgement of the neck veins. Hoarseness and vocal cord paralysis suggests a recurrent laryngeal nerve palsy.

Diagnostic approach

The diagnostic approach aims to confirm the presence of a thyroid nodule, assess the functional status of the gland and identify the underlying pathology.

Investigations

The investigation of a solitary thyroid nodule should include a biochemical assessment of the functional status of the thyroid, a thyroid ultrasound, isotope scanning and fine-needle aspiration cytology of the nodule (**Figure 4.15**).

Biochemical assessment

Thyroid function tests are performed. Thyroid anti-thyroglobulin and anti-microsomal antibodies are increased in thyroiditis. If there is a family history suggestive of medullary carcinoma, measure the serum calcitonin level. If there is a suspicion of multiple endocrine neoplasia type 2 syndrome, the patient needs 24-hour urinary catecholamine estimation to exclude a phaeochromocytoma prior to surgery Surgery in the presence of an undiagnosed phaeochromocytoma can result in life-threatening hypertension.

Ultrasound

An ultrasound scan can define whether a lesion is a truly solitary nodule or a dominant nodule in nodular goitre. It also distinguishes solid and cystic lesions. There are no reliable ultrasound criteria to distinguish benign and malignant lesions. However, features that suggest malignancy include

- Reduced echogenicity
- Microcalcification

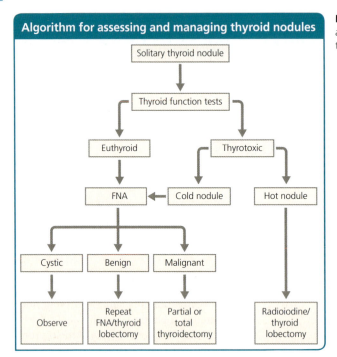

Figure 4.15 Algorithm for the assessment and management of thyroid nodules.

- Irregular margins
- An increased blood flow on Doppler ultrasonography.

Isotope scanning

This technique cannot differentiate benign and malignant nodules. Most solitary thyroid nodules are cold. The majority of cancers arise in cold nodules, with the risk of cancer in a cold nodule being about 10%. The risk of tumour in a hot nodule is negligible.

Fine-needle aspiration cytology

This is an important investigation of the solitary thyroid nodule as it will differenti-ate benign from malignant causes in 95% of patients. Possible cytopathological diagnoses are benign, malignant, suspicious and inadequate. Fine-needle aspiration cytology can distinguish benign and malignant tumours, except for patients with follicular neoplasms in whom FNA can not differentiate an adenoma from a carcinoma. The diagnosis of a follicular carcinoma requires evidence of capsular invasion which cannot be assessed with FNA alone. A definitive result on fine-needle aspiration cytology allows surgery to be avoided in those with minimally symptomatic benign disease and appropriate surgical management of thyroid neoplasms.

Thyroid neoplasms

Thyroid tumours are classified as either benign of malignant (**Table 4.7**). The most common malignant tumours are papillary and follicular carcinomas.

Benign thyroid neoplasms

Most benign thyroid tumours are follicular adenomas. Papillary adenomas are rare, and

Classification of thyroid tumours	
Benign	Malignant
Follicular adenoma	Papillary carcinoma
Teratoma	Follicular carcinoma
	Medullary carcinoma
	Lymphoma
	Squamous cell carcinoma
	Metastatic

Table 4.7 Classification of thyroid tumours

Comparison of papillary and follicular tumours	
Papillary	Follicular
Multifocal	Solitary
Unencapsulated	Encapsulated
Lymphatic spread	Haematogenous spread
Metastasises to regional nodes	Metastasises to lung, brain and bone

Table 4.8 Comparison of papillary and follicular tumours

all papillary tumours should be considered to be potentially malignant.

Follicular adenoma

Approximately 85% of follicular lesions are benign and 15% are malignant. They are encapsulated, smooth, discrete lesions with either a glandular or an acinar pattern.

Unfortunately, follicular adenomas cannot be differentiated from carcinoma on fine-needle aspiration cytology alone. The diagnosis requires histological assessment to exclude capsular invasion, and surgery is required for all follicular lesion.

Toxic adenoma

These account for 5% of all cases of thyrotoxicosis. The female to male ratio is 9:1. Most clinical presentations are with either a thyroid nodule (50%) or thyrotoxicosis (40%). Radioisotope scanning shows a hot nodule. Treatment is by thyroid lobectomy. Postoperative management will require T_4 replacement therapy until the suppressed gland returns to normal.

Malignant thyroid tumours

Differentiated thyroid cancer accounts for 80% of thyroid neoplasms. The female to male ratio is approximately 4:1. Malignant thyroid tumours usually present as a solitary thyroid nodule in a young or middle-aged adult. Papillary and follicular tumours have different characteristics (**Table 4.8**).

Red flag signs for thyroid cancer are:

- Male gender
- Extremes of age (<20 or >65 years)
- Rapid growth
- Symptoms of local invasion (pain, hoarseness)
- A history of irradiation of the neck
- A family history of thyroid carcinoma

Papillary tumours

Most papillary tumours are less than 2 cm in diameter at presentation. Approximately 50% are multicentric with a simultaneous tumour in the contralateral lobe. Early spread occurs to the regional lymph nodes.

Total thyroidectomy is the surgical procedure of choice. Many tumours are TSH dependent so TSH suppression with postoperative T_4 replacement is appropriate. If nodal metastases are present, a neck dissection is also required.

Follicular tumours

Follicular adenoma and follicular carcinomas cannot be differentiated by fine-needle aspiration cytology alone. The treatment of all follicular neoplasms is thyroid lobectomy, and a frozen section is analysed. If the frozen section confirms a follicular carcinoma, a total thyroidectomy should be performed during the same anaesthetic. If the frozen section confirms an adenoma, no further surgery required.

All patients require suppressive T_4 therapy.

Anaplastic carcinoma

These account for fewer than 5% of all thyroid malignancies. They occur in the elderly and are usually an aggressive tumour. Death often occurs within 6 months.

Local infiltration causes dyspnoea, hoarseness and dysphagia. Incision biopsy should be avoided as it often causes uncontrollable local spread. Thyroidectomy is seldom feasible. Radiotherapy and chemotherapy are important modes of treatment in the palliation of symptoms.

Thyroid lymphoma

This tumour accounts for 2% of all thyroid malignancies. It often arises in a thyroid gland in a patient with Hashimoto's thyroiditis or non-Hodgkin's B-cell lymphoma. It presents as a goitre, and the diagnosis is often be made by fine-needle aspiration cytology.

Radiotherapy is the treatment of choice. The prognosis is good, with the 5-year survival rate often being more than 85%.

Medullary carcinoma

This carcinoma accounts for 8% of all thyroid malignancies. It arises from the parafollicular C cells.

About 20% of cases are familial with an autosomal dominant inheritance and almost complete penetrance. It may occur as part of multiple endocrine neoplasia syndrome types 2a and 2b. At-risk patients can be identified by looking for a mutation in the RET proto-oncogene. These patients should then be offered prophylactic thyroidectomy. Sporadic cases usually have unilateral disease.

Medullary carcinoma metastasises to the regional nodes and also, via the blood, to the bone, liver and lung. About 50% of patients have lymph node metastases at presentation. The tumours produce calcitonin so serum calcitonin levels are used in follow-up to monitor for the presence of metastatic disease. Total thyroidectomy is the treatment of choice.

Management

Thyroid tumours are managed by removal of the involved lobe or the whole thyroid gland.

Surgery

The role of total thyroidectomy and thyroid lobectomy in the management of differentiated tumours is controversial. In the hands of an experienced surgeon, complications are rare after thyroidectomy. The complications of thyroidectomy include:

- Haemorrhage
- Respiratory obstruction
- Recurrent laryngeal nerve palsy
- Hypocalcaemia
- Pneumothorax
- Air embolism
- Recurrent hyperthyroidism
- Hypothyroidism

It is important to preserve the recurrent laryngeal nerves and parathyroid glands to avoid hoarseness or stridor and hypocalcaemia, respectively.

> **Haemorrhage following thyroidectomy can cause acute airway obstruction.** Immediate opening of the wound on the ward can therefore be life-saving.

Thyroiditis

Thyroiditis is inflammation of the thyroid gland. It results from viral or bacterial infection or autoimmune disease.

de Quervain's thyroiditis

de Quervain's thyroiditis (granulomatous or subacute thyroiditis) is believed to be caused by a viral infection. It presents with a painful swelling of one or both thyroid lobes, usually associated with malaise and fever. Patients often have clinical features of mild hyperthyroidism, and the free T_4 level is usually raised.

It is a self-limiting illness with spontaneous recovery. In the long term, 5% of patients develop mild hypothyroidism. Symptomatic improvement can occur with anti-inflammatory drugs. Steroids hastens resolution in those with severe symptoms.

Hashimoto's thyroiditis

Hashimoto's thyroiditis (lymphomatous thyroiditis) is an autoimmune disease. It produces diffuse swelling of thyroid gland. Histologically, the thyroid is infiltrated with lymphocytes and plasma cells. Serum anti-thyroglobulin and anti-microsomal antibody levels are raised. Patients eventually become hypothyroid.

T4 replacement therapy suppresses TSH section and reduces the size of the thyroid gland. Surgery is rarely required. In the long term, the risk of thyroid lymphoma is increased.

Riedel's thyroiditis

Riedel's thyroiditis (acute fibrous thyroiditis) is a rare disease but is important because it clinically mimics malignancy.

Histologically, a diffuse inflammatory infiltrate occurs throughout the thyroid gland and may extend beyond the capsule into the adjacent structures. Riedel's thyroiditis is associated with sclerosing cholangitis and retroperitoneal and mediastinal fibrosis.

Surgery is rarely required, but division of the isthmus may be necessary to decompress the trachea.

Acute suppurative thyroiditis

Acute suppurative thyroiditis is caused by a bacterial or fungal infection. It produces an acutely inflamed thyroid gland. The diagnosis is confirmed by fine-needle aspiration cytology. Treatment is with intravenous antibiotics.

Parathyroid conditions

Hyperparathyroidism is the increased production of parathyroid hormone by the parathyroid glands. It can be primary, secondary or tertiary.

Primary hyperparathyroidism is due to an autonomous overproduction of parathyroid hormone by the parathyroid glands.

Secondary hyperparathyroidism is a reactive increase in parathyroid hormone production to compensate for hypocalcaemia, usually as a result of chronic renal failure.

Tertiary hyperparathyroidism is a condition in which reactive parathyroid hyperplasia results in a hypersecretion of parathyroid hormone despite correction of the underlying imbalance in calcium homeostasis.

Epidemiology

Hyperparathyroidism is a common disorder and affects approximately one in 1000 of the population. It affects one in 500 women over the age of 45 years.

Aetiology

Primary hyperparathyroidism can be due a parathyroid adenoma (85%), a parathyroid hyperplasia (15%) or rarely a parathyroid carcinoma (<1%).

Clinical features

Most patients with hyperparathyroidism are asymptomatic, and most cases are identified when hypercalcaemia is detected on testing for other conditions. The clinical features of hyperparathyroidism are shown in **Table 4.9**. The symptoms are often vague and non-specific.

Clinical features of hyperparathyroidism	
System	Symptoms and signs
General	Polydipsia, weight loss
Cardiovascular	Hypertension, heart block
Musculoskeletal	Bone pain, pathological fractures
Gastrointestinal	Anorexia, nausea, constipation
Neurological	Depression, lethargy, weakness, psychosis

Table 4.9 Clinical features of hyperparathyroidism

The symptoms of hypercalcaemia can be remembered as 'bones, stone, abdominal groans and psychic moans'.

Causes of hypercalcaemia	
Causes	Examples
Endocrine	Primary hyperparathyroidism, thyrotoxicosis
Malignant	Bone metastases, ectopic parathyroid hormone production
Granulomatous disease	Sarcoidosis, tuberculosis
Metabolic	Familial hypercalciuric hypercalcaemia, renal failure
Drug induced	Thiazide diuretics, vitamin D toxicity, lithium, milk alkali syndrome
Other	Immobilization, aluminium toxicity

Table 4.10 Causes of hypercalcaemia

Diagnostic approach

The clinical context in which hypercalcaemia occurs might suggest an obvious underlying cause. If there is no obvious cause, primary hyperparathyroidism is the most likely diagnosis and biochemical investigations will be undertaken to identify the underlying cause.

Investigations

Serum corrected calcium and parathyroid hormone levels are both increased in primary hyperparathyroidism. About 75% of patients with primary hyperparathyroidism have hypercalciuria and 50% have hypophosphataemia. There may also be a mild hyperchloraemic acidosis. In secondary hyperparathyroidism, the serum parathyroid hormone is increased but the calcium level is either normal or low.

The causes of hypercalcaemia are shown in Table 4.10.

Management

The management of hyperparathyroidism depends on the severity of the hypercalcaemia and the underlying cause.

Surgery

The management of patients with mild symptomatic hypercalcaemia or a lack of symptoms is controversial. Some physicians recommend simple observation while others prefer early surgical intervention. The clear indications for surgery in hyperparathyroidism are significant symptoms, a corrected calcium of more than 2.8 mmol/L and complications associated with hypercalcaemia.

Surgery for a parathyroid adenoma involves a parathyroidectomy. Preoperatively, methylene blue is infused intravenously over a period of about 1 hour. This selectively stains the parathyroid glands. Normal glands stain pale green. Pathological glands stain dark blue or black. If a parathyroid adenoma and one normal gland are identified, the adenoma is removed and no further surgery is required. If parathyroid hyperplasia is found, all four glands should be removed and one gland transplanted into a marked forearm site so that the site is documented in case there are future pathological changes in the gland.

Adrenal conditions

Adrenal conditions result from an overproduction of hormones from either the adrenal medulla (catecholamines) or the adrenal cortex (cortisol, aldosterone).

Phaeochromocytomas

Phaeochromocytomas are neuroendocrine tumours, usually of the adrenal medulla. Extraadrenal neuroendocrine tumours are called paraganglionomas. Most secrete adrenaline/epinephrine but some secrete noradrenaline/norepinephrine and dopamine. The clinical features are due to intermittent catecholamine excess.

> Of all phaeochromocytomas, 10% are malignant, 10% are bilateral and 10% are extra-adrenal.

Clinical features

The symptoms of a phaeochromocytoma are often sporadic and paroxysmal. Attacks last minutes or hours and occur at variable intervals. The clinical features include hypertension, palpitations, tachycardia, chest pain and sweating. Long-term effects include hypovolaemia and cardiomyopathy.

Phaeochromocytomas are associated with multiple endocrine neoplasia syndrome type 2, neurofibromatosis and Von Hippel–Lindau syndrome.

> Von Hippel–Lindau syndrome is a rare, autosomal dominant condition that predisposes individuals to both benign and malignant tumours. The most common tumours are retinal hemangioblastomas, clear cell renal carcinomas, phaeochromocytomas and pancreatic neuroendocrine tumours.

Investigations

To confirm the diagnosis of a phaeochromocytoma, it is necessary to demonstrate a catecholamine excess by measuring 24-hour urinary vannilyl mandelic acid, 24-hour urinary total catecholamines and serum adrenaline/epinephrine or noradrenaline/norepinephrine. Tumours can be localised using abdominal CT, MRI or meta-iodobenzylguanidine scanning.

Management

The clinical features of a phaeochromocytoma cannot be controlled in the long term by drugs alone. Adrenalectomy is invariably necessary after careful preoperative preparation. Surgery for a phaeochromocytoma requires a close liaison between the surgeon and the anaesthetist.

Preoperative preparation requires alpha-blockade with phenoxybenzamine for at least 2 weeks before surgery. Beta-blockade should be performed after alpha-blockade. Beta-blockade without alpha-blockade risks a hypertensive crisis. Preoperative hypovolaemia should be corrected.

As the tumour releases catecholamines, potential intraoperative problems include hypertension associated with handling of the tumour, and hypotension following devascularisation of the tumour. Tight intraoperative control of blood pressure is necessary and is achieved with fluids, nitroprusside and dopamine infusions.

Cushing's syndrome

Cushing's syndrome is due to cortisol excess resulting from either primary (20%) or secondary (80%) adrenal disease (**Table 4.11**). Cushing's disease is the syndrome that occurs as a result of an ACTH-secreting pituitary microadenoma.

Clinical features

The clinical features of Cushing's syndrome are shown in **Table 4.12**. Weight gain is common, particularly over the face, supraclavicular region and upper back. Skin changes include abdominal striae and easy bruising. Progressive proximal muscle weakness means that patients have difficulty climbing stairs, getting out of low chairs and raising their arms.

Causes of Cushing's syndrome	
Primary	Secondary
Adrenal adenoma	Cushing's disease
Adrenal carcinoma	Ectopic ACTH production
Adrenal cortical hyperplasia	
The most common malignancies associated with ectopic adrenocorticotrophic hormone (ACTH) production are small cell carcinoma of the lung, carcinoid tumours and medullary carcinoma of the thyroid.	

Table 4.11 Causes of Cushing's syndrome

Clinical features of Cushing's syndrome	
Symptoms	Signs
Weight gain	Truncal obesity
Menstrual irregularity	Plethora
Hirsutism in women	Moon face
Headache	Hypertension
Thirst	Bruising
Back pain	Striae
Muscle weakness	Buffalo hump
Abdominal pain	Acne
Lethargy and depression	Osteoporosis

Table 4.12 Clinical features of Cushing's syndrome

New-onset hypertension and diabetes mellitus, difficulty with wound healing, an increased number of infections and osteoporotic fractures also occur (**Figure 4.16**). In women there may be menstrual irregularities, amenorrhea, infertility and decreased libido. A decrease in libido and impotence can occur in men. Psychological problems such as depression, cognitive dysfunction and emotional lability are common.

In Cushing's disease, the presenting clinical features arise from either the endocrine effects or from pressure on adjacent structures. Pituitary tumours press on the optic chiasma, resulting in visual changes include bitemporal hemianopia, third cranial nerve palsy and proptosis.

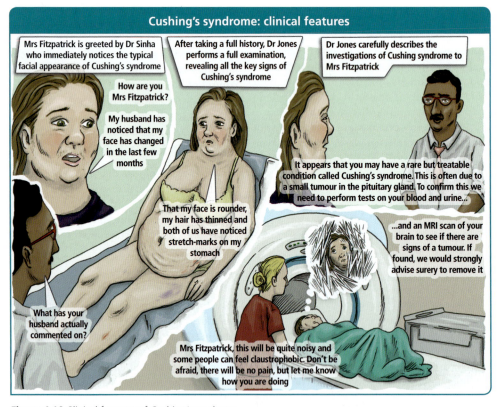

Figure 4.16 Clinical features of Cushing's syndrome.

The clinical features of Cushing's syndrome develop very slowly. The changes in appearance are often noticed by those close to the patients rather than by the patients themselves.

The main clinical features of steroid excess can be summarised using the mnemonic CUSHINGOID:

- Cataracts
- Ulcers
- Skin – bruising, striae
- Hypertension, hirsutism and hyperglycaemia
- Infections
- Necrosis – avascular necrosis of the femoral head
- Glycosuria
- Osteoporosis
- Immunosuppression
- Diabetes

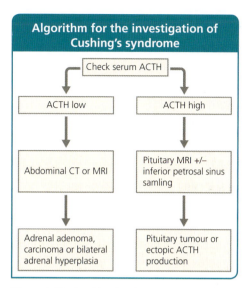

Figure 4.17 Algorithm for the investigation of Cushing's syndrome.

Diagnostic approach

The clinical presentation often does not identify the cause of the Cushing's syndrome. The aim of the investigations is therefore to provide biochemical confirmation of the diagnosis, identify the site of the pathological lesion and confirm the nature of the pathology.

Investigations

The diagnosis of Cushing' syndrome can be confirmed by finding an increased 24-hour urinary free cortisol level. The anatomical site of lesion (adrenal, pituitary or ectopic) can usually be identified by a combination of serum ACTH measurements and imaging (Figure 4.17). The serum ACTH will be low in adrenal disease, and high when there is pituitary overproduction or ectopic production of ACTH.

Imaging

This is vital in order to identify the site of the pathological lesion. MRI of the pituitary has a high sensitivity for identifying pituitary microadenomas but is not 100% predictive. If diagnostic doubt exists, sampling of bilateral inferior petrosal sinus for ACTH may prove diagnostic. Abdominal CT allows the identification of adrenal pathology, and somatostatin scintigraphy may identify sites of ectopic hormone production.

Management

Cushing's disease is best managed by transphenoidal microadenectomy, in which the pituitary microadenoma is removed through the nasal sinuses. The success rate is approximately 90%. If pituitary surgery fails, bilateral adrenalectomy should be considered. However, 25% patients undergoing bilateral adrenalectomy develop Nelson's syndrome.

Patients with adrenal adenomas require adrenalectomy. This can be performed either laparoscopically or via open surgery.

Nelson's syndrome is due to rapid enlargement of a pituitary adenoma following the removal of both adrenal glands. Adrenalectomy eliminates the production of cortisol, and the lack of negative feedback allows any pre-existing pituitary adenoma to grow unchecked.

Conn's syndrome

An excess secretion of aldosterone (aldosteronism) can be:

- Primary due to primary pathology of the adrenal gland
- Secondary to a reduction in plasma volume and the resulting increase in angiotensin production

Conn's syndrome is primary hyperaldosteronism due to an aldosterone-producing adenoma (50%), bilateral idiopathic hyperplasia (40%) or an aldosterone-secreting adrenal carcinoma. The most common causes of secondary hyperaldosteronism are cirrhosis, nephrotic syndrome and cardiac failure.

Epidemiology

Conn's syndrome usually occurs in patients aged 30–60 years and accounts for 1% of cases of hypertension.

Clinical features

Conn's syndrome presents with hypertension that often responds poorly to treatment. Biochemically, there is usually a hypokalaemic alkalosis.

> A diagnosis of Conn's syndrome should be suspected in a patient with newly diagnosed hypertension who has a low serum potassium level.

Investigations

Investigations are needed to confirm primary hyperaldosteronism and to localise the pathology. The diagnosis depends on demonstrating a reduced serum potassium level, increased urinary potassium excretion and increased plasma aldosterone.

Abdominal MRI can demonstrate 80% of adrenal adenomas. Assessment of the function of an adrenal lesion may require isotope (NP59) scanning or renal vein sampling for aldosterone.

Management

If an adrenal adenoma is demonstrated, adrenalectomy is the treatment of choice. Patients may requires preoperative spironolactone to increase their serum potassium level reducing the risk of intraoperative arrhythmias. The blood pressure returns to normal after surgery in 70% of patients.

Multiple endocrine neoplasia

The term 'multiple endocrine neoplasia' describes several distinct endocrine syndromes that result from tumours of the endocrine glands. The tumours are either malignant or benign. Tumours of non-endocrine tissues also occur. The features of the multiple endocrine neoplasia syndromes are shown in **Table 4.13**.

Features of MEN syndromes		
MEN syndrome type 1	MEN syndrome type 2a	MEN syndrome type 2b
Hyperparathyroidism	Medullary thyroid carcinoma	Medullary thyroid carcinoma
Pancreatic islet cell tumours	Phaeochromocytoma	Phaeochromocytoma
Pituitary tumours	Hyperparathyroidism	Multiple mucosal neuromas
Thyroid adenoma		Ganglioneuromatosis of the gut
Adrenal adenoma		Marfanoid appearance
Carcinoid tumours		

The pancreatic islet cell tumours of multiple endocrine neoplasia (MEN) syndrome type 1 are gastrinoma (60%), insulinoma (10%), VIPoma and glucagonoma.

Table 4.13 Features of multiple endocrine neoplasia syndromes

Carcinoid tumours

Carcinoid tumours are neuroendocrine lesions of the gastrointestinal tract that arise from amine precursor uptake and decarboxylation (APUD) cells. APUD cells produce 5-hydroxyindoleacetic acid, a metabolite of serotonin.

The tumours are most commonly found in the appendix (30%) and small bowel (20%). Carcinoid syndrome occurs when they metastasise, particularly to the liver and specific clinical features develop.

Clinical features

Carcinoid tumours often present late with very vague clinical features. The most common symptom is right-sided abdominal discomfort that may have been present for a number of years prior to diagnosis. Previous investigations have often been normal. The diagnosis is often made only after urgent surgery for intestinal obstruction.

The symptoms of carcinoid syndrome include diarrhoea and flushing. The flushing affects the face and is often precipitated by alcohol or chocolate. Palpitations and hypotension also occur. The abdominal examination is often normal, but an abdominal mass or hepatomegaly may be present. Other clinical features include telangiectasia, pellagra and tricuspid regurgitation.

Investigations

The diagnosis is confirmed by finding increased 5-hydroxyindoleacetic acid levels in a 24-hour urine specimen. Plasma chromogranin A levels may be increased. Radiological investigations are rarely helpful. An ultrasound occasionally demonstrates an abdominal mass or liver secondaries. [111]Indium-octreotide scintigraphy will identify a primary or secondary tumour.

Management

In patients presenting with intestinal obstruction, the diagnosis is often made following histological examination of the resected primary tumour. Symptomatic carcinoid syndrome can often be improved by the use of a somatostatin analogue (e.g. octreotide).

The prognosis of carcinoid tumours is better than that of adenocarcinomas at similar sites. For surgically resectable tumours, 10-year survival rates of more than 60% have been reported.

Appendiceal carcinoid tumours

Carcinoids are the most common tumour of the appendix. They are an incidental finding in 0.5% of appendicectomy specimens and account for 85% of all appendiceal tumours. Most occur at the tip of the appendix and are small: 80% of tumours are less than 1 cm in diameter.

Appendicectomy is adequate treatment if the tumour is less than 1 cm in diameter. Right hemicolectomy should be considered for tumours bigger than 1 cm. The prognosis is good, with 5-year survival rates of more than 90%.

Answers to starter questions

1. A hormone is a blood borne messenger which is produced by one organ, secreted into the blood stream and carried to other parts of the body. Only those organs that have receptors for a hormone are able to respond to it. Hormones have a short half-life and are rapidly destroyed. Their levels are controlled by complex feedback mechanisms, often involving the pituitary gland. In health the levels are closely regulated. In disease states the feedback mechanism is deranged and under-or over-production of a hormone occurs.

2. Endocrine tumours present as a result of the local effects of the tumour within the gland or the systemic effects of over or under-production of a particular hormone. Small tumours, even benign lesions, sometimes have a dramatic clinical presentation as a result of local anatomical consequences or the resulting endocrine derangement. Small benign pituitary adenomas can compress the optic chiasm resulting in visual field defects. Small benign phaeochromocytomas sometimes present with severe hypertension as a result of catecholamine over-production.

3. Thyroid disease usually presents with symptoms resulting from either an alteration in thyroid status or as a result of change in the thyroid gland. A generalised enlargement of the thyroid gland is known as a goitre. Thyroid cancer often presents as a solitary nodule within the thyroid gland. Examination often shows a non-tender lump in one lobe of the gland. Symptoms and signs that suggest malignancy include a firm, fixed lump, hoarseness and cervical lymphadenopathy.

4. The recurrent laryngeal nerves are branches of the vagus nerves that supply the intrinsic muscles of the larynx. They ascend in the neck, between the oesophagus and the trachea and are closely related to the lobes of the thyroid gland. It is important to positively identify the recurrent laryngeal nerves during thyroid surgery as inadvertent damage can result in hoarseness and stridor.

5. Primary hyperparathyroidism is due to autonomous overproduction of parathyroid hormone by the parathyroid glands. Secondary hyperparathyroidism is a reactive increase in parathyroid hormone production to compensate for a hypocalcaemia, usually as a result of chronic renal failure. In primary hyperparathyroidism, the serum corrected calcium and PTH are both increased. In secondary hyperparathyroidism the serum PTH is increased but the calcium will be either normal or low.

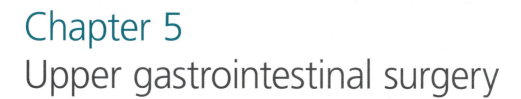

Chapter 5
Upper gastrointestinal surgery

Introduction 91
Case 3 Epigastric pain and
        weight loss 92
Core sciences 94
History, examination and
investigation. 98

Gastro-oesophageal reflux 100
Achalasia 101
Peptic ulcer disease 102
Oesophageal cancer 104
Gastric cancer 106

Starter questions

Answers to the following questions are on page 109.

1. How does the blood supply of the gastrointestinal tract relate to its embryology?
2. Why is it important that oesophageal manometry and pH studies are performed in patients with gastro-oesophageal reflux disease being considered for surgery?
3. Is *Helicobacter pylori* a parasite or a commensal organism?
4. Why is the prognosis for oesophageal and gastric cancer so poor?
5. How do tumours of the small bowel differ from those of the stomach?

Introduction

The upper gastrointestinal tract comprises the oesophagus, stomach and small intestine. The focus of surgery for disease in this region has changed significantly over the past few decades. Until recently, elective and emergency surgery for peptic ulcer disease was common. However, with the advent of H2 receptor antagonists and pro-ton pump inhibitors, the need for elective surgery for peptic ulcer disease has all but disappeared. Most upper gastrointestinal surgery in the 21st century is performed for malignant disease. Unfortunately, both oesophageal and gastric adenocarcinoma often present late and, even following surgery, the prognosis is poor.

Case 3 Epigastric pain and weight loss

Presentation

A 75-year-old man, Mr George Johnson, presents to his general practitioner with a 3-month history of persistent epigastric pain. Over this time, he has lost 7 kg in weight.

Initial interpretation

Abdominal pain and weight loss in an elderly man is highly suggestive of an underlying gastrointestinal malignancy. Subsequent assessment and investigation aims to confirm or exclude a neoplastic process.

History

George has noticed that his health has been deteriorating for several weeks. He first noticed intermittent epigastric pain after eating. Over time, the pain has increased in severity and become more persistent. He has resorted to eating smaller meals. He feels tired and lethargic. He has lost weight and his clothes feel looser.

Interpretation of history

Increasing and refractory epigastric pain associated with symptoms of malignancy, such as malaise and weight loss is highly suggestive of a gastric carcinoma. Other common abdominal malignancies that present in a similar fashion are cancers of the colon and pancreas.

Further history

George has noticed no change in his bowel habit. He was previously very fit and healthy and is not taking any regular

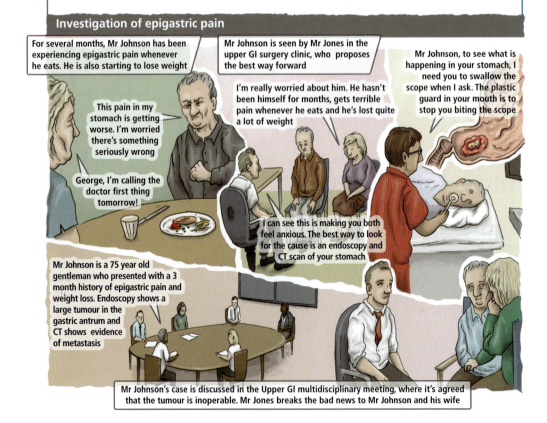

Investigation of epigastric pain

For several months, Mr Johnson has been experiencing epigastric pain whenever he eats. He is also starting to lose weight

Mr Johnson is seen by Mr Jones in the upper GI surgery clinic, who proposes the best way forward

Mr Johnson, to see what is happening in your stomach, I need you to swallow the scope when I ask. The plastic guard in your mouth is to stop you biting the scope

This pain in my stomach is getting worse. I'm worried there's something seriously wrong

I'm really worried about him. He hasn't been himself for months, gets terrible pain whenever he eats and he's lost quite a lot of weight

George, I'm calling the doctor first thing tomorrow!

I can see this is making you both feel anxious. The best way to look for the cause is an endoscopy and CT scan of your stomach

Mr Johnson is a 75 year old gentleman who presented with a 3 month history of epigastric pain and weight loss. Endoscopy shows a large tumour in the gastric antrum and CT shows evidence of metastasis

Mr Johnson's case is discussed in the Upper GI multidisciplinary meeting, where it's agreed that the tumour is inoperable. Mr Jones breaks the bad news to Mr Johnson and his wife

Case 3 *continued*

medication. He has not needed to consult his general practitioner for several years.

Examination

On examination, George is thin and cachectic. He appears anaemic but is not jaundiced. There is a palpable lymph node is the left supraclavicular fossa. Inspection of the abdomen shows a fullness in the epigastrium. Palpation confirms a non-pulsatile epigastric mass. There is no hepatomegaly and no shifting dullness or a fluid thrill to suggest the presence of extensive ascites.

Interpretation of findings

Anaemia and cachexia resulting from malnutrition suggest a malignant process. The palpable node in the supraclavicular fossa (Virchow's node) is almost pathognomic of a gastric carcinoma. The non-pulsatile epigastric mass helps to confirm the clinical suspicion of a gastric carcinoma.

Investigations

A full blood count shows that George is anaemic (a haemoglobin level of 89 g/L). A blood film shows the anaemia is hypochromic and microcytic, suggesting that the cause is iron deficiency. The results of liver function tests are normal.

George is referred to a gastroenterologist at the local hospital and undergoes an upper gastrointestinal endoscopy. This shows a large fungating tumour in the antrum of the stomach (**Figure 5.1**). A biopsy taken during the endoscopy shows an adenocarcinoma of the stomach. George is referred to a upper gastrointestinal surgeon who arranges an abdominal CT scan to stage the adenocarcinoma. This shows a small volume of ascites, large lymph nodes in the porta hepatis and secondary deposits within the liver.

Diagnosis

This elderly patient has carcinoma of the stomach, confirmed by an endoscopic biopsy. Like many patients, George presented with vague symptoms and, by the time of his diagnosis, had metastatic disease.

The surgeon regards the tumour as inoperable. George is too frail to tolerate palliative chemotherapy. His health continues to deteriorate and he dies peacefully at home 4 months later.

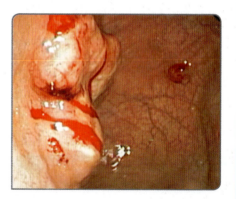

Figure 5.1 Endoscopic appearance of gastric carcinoma.

Core sciences

Embryology

Embryologically, the gastrointestinal tract is divided into three sections:

- The foregut extends from the oesophagus to the ampulla of Vater in the second part of the duodenum
- The midgut starts at the ampulla of Vater and continues to the junction of mid and distal transverse colon
- The hindgut consists of the distal colon and upper rectum

Each section has its own blood supply and venous and lymphatic drainage. The blood supply to the foregut, midgut and hindgut arises from the coeliac axis, superior mesenteric artery and inferior mesenteric artery, respectively.

Anatomy

The wall of the gastrointestinal tract from the oesophagus to the anal canal contains four basic layers (**Figure 5.2**). The innermost layer is the mucosa, which lines the lumen of the gut. The mucosa consists of three layers:

- The epithelium lines the lumen and is simple columnar in type

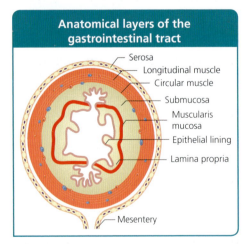

Anatomical layers of the gastrointestinal tract

- Serosa
- Longitudinal muscle
- Circular muscle
- Submucosa
- Muscularis mucosa
- Epithelial lining
- Lamina propria
- Mesentery

Figure 5.2 Anatomical layers of the gastrointestinal tract.

- The lamina propria is the loose connective tissue below the epithelium. It contains capillaries and lymphoid tissue
- Under the lamina propria is a thin layer of smooth muscle known as the muscularis mucosa

The functions of the mucosa include:

- The secretion of mucus and enzymes
- The release of hormones into the plasma
- Protection against infectious disease
- The absorption of the end products of digestion

The submucosa lies outside the mucosa. It is made up of connective tissue containing blood and lymphatic vessels and nerve fibres.

Outside the submucosa is the smooth muscle layer that is responsible for peristalsis and segmentation of the gut. It is divided into two layers: an inner circular layer and an outer longitudinal layer. At specific locations (e.g. the pylorus), the circular layer thickens to form sphincters. These control to some extent the passage of materials through the gut.

The serosa is the outermost layer of the gut and intraperitoneal organs. It is also known as the visceral peritoneum. It consists of simple squamous epithelium overlying thin areolar connective tissue.

The oesophagus has an adventitia (i.e. a firm fibrous layer) rather than a serosa that firmly supports the organ.

Anatomy of the oesophagus

The oesophagus is about 25 cm long in adults and is classified into cervical, thoracic and intra-abdominal sections. It starts at the lower edge of pharynx, at the level of the C6 vertebra, and ends at the cardia of the stomach, which lies within the abdomen. The oesophagus passes through the diaphragm at the level of the T10 vertebra.

The oesophagus is lined by non-keratinising stratified squamous epithelium. In the transition zone at the gastro-oesophageal junction, the lining becomes columnar epithelium.

The blood supply arises from the inferior thyroid artery and the oesophageal branch of the left gastric artery.

The venous drainage is into both the portal and systemic systems. As a result, there is a portosystemic anastomosis in the lower oesophagus between the oesophageal branch of the left gastric vein and tributaries of the azygos vein.

> As result of the portosystemic anastomosis in the lower oesophagus, oesophageal varices develop if the portal venous system pressure is raised.

Although there is no anatomical sphincter at the lower end of the oesophagus, there is a functional sphincter mechanism to prevent gastro-oesophageal reflux. This is made up of the basal tone in the muscle and the pressure difference between the abdominal cavity and the lumen of the oesophagus. Several external mechanical factors also help to prevent reflux:

- A flap valve mechanism in the oesophageal mucosa
- The cardio-oesophageal angle forming an acute angulation between the stomach and oesophagus
- Diaphragmatic pinchcock causing external pressure on the oesophagus
- Mucosal rosette increasing the apposition of the oesophageal mucosa
- The phreno-oesophageal ligament lying across the front of the oesophagus
- Abdominal pressure transmitted across the oesophageal wall

Anatomy of the stomach

The stomach is described as being composed of several regions (**Figure 5.3**):

- Lesser curvature
- Greater curvature
- Fundus
- Incisura angularis
- Body
- Pylorus

The lesser omentum connects the lesser curve of the stomach to the liver. The greater omentum is connected to the greater curve of

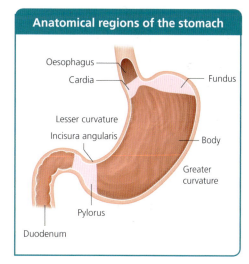

Figure 5.3 Anatomical regions of the stomach

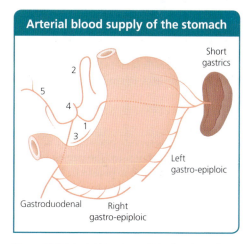

Figure 5.4 Arterial blood supply to the stomach. ① Splenic. ② Left gastric. ③ Right gastric. ④ Coeliac axis. ⑤ Common hepatic.

the stomach lies anterior to the small bowel and folds back on itself to join the transverse colon.

Blood supply

Five main arteries supply the stomach (**Figure 5.4**):

- The left gastric artery arises from the coeliac axis
- The right gastric artery arises from the common hepatic artery
- The right gastro-epiploic artery arises from the gastroduodenal artery

- The left gastro-epiploic artery arises from the splenic artery
- The short gastric arteries are branches of the splenic artery

Lymphatic drainage

The stomach drains into four groups of nodes:

- Hepatic group
- Subpyloric group
- Gastric group
- Pancreatico-lienal group

Histology

The gastric mucosa is simple columnar epithelium with numerous invaginations known as gastric pits. The gastric pits lead into the gastric glands, which secrete the gastric juice. Four types of cell are found in the gastric mucosa:

- The mucous cells secrete acidic mucus
- The parietal cells secrete hydrochloric acid and intrinsic factor. Intrinsic factor is a glycoprotein responsible for the absorption of vitamin B12 in the terminal ileum
- The chief cells secrete pepsinogen, an inactive form of pepsin. The pepsinogen is initially activated to pepsin by hydrogen ions in the acidic environment of the stomach. It is then activated by the pepsin that is being produced. Pepsin is an enzyme responsible for the digestion of proteins to peptides
- The neuroendocrine cells secrete multiple hormones into the plasma. The most important of these is gastrin. Gastrin is a peptide hormone that increases gastric motility.

The vagus nerve

Both the left and right vagus nerves enter the abdomen through the oesophageal hiatus. The left vagus nerve passes on to the anterior wall of the stomach, and the right vagus nerve passes on to the posterior wall of the stomach. The anterior vagus runs along the lesser curvature. The nerve of Latarjet arises from the anterior vagus nerve and supplies the pylorus. The posterior vagus supplies the coeliac ganglion providing parasympathetic intervention of the stomach and small bowel.

Anatomy of the small intestine

The small intestine is about 5 m long and is the longest part of the alimentary canal. It is divided into three anatomical regions: the duodenum, jejunum and ileum.

Duodenum

The duodenum is approximately 25 cm long and is C shaped. It is classified into four parts:

- The first part is a continuation of the pylorus and runs transversely
- The second part runs vertically in front of the hilum of the right kidney
- The third part runs horizontally below the pancreas
- The fourth part runs upwards to the duodenojejunal junction

All except the first part of the duodenum lie retroperitoneally. The ligament of Treitz connects the duodenojejunal flexure, the junction between the duodenum and jejunum, to the right crus of the diaphragm.

The duodenal papilla is located on the medial wall of the second part of the duodenum. It is the site of entry of the common bile duct and pancreatic duct.

The blood supply of the duodenum is from two arteries: the superior pancreaticoduodenal artery, a branch of the gastroduodenal artery, and the inferior pancreaticoduodenal artery, a branch of the superior mesenteric artery. The venous drainage is into the portal and superior mesenteric veins.

Lymph drains to the coeliac and superior mesenteric nodes.

Jejunum and ileum

The jejunum begins at the duodenojejunal junction and is about 2.4 m long. It continues into the ileum, which measures about 3.6 m and ends at the ileocaecal valve. The ileum is connected to the posterior abdominal wall by the small bowel mesentery.

The blood supply is from the superior mesenteric artery, branches of which form arcades within the mesentery. The lower part of the ileum is supplied by the ileocolic artery. The venous drainage is into the superior mesenteric vein. The lymphatic drainage is into the superior mesenteric nodes.

Histology

The small intestine is highly modified to absorb fluid and nutrients. Three features increase the surface area:

- Plicae circulares, which are permanent deep folds of the mucosa and submucosa
- Villi, which are finger-like extensions of the mucosa
- Microvilli, which are projections of the plasma membrane of each absorptive epithelial cell

The small intestine is lined with simple columnar epithelium containing goblet cells. The epithelium shows invaginations known as intestinal glands or crypts of Lieberkühn. These contain absorptive cells and neuroendocrine cells that produce hormones (e.g. vasoactive intestinal polypeptide).

The submucosa is the remainder of the gastrointestinal tract in the proximal duodenum and terminal ileum. The submucosa in the proximal duodenum contains alkaline mucous glands (Brunner's glands), and the submucosa of the terminal ileal contains Peyer's patches, which are aggregates of lymphoid tissue that form part of the gut-associated immune system.

Physiology

The gastrointestinal tract is primarily involved in digesting food for absorption into the body. The function of the various parts of the gastrointestinal tract is shown in **Table 5.1**. An important contribution to digestion is made by enzymes, which are

Major functions of the gastrointestinal tract	
Organ	Function
Mouth	Ingestion of food, mastication, initiation of digestion, swallowing
Pharynx and oesophagus	Propulsion
Stomach	Mechanical breakdown, digestion, absorption
Small intestine	Mechanical breakdown, digestion, absorption
Large intestine	Absorption, propulsion, defaecation

Table 5.1 Major functions of the gastrointestinal tract

Import enzymes involved in digestion	
Organ	Break down
Salivary amylase	Starch into small polysaccharides and maltose
Pepsin	Proteins into small polypeptides
Pancreatic amylase	Starch into polysaccharides and disaccharides
Lipase	Fats into glycerol and fatty acids
Aminopeptidase	Small polypeptides into amino acids

Table 5.2 Important enzymes involved in digestion

specific catalysts involved in the breakdown of biological molecules. The main enzymes involved in digestion are shown in **Table 5.2**.

The smooth muscle of the gastrointestinal tract has its own inherent activity independent of its innervation but modulated by the autonomic nervous system, especially the parasympathetic nervous system. Parasympathetic efferent fibres synapse in ganglia that are located in nerve plexuses in the wall of the gastrointestinal tract. Postganglionic fibres then supply the mucosal glands and smooth muscle. The submucosal plexus is known as Meissner's plexus. The plexus between the two layers of the muscularis mucosa is known as Auerbach's plexus.

History, examination and investigation

Patients with upper gastrointestinal disease often present with vague symptoms and no abnormal findings on abdominal examination. The common symptoms and signs of upper gastrointestinal disease are shown in **Table 5.3**.

History

Upper gastrointestinal disease often presents with heartburn, dysphagia or dyspepsia.

Heartburn

Heartburn is a burning retrosternal sensation, discomfort or pain. It results from the regurgitation of acid or bile into the oesophagus and occasionally occurs in healthy individuals. The pain may radiate to the neck and is often associated with an acid or bitter taste in the mouth that is known as water brash.

Dysphagia

Dysphagia is difficulty with swallowing and can occur with either solids or liquids, or both. The patient often describes it as food 'sticking' after swallowing. The symptoms may be progressive, initially with solids and then with liquids. It may be associated with a regurgitation of undigested food.

Dysphagia usually results from obstruction at the lower end of the oesophagus. It is caused by extrinsic or intrinsic mechanical oesophageal compression or neuromuscular problems (**Table 5.4**).

Causes of dysphagia	
Cause	Examples
Intrinsic compression	Benign stricture, oesophageal carcinoma, bolus obstruction, achalasia, diffuse oesophageal spasm
Extrinsic compression	Carcinoma of the bronchus, thoracic aortic aneurysm, goitre
Neuromuscular	Multiple sclerosis, systemic sclerosis, Chagas' disease, autonomic neuropathy

Table 5.4 Causes of dysphagia

Dyspepsia

Dyspepsia refers to epigastric discomfort or 'indigestion'. It is often chronic and recurrent. The pain is rarely severe and rarely radiates from the epigastrium. Depending on the underlying cause, the symptoms may be precipitated or relieved by food. It is often associated with nausea and a sensation of bloating.

Dyspepsia may be a sign of upper gastrointestinal pathology, particularly in those over 50 years of age. Functional dyspepsia is the occurrence of the symptom without any evidence of organic disease. It has been estimated to occur in 15% of the adult population.

Examination

There are often no abnormal findings on an abdominal examination of a patient with upper gastrointestinal disease. Patients with advanced oesophageal or gastric malignancy are invariably thin, anaemic and cachectic. There may be a palpable lymph node in the supraclavicular fossa. A non-pulsatile epigastric mass may be seen in those with advanced gastric cancer.

Investigation

The investigation most commonly used in upper gastrointestinal disease is upper gas-

Symptoms and signs of upper gastrointestinal disease	
Symptoms	Signs
Dysphagia	Anaemia
Heartburn	Epigastric mass
Dyspepsia	Supraclavicular node (Virchow's node)
Epigastric pain	

Table 5.3 Common symptoms and signs of upper gastrointestinal disease

trointestinal endoscopy. In patients with potential gastro-oesophageal reflux disease (GORD), a functional assessment of the lower oesophageal sphincter may prove useful. This is done using oesophageal manometry and pH monitoring.

> **So that gastric carcinoma can be detected as early as possible,** upper gastrointestinal endoscopy should be considered in all patients over 40 years of age who have a new onset of dyspeptic symptoms.

Upper gastrointestinal endoscopy

Upper gastrointestinal endoscopy is a diagnostic and possibly a therapeutic procedure in a small number of patients. It allows the upper gastrointestinal tract to be visualised as far as the second part of the duodenum. It is used in the assessment of:

- Dyspepsia
- Dysphagia
- Gastrointestinal bleeding
- Anaemia
- Gastroesophageal reflux

Ideally, the patient should be 'nil by mouth' for 6 hours prior to the procedure, allowing any gastric residue to empty from the stomach into the intestine. The endoscopy is conducted under intravenous sedation or following topical local anaesthesia of the pharynx. Interventional procedures that can be performed during the procedure include:

- Endoscopic biopsy
- Injection of adrenaline into a bleeding peptic ulcer
- Application of small rubber bands to oesophageal varices
- Dilation of an oesophageal stricture
- Removal of foreign bodies such as a food bolus or false teeth
- Insertion of self-expanding stent across a malignant stricture
- Photodynamic therapy of oesophageal tumours

Upper gastrointestinal endoscopy is a relatively safe procedure, but the risk of complications increases if an additional procedure is performed. Complications include aspiration, bleeding and gastrointestinal perforation.

Endoscopic ultrasound

This is the combined use of endoscopy and ultrasound to obtain images of the upper gastrointestinal tract. It is used to assess the wall of the oesophagus, stomach and duodenum, as well as adjacent structures and organs (e.g the pancreas). The blood supply to organs can be measured if endoscopic ultrasound is combined with Doppler imaging. Endoscopic biopsies of lesions deep in the wall of the gastrointestinal tract or pancreas and liver can be taken under endoscopic guidance.

Oesophageal pH studies and manometry

Oesophageal pH measurement and manometry is most commonly used in the preoperative assessment of patients with GORD. It is also used in the diagnosis of achalasia (see page 101).

Manometry

Manometry is used to evaluate the motor function of the oesophagus. A pressure transducer is inserted into the oesophagus via the nose measuring the oesophageal pressure at several points a few centimetres apart. The pressure wave within the oesophagus is then measured during swallowing. The assessment is repeated at various levels within the oesophagus as the transducer is withdrawn.

Oesophageal pH studies

The position of the lower oesophageal sphincter must first be identified by manometry. A pH probe is then inserted, via the nose, to a set distance (usually 4 cm) above the lower oesophageal sphincter. The probe is left in place for 24 hours, constantly recording the pH within the oesophagus. The patient is asked to record when they experience heartburn and this is subsequently correlated with the pH measurements.

oesophageal spasm, oesophageal carcinoma, scleroderma and Chagas' disease.

Diagnostic approach

A chest radiograph may show widening of the mediastinum, an air–fluid level behind the heart, and absence of the gas bubble that is usually seen in the gastric fundus. A barium swallow may show oesophageal dilatation, with a food residue, small and ineffective oesophageal contractions and a 'rat tail' appearance of the distal oesophagus (**Figure 5.7**).

Oesophageal manometry shows an absent primary peristaltic wave and non-propulsive tertiary contractions.

It is essential to exclude a diagnosis of oesophageal cancer and an endoscopy is essential to exclude 'pseudoachalasia' due to a submucosal oesophageal carcinoma. Endoscopy in a patient with achalasia will also show a tight lower oesophageal sphincter that relaxes with gentle pressure.

Management

The management of achalasia is either balloon dilatation or cardiomyotomy.

Balloon dilatation

A balloon is placed across the lower oesophageal sphincter and inflated to 300 mmHg for 3 minutes. With this approach, 60% of patients are free of dysphagia at 5 years. The procedure may need to be repeated on

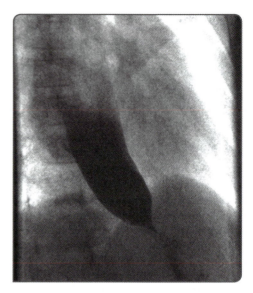

Figure 5.7 Barium swallow showing the 'rat tail' appearance of achalasia

several occasions if symptoms recur. There is a 3% risk of oesophageal perforation after balloon dilatation.

Surgery

In a cardiomyotomy, the muscle fibres of the lower oesophagus are incised down to the mucosa along an 8–10 cm length of oesophagus. Surgery can be performed laparoscopically. After this procedure, 85% of patients are free from dysphagia. About 10% develop oesophageal reflux and 3% develop a peptic stricture.

Peptic ulcer disease

Peptic ulcer disease is defined as the presence of complete, established deficits in the columnar mucosa of the lower oesophagus, stomach or duodenum.

Epidemiology

The number of hospital admissions for uncomplicated peptic ulcer disease is falling. Elective surgery is now less common owing to the use of drugs that reduce gastric acid production. However, the incidence of complications of peptic ulcer disease,

such as bleeding and perforation, remains unchanged due to the increased use of anti-inflammatory drugs in elderly individuals. Bleeding and perforation are still associated with a mortality of more than 10%.

Aetiology

The most important aetiological factors include:

- *Helicobacter pylori* infection
- Drugs – non-steroidal anti-inflammatory drugs

- Smoking and alcohol
- Male sex
- High acid production in the stomach

Helicobacter pylori is a urease-producing, Gram-negative spiral flagellated bacterium. To avoid the acidic stomach environment, it burrows through the mucous lining of the stomach and can irritate the epithelium. It is found in 90%, 70% and 60% of patients with duodenal ulceration, gastric ulceration and gastric cancer, respectively.

> **About 80% of people in whom *H. pylori* is found are asymptomatic.** It is endemic in the developing world and its prevalance seems to decrease as countries develop.

Clinical features

Duodenal and gastric ulcers can present differently (**Table 5.5**). Duodenal ulcers usually present with epigastric pain that is worse during fasting and is relieved by food. The symptoms may be worse at night, and the pain often follows a relapsing and remitting course. Gastric ulcers often present with epigastric pain that is worse on eating. Patients with either duodenal or gastric

Distinguishing features of gastric and duodenal ulcers		
Feature	Gastric ulcer	Duodenal ulcer
Site	Epigastrium	Epigastrium
Onset	Soon after eating	Hours after eating / Nocturnal pain
Relieving factors	Vomiting	Eating
Precipitating factors	Eating	Missing a meal
Periodicity	Every 2–3 months	Every 4–6 months
Duration of attack	Day or weeks	Weeks or months
Weight loss	Significant weight loss	Minimal weight loss

Table 5.5 Distinguishing features of gastric and duodenal ulcers

ulcers may also present with iron-deficiency anaemia or an acute complication such as an upper gastrointestinal bleed or perforation (see Chapter 10).

Diagnostic approach

Patients presenting with symptoms suggestive of peptic ulcer disease must undergo an upper gastrointestinal endoscopy. If an ulcer is identified, *H. pylori* infection is sought.

Investigations

The diagnosis can be confirmed by upper gastrointestinal endoscopy. Proximal gastric ulcers (type 1) are most commonly found on the lesser curve and antrum of the stomach. Distal gastric and duodenal ulcers (type 2) are found in the pre-pyloric region or duodenum. Type 2 ulcers are four times as common as type 1 ulcers.

Helicobacter pylori can be detected by a rapid urease test performed on an endoscopic biopsy specimen. In this test, urease produced by the bacteria breaks down urea to ammonia, increasing pH detected by a colour change of an indicator dye.

Management

Most patients can be managed with medication, so elective surgery for peptic ulcer disease is rarely required.

Medication

Helicobacter pylori can be eradicated in 80% patients using 1 week of triple antibiotic therapy. Various drug combinations have been described, including amoxicillin, clarithromycin, metronidazole and omeprazole. Short-term recurrence is infrequent. There is currently no clear information on long-term recurrence rates.

Surgery

The indications for surgery in duodenal ulceration are:

- Persistence of the symptoms despite adequate medical treatment
- Acute upper gastrointestinal haemorrhage

- Perforated peptic ulcer disease
- Obstruction due to pyloric stenosis as a result of scarring around ulcers in the distal gastric antrum, close to the pylorus

Upper gastrointestinal haemorrhage and perforated peptic ulcer disease present as emergencies and often require urgent surgery (see Chapter 10). The aim of elective surgery is to cure the predisposition to ulcer formation with the lowest risk of recurrence and complications. This usually involves resection of the acid-producing region of the stomach (by partial gastrectomy or antrectomy) or elimination of the cephalic phase of acid production by dividing the vagus nerves (vagotomy).

Prognosis

Proton pump inhibitors produce healing in 90% of peptic ulcers after 2 months of treatment. Recurrence is infrequent when long-term maintenance therapy is needed. The complications following gastrectomy are shown in **Table 5.6**.

Pyloric stenosis

Pyloric stenosis is narrowing of the outflow of the stomach as a result of scarring of the pylorus. This is often caused by pre-pyloric or proximal duodenal ulceration. This complication of peptic ulceration is a completely

Postgastrectomy complications

Complication	Cause
Diarrhoea	Reduced intestinal transit times
Dumping	Reactive hypoglycaemia due to early transit of carbohydrate into the small intestine
Bilious vomiting	Reflux of bile into a gastric remnant
Vitamin B_{12} deficiency	Removal of the site of intrinsic factor production in the stomach
Iron deficiency	Reduced gastric acid production impairing iron absorption
Recurrent ulceration	Failure to correct the underlying ulcer tendency

Table 5.6 Postgastrectomy complications

different condition to infantile pyloric stenosis seen in children.

It usually presents with vomiting of undigested food, weight loss, epigastric pain and dehydration. The abdomen is distended, and there may be visible peristalsis and a succussion splash (see page 32).

Biochemical assessment may show a hypochloraemic, hypokalaemic metabolic alkalosis. Endoscopy will confirm the diagnosis and may allow balloon dilatation of the stricture. If this fails, the patient undergoes either gastrojejunostomy or proximal gastric vagotomy with duodenoplasty.

Oesophageal cancer

Approximately 90% of oesophageal cancers are squamous cell carcinomas. They usually occur in the upper or middle third of the oesophagus. About 10% are adenocarcinomas, and these usually occur in the lower third of the oesophagus.

Epidemiology

Oesophageal cancer is the sixth leading cause of cancer death worldwide and has a clear association with social deprivation. Its incidence varies between countries and in different ethnic groups and populations. The incidence is high in Transkei, areas of

Northern China and around the Caspian sea. It accounts for about 7000 deaths per year in the UK.

Aetiology

Although the exact cause of oesophageal cancer is not known, several factors are thought to increase its risk of developing. Smoking and alcohol are known risk factors. The development of Barrett's oesophagus (see page 106). significantly increases the risk of cancer. The risk factors for squamous cell oesophageal carcinoma and adenocarcinoma of the stomach are shown in **Table 5.7**.

Risk factors for oesophageal and gastric cancer	
Oesophageal	Gastric
Alcohol and tobacco	A diet low in vitamin C
A diet high in nitrosamines	Blood group A
Aflatoxins	Pernicious anaemia
Trace element deficiency – e.g. molybdenum	Hypogammaglobulinaemia
Vitamin deficiencies – e.g. Vitamins A and C	Post gastrectomy
Achalasia	
Coeliac disease	
Genetic – tylosis	

Table 5.7 Risk factors for oesophageal and gastric cancer

Tylosis is an inherited condition characterised by thickening of the skin of the hands and feet, and the development of oesophageal cancer in early adult life. It is caused by a mutation in the *RHBDF2* gene and is inherited in an autosomal dominant pattern.

Clinical features

The classical clinical presentation of oesophageal carcinoma is progressive dysphagia, first with solids and then with liquids. Respiratory symptoms may occur from two causes: an overspill of fluid or solids into the respiratory tract, and the formation of a tracheo-oesophageal fistula – a communication between the trachea and oesophagus. Weight loss is usually a prominent feature.

Diagnostic approach

All patients with dysphagia should be investigated by endoscopy as they may have an oesophageal malignancy.

Investigations

The diagnosis can be confirmed by endoscopy with biopsy. Resectability and fitness for surgery are assessed by:

- CT scanning
- Lung function tests
- Endoscopic ultrasound
- Bronchoscopy
- Laparoscopy

Most tumours are irresectable and incurable at presentation.

Management

Surgery is the mainstay of treatment for adenocarcinomas as they are not radiosensitive. Squamous cell carcinomas can be treated with either surgery or radiotherapy.

Surgery

Oesophagectomy is the treatment of choice for oesophageal carcinoma. However, fewer than 50% of patients are suitable for potentially curative treatment. It is advisable to carry out treatment in centres that regularly perform the operation and have a low operative mortality.

The surgical approach depends on the site of the tumour (**Table 5.8**). All or part of the oesophagus is removed. The stomach or small bowel is then anastomosed to the remaining oesophagus in either the abdomen or the neck.

Complications of oesophagectomy include:

- Chest infection or pleural effusion
- Anastomotic leak
- Chylothorax
- Recurrent laryngeal nerve damage
- Benign anastomotic stricture

Palliative treatment

In patients with inoperable disease, the aim of palliative treatment is to relieve the obstruction and dysphagia with minimal

Surgical approaches to the oesophagus	
Site of tumour	Approach
Upper and middle thirds	Transhiatal oesophagectomy Transthoracic oesophagectomy
Lower third	Total gastrectomy via a thoracoabdominal approach

Table 5.8 Surgical approach to the oesophagus depending on the site of the tumour

morbidity. This may be achieved by oesophageal intubation or stenting.

Intubation is guided by endoscopy or radiology. A rigid plastic tube (e.g. an Atkinson tube) can be placed endoscopically but requires dilatation of the oesophagus and tumour before it can be inserted, with a risk of oesophageal perforation. Self-expanding stents do not require pre-dilatation, are safer and their use has increased significantly. Complications of stents and tubes include oesophageal perforation, displacement or migration of the tube, and blockage of the tube if the tumour grows into or over it.

Endoscopic laser ablation produces good palliation but may need to be repeated every 4–6 weeks and is also associated with a risk of oesophageal perforation.

Squamous carcinomas are radiosensitive. Radiotherapy may produce some palliation but carries the risk that a tracheo-oesophageal fistula will be formed.

Prognosis

Fewer than 40% of those undergoing 'curative' treatment survive for 1 year. The 5-year survival is very poor – 20% or less.

Barrett's oesophagus

Barrett's oesophagus is a columnar cell lining of the distal oesophagus due to intestinal metaplasia of the distal oesophageal mucosa (i.e. change of the epithelial lining from squamous to columnar type). It is caused by gastro-oesophageal reflux and is seen in about 10% of patients with chronic GORD. Bile reflux seems to be an important aetiological factor.

Barrett's oesophagus is a premalignant condition that can progress to dysplasia and adenocarcinoma. It increases the risk of malignancy 30-fold. Approximately 1% of patients with Barrett's oesophagus progress to carcinoma each year.

> **The normal oesophagus is lined by non-keratinising squamous epithelium.** A transition to columnar epithelium occurs at the gastro-oesophageal junction in healthy individuals.

Clinical features

Barrett's oesophagus is usually asymptomatic, being recognised as an incidental finding on endoscopy. It appears as 'velvety' epithelium extending more than 3 cm above the gastro-oesophageal junction. The significance of 'short segment' Barrett's, i.e. less than 3 cm in length, is unclear.

Management

Most patients whose Barrett's oesophagus is identified incidentally on endoscopy are started on life-long acid suppression.

Surgery

Anti-reflux surgery may reduce the progression to dysplasia and cancer. Endoscopic mucosal ablation, which is usually achieved using photosensitisers and laser therapy may also reduce progression.

Prognosis

The role of endoscopic surveillance in patients with Barrett's oesophagus is controversial. The aim of surveillance is to detect dysplasia before it progresses to carcinoma. However, about 40% of patients with dysplasia already have a focus of adenocarcinoma. Oesophagectomy for oesophageal dysplasia has an 80% 5-year survival.

Gastric cancer

A high index of suspicion for a diagnosis of gastric cancer is required so that the diagnosis is not missed. Most patients present late and are not suitable for radical surgery.

Epidemiology

Gastric cancer is one of the most common causes of cancer deaths worldwide. It accounts for 7000 deaths per year in the UK.

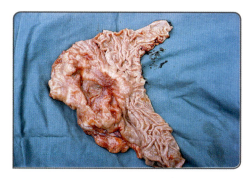

Figure 5.8 Gross pathological specimen of a gastric carcinoma.

The incidence increases with age, and the male-to-female ratio is 2:1.

Despite an overall decline in the incidence rate of gastric cancer, several countries, including the UK, have seen an increase in the incidence of adenocarcinomas of the gastric cardia, sometimes referred to proximal gastric cancers.

Aetiology

Macroscopically, tumours vary in appearance. Most are adenocarcinomas.

Malignant gastric ulcers typically have raised everted edges and sometimes have a necrotic base (**Figure 5.8**). Linitis plastica is a diffusely infiltrating tumour of the mucosa and submucosa with marked fibrosis. This leads to a shrunken, thickened stomach that fails to distend. Anaplastic signet-ring tumours, with a typical histological appearance, have a poor prognosis.

Spread is typically via the lymphatics or portal system. It can occur via the peritoneal cavity to the ovaries, where the secondaries are known as Krukenberg tumours. The risk factors for gastric cancer are shown in **Table 5.7**.

Clinical features

New-onset dyspepsia in patients over the age of 50 years suggests gastric carcinoma, as does any dyspepsia that fails to respond to treatment. Weight loss and an epigastric mass are late and worrying signs. Some patients will develop an iron deficiency anaemia. Dysphagia and early postprandial vomiting occur with proximal obstructing tumours.

Late postprandial vomiting, especially of altered food and with no bile, suggests gastric outlet obstruction.

> **Gastric cancer can be difficult to diagnose** as the initial symptoms are often vague, non-specific and easily mistaken for those of other, less serious conditions, such as peptic ulcer disease which is far more common.

Diagnostic approach

It is recommended that all patients over the age of 40 years who have new-onset dyspepsia undergo an upper gastrointestinal endoscopy.

Investigations

Upper gastrointestinal endoscopy will confirm the diagnosis, site and extent of a tumour.

The tumour is staged using a combination of preoperative investigations and intraoperative assessment:

- Endoscopic ultrasound may allow an assessment of how far the tumour has penetrated the wall of the oesophagus
- Abdominal CT allows an assessment of nodal spread and the extent of metastatic disease
- Laparoscopy shows peritoneal seedlings
- Peritoneal lavage allows free tumour cells to be detected

Management

Surgery offers the only prospect of curing gastric carcinoma.

Surgery

A tumour is resectable if it is confined to the stomach or if only the N1 (<3 cm from the tumour) or N2 (>3 cm from the tumour)lymph nodes are involved. However, surgery may palliate patients' symptoms even if the disease is incurable.

Tumours of the gastric antrum may be suitable for a partial gastrectomy, usually with a Polya reconstruction (**Figure 5.9**). Other tumours are treated by a total gastrectomy with oesophagojejunal anastomosis and roux-en-Y biliary diversion (**Figure 5.10**).

Partial gastrectomy with Polya reconstruction

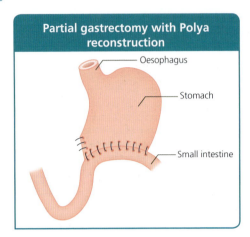

Figure 5.9 Partial gastrectomy with Polya reconstruction.

Total gastrectomy with roux-en-Y reconstruction

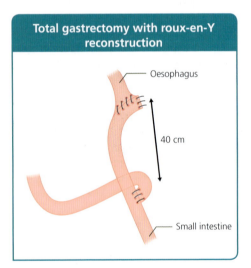

Figure 5.10 Total gastrectomy with roux-en-Y reconstruction.

Resection of the tumour and N1 nodes is regarded as a D1 gastrectomy. If the tumour and N2 nodes are resected, this is regarded as a D2 gastrectomy. A D2 gastrectomy is associated with increased postoperative mortality but may have improved long-term survival.

The results of adjuvant chemotherapy after surgery are disappointing. Chemoradiotherapy may reduce the risk of relapse and improve survival.

Prognosis

The prognosis is generally very poor, with a 5-year survival rate of approximately 5%.

Gastrointestinal stromal tumours

Gastrointestinal stromal tumours arise from non-epithelial and non-lymphoid tissues in the gastrointestinal tract. They can be benign, malignant or of indeterminate potential.

Leiomyosarcomas are a form of gastrointestinal stromal tumour that accounts for 2–3% of all gastric tumours. They arises from the smooth muscle of the stomach wall. Lymphatic spread is rare. About 75% of patients with leiomyosarcomas present with an upper gastrointestinal bleed, and 60% have a palpable abdominal mass on examination. The diagnosis can be confirmed by upper gastrointestinal endoscopy and CT scanning. Partial gastrectomy may allow adequate resection. The 5-year survival is approximately 50%.

Gastric lymphoma

The stomach is the most common extranodal primary site for non-Hodgkin's lymphoma.

Gastric lymphoma accounts for approximately 1% of gastric malignancies. The clinical presentation is very similar to that of gastric carcinoma. About 70% of tumours are resectable, and the 5-year survival is approximately 25%. Adjuvant radiotherapy and chemotherapy reduce the risk of recurrence and increase survival.

Sister Mary Joseph nodule

A Sister Mary Joseph nodule usually presents as a firm, red, non-tender nodule in the umbilicus. It is often associated with advanced intra-abdominal malignancy as it results from a spread of tumour within the falciform ligament.

About 90% of tumours are adenocarcinomas, the most common primary sites being the stomach and ovary. The primary tumour is almost invariably inoperable.

Answers to starter questions

1. Embryologically the gastrointestinal tract is divided into three parts. The foregut extends from the gastroesophageal junction to the second part of the duodenum. The midgut extends from the duodenum to the mid-transverse colon. The hindgut extends from the transverse colon to the lower rectum. The blood supply to each is derived from coeliac axis, superior mesenteric artery and inferior mesenteric artery respectively. Knowledge of this embryology is important when considering the extent of surgical resections.

2. Gastro-oesophageal reflux disease presents with heartburn and indigestion. These symptoms are common in the normal population and there is a poor correlation between the severity of the symptom and objective evidence of oesophagitis. In patients being considered for surgery, it is important to obtain objective evidence of failure of the lower oesophageal sphincter and the presence of reflux. The function of the lower oesophageal sphincter can be assessed by oesophageal manometry and the presence of reflux by oesophageal pH studies. When objective evidence of reflux is demonstrated before surgery, the outcome of a surgery is improved.

3. *Helicobacter pylori (H. pylori)* is a urease-producing gram-negative spiral flagellated bacterium. It is found in 20% of the normal population and in 90%, 70% and 60% of patients with duodenal ulceration, gastric ulceration and gastric cancer respectively. The majority of people who have *H. pylori* are asymptomatic. It is endemic in the developing world and its prevalence seems to decrease with development. The fact that most people infected with *H. pylori* never develop symptoms has led many to argue that it is a commensal organism of the gastrointestinal tract.

4. Tumours of the oesophagus and stomach spread early to the locoregional lymph nodes and may also metastasise to the liver or within the peritoneal cavity before they cause symptoms. The symptoms they cause may be minimal and often mimic benign disease. As a result, patients with either dysphagia or dyspepsia often tolerate their symptoms for an extensive period of time before they seek medical advice or are referred. By the time they are investigated, tumours have often spread and are not suitable for a curative surgical resection.

5. Primary tumours of the small bowel are rare in comparison to those in the remainder of the gastrointestinal tract. The majority of gastric carcinomas are adenocarcinomas. The majority of small bowel tumours arise from either the neuroendocrine cells or small bowel lymphatics causing either carcinoid tumours or lymphomas respectively. Adenocarcinoma of the small bowel are uncommon but they do occur as part of the hereditary polyposis syndromes. The reason for this regional variation is unclear.

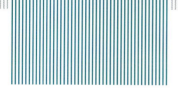

Chapter 6
Colorectal surgery

Introduction.	111	Intestinal stomas	124
Case 4 Groin lump	112	Enterocutaneous fistulae	124
Case 5 Change in bowel habit	113	Inflammatory bowel disease	125
Core science	115	Diverticular disease	129
History, examination and		Colorectal polyps	130
investigation	118	Colorectal cancer	131
Abdominal wall hernias	121	Perianal conditions	134

Starter questions

Answers to the following questions are on page 138.

1. What are the anatomical differences between a direct and indirect inguinal hernia?
2. Why are enterocutaneous fistulas so difficult to manage?
3. Why do colonic diverticulae occur?
4. How does the clinical presentation of colorectal cancer depend on the site of the tumour?
5. Why is emergency presentation of colorectal cancer associated with a worse outcome than elective surgery?
6. Why is it important to understand the anatomy of the anal canal when managing perianal sepsis?

Introduction

Colorectal surgery treats diseases of the colon, rectum and anal canal. Patients present to either a physician or a surgeon with either local symptoms directly related to the gastrointestinal tract or systemic manifestations of the disease. Not all patients require surgical intervention. However, for those who do, a clear understanding of the anatomy of the colon, rectum and anal canal is essential to understand the nature of the procedures performed.

Case 4 Groin lump

Presentation

A 70-year-old man, Mr William Blythe, presents to his general practitioner with a 3-week history of a painful lump in his right groin (**Figure 6.1**).

Initial interpretation

The most common cause of a groin lump in an elderly man is an inguinal or a femoral hernia. Inguinal hernias are more common than femoral hernias. Other less common causes of groin lumps include a saphena varix (dilatation of the long saphenous vein at its junction with the femoral vein), a femoral artery aneurysm and an enlarged inguinal or femoral lymph node

History

William first noticed the lump after moving some furniture. The lump was uncomfortable and slightly tender. It reduced

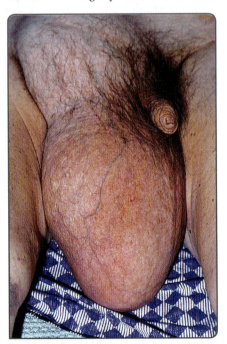

Figure 6.1 Right inguinoscrotal hernia.

in size with gentle pressure and eventually disappeared. However, it recurred on several occasions over the intervening 3 days. William has no abdominal symptoms of note. In particular, he has no abdominal pain, vomiting or abdominal distension. His bowels have continued to be open regularly.

Interpretation of history

A groin lump that is reducible is highly suggestive of an uncomplicated hernia. A hernia that is irreducible suggests the presence of complications.

Further history

William is otherwise fit and well with no significant past medical history.

Examination

An examination of William while he is standing shows the lump in the right groin. It is arising above and lateral to the public tubercle. When William coughs, the lump increases in size (i.e. it shows a cough impulse). When he is lying down, the lump reduces in size. It disappears with gentle pressure. There is no scarring or distension of the abdomen.

Palpation of the abdomen shows no masses, and the bowel sounds are normal.

Interpretation of findings

A groin lump that increases in size on standing, has a cough impulse, reduces in size on lying down and eventually disappears indicates an inguinal hernia.

Inguinal hernias are direct (arising through the posterior wall of the inguinal canal) or indirect (arising within the spermatic cord). Direct inguinal hernias reduce to a point above and lateral to the pubic tubercle. Indirect hernias reduce to a point below and medial to the pubic tubercle (**Figure 6.2**).

Case 4 *continued*

Direct versus indirect inguinal hernia

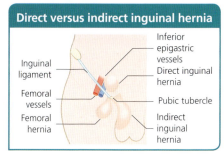

Figure 6.2 Direct versus indirect inguinal hernia.

Complications of hernias included irreducibility and strangulation. Strangulated hernias are painful, irreducible and associated with the symptoms and signs of intestinal obstruction. Williams's hernia is reducible with no features of strangulation.

Investigations

An uncomplicated hernia is a clinical diagnosis and does not require investigation. If there is doubt regarding the diagnosis, an ultrasound or CT scan may help to confirm it.

Diagnosis

William has a reducible direct inguinal hernia. The risk of strangulation is low,

and there would be no need for surgical intervention if William had no symptoms. However, William's hernia is painful and he is keen to consider surgery. He is therefore referred to the general surgery service at his local hospital.

The surgeon confirms the presence of a hernia and offers to repair it as a day case. During the operation, the hernia is reduced and the posterior wall of the inguinal canal is reinforced with a synthetic mesh – a Lichtenstein hernia repair (**Figure 6.3**). William makes an uncomplicated recovery from his surgery and is advised to avoid heavy lifting for a month.

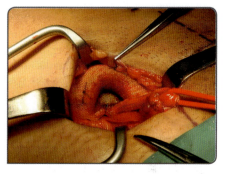

Figure 6.3 Repair of an inguinal hernia using a tension-free mesh (Lichtenstein repair).

Case 5 Change in bowel habit

Presentation

A 64-year-old woman, Mrs Georgina Taylor, presents to her general practitioner with a 2-month history of a change in bowel habit. She has noticed that she has become constipated, with increasing difficulty passing stools.

Initial interpretation

Constipation is a common symptom affecting all age groups. Causes include a change in diet, dehydration or a side effect of medication. However, it can also be the presenting symptom of colorectal disease. Assessment aims to identify those patients needing urgent investigation.

Case 5 *continued*

History

Over the preceding 2 months, Georgina has noticed that her bowel habit has changed from a regular pattern of once per day to going several days without passing a stool, followed by the occasional day when she passes a stool several times in one day.

Interpretation of history

A change in bowel habit in a woman of this age raises the suspicion of a colorectal cancer.

Further history

Georgina feels that her bowel is not completely empty after passing a stool. She has noticed that her stools are occasionally covered in mucus and that she has had occasional spots of rectal bleeding. There has been no recent change in her diet and she is not taking any regular medication. She has no abdominal pain but she has observed that her abdomen appears distended. She has had no previous abdominal surgery. Her father died at the age of 70 years from bowel cancer.

Examination

On examination, there is no evidence of surgical scars on the abdomen. The abdomen appears distended. Palpation shows no obvious masses or areas of tenderness. There is no evidence of a groin hernia. The bowel sounds are normal. Rectal examination shows an ulcerating mass at the tip of the examining finger.

Interpretation of findings

A change in bowel habit associated with the passage of mucus and blood per rectum is highly suggestive of the presence of a rectal carcinoma. The sensation of incomplete emptying of the rectum (tenesmus) is suggestive of a rectal lesion activating the rectal muscle wall stretch receptors. The finding of an ulcerating rectal lesion on digital examination adds further support to the diagnosis.

Investigations

Rapid access to a colorectal surgeon at the local hospital is arranged, and he confirms the clinical findings. The tumour does not appear to be fixed to the pelvis. A few days later, Georgina undergoes a colonoscopy. This shows a malignant ulcer 10 cm from the anal margin (**Figure 6.4**). An endoscopic biopsy is taken. The remainder of the colon is normal.

Diagnosis

The biopsy shows a poorly differentiated adenocarcinoma, confirming the diagnosis of a rectal carcinoma. An MRI scan confirms that the tumour is localised to the rectal wall. A CT scan of the thorax, abdomen and pelvis shows that the tumour is localised to the pelvis with no evidence of metastatic spread.

After bowel preparation, Georgina undergoes a laparoscopically assisted anterior resection (removal of the sigmoid colon and upper rectum) with a primary anastomosis between the descending colon and the remaining rectum, and a defunctioning

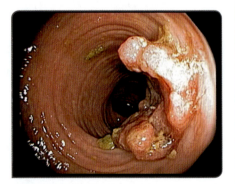

Figure 6.4 Endoscopic appearance of a rectal carcinoma.

Case 5 *continued*

loop ileostomy. A defunctioning ileostomy diverts bowel contents away from the anastomosis. Once the anastomosis has healed the ileostomy can be reversed. She makes a rapid and uncomplicated recovery from the surgery. Histology of the colon and rectum shows that the tumour is confined to the rectal wall, and there is no evidence of spread to the lymph nodes. She requires no adjuvant therapy.

Core science

The inguinal canal

The inguinal canal is an oblique passage through the lower abdominal wall that contains the spermatic cord in men (**Figure 6.5**) and the round ligament of the uterus in women.

Boundaries of the inguinal canal

The lateral boundary of the inguinal canal is the deep inguinal ring. It is an opening in the fascia transversalis about 1 cm above

Inguinal canal anatomy

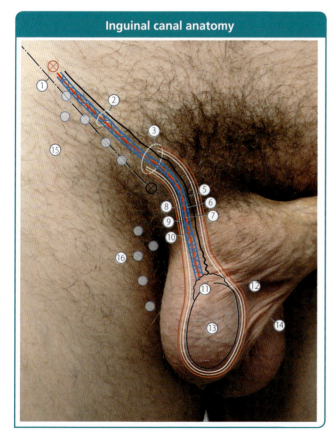

Figure 6.5 Anatomy of the inguinal canal. ① inguinal ligament; ② spermatic cord in the inguinal canal; ③ spermatic cord emerging from superficial inguinal ring; ⑤ pampiniform plexus; ⑥ testicular artery; ⑦ external spermatic fascia; ⑧ cremasteric fascia (external oblique); ⑨ cremasteric fascia (internal oblique); ⑩ internal spermatic fascia (transversalis fascia); ⑪ epididymis (head); ⑫ skin of scrotum; ⑬ testicle (surrounded by the tunica vaginalis); ⑭ , midline scrotal raphe; ⑮ horizontal group of lymph nodes; ⑯ vertical group of lymph nodes; ⊗ position of deep inguinal ring; ⊗ pubic tubercle.

Boundaries of the inguinal canal

Boundary	Structure
Anterior	External oblique aponeurosis, reinforced in the lateral third by the internal oblique muscle
Posterior	Fascia transversalis, reinforced in the medial third by the conjoint tendon
Roof	Arched fibres of the conjoint tendon
Floor	Inguinal ligament – lower border of the external oblique aponeurosis
Medial	Superficial inguinal ring
Lateral	Deep inguinal ring

Table 6.1 Boundaries of the inguinal canal

the inguinal ligament, midway between the anterior superior iliac spine and the symphysis pubis. It lies just lateral to the inferior epigastric vessels.

The medial boundary of the inguinal canal is the superficial inguinal ring. This a triangular defect in the external oblique aponeurosis that overlies the pubic crest. The pubic crest forms the base of the opening. The other boundaries of the inguinal canal are shown in **Table 6.1**.

Contents of the inguinal canal

In both men and women, the inguinal canal contains the ilioinguinal nerve. In men, it also contains the spermatic cord. Each layer of the anterior abdominal wall gives rise to a layer of the spermatic cord. From the inside to the outside, these are:

- The internal spermatic fascia, from the fascia transversalis
- The cremasteric fascia, from the internal oblique muscle
- The external spermatic fascia, from the external oblique muscle

The femoral sheath and canal

The femoral sheath is a prolongation of the transversalis fascia below the inguinal ligament in front of the femoral vessels (**Figure 6.6**).

Anatomy of the femoral canal

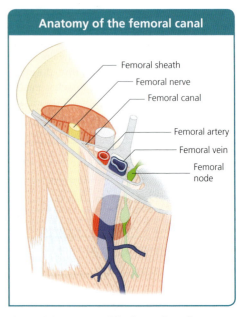

Figure 6.6 Anatomy of the femoral canal.

The lateral and medial compartments contain the femoral artery and femoral vein, respectively. The medial compartment is called the femoral canal and also contains lymphatic vessels and a lymph gland. The anatomical boundaries of the femoral canal are as follows:

- Anterior – inguinal ligament
- Posterior – pectineal ligament
- Medial – lacunar ligament
- Lateral – femoral vein

Anatomy of the large intestine

The large intestine begins at the caecum and ends at the beginning of the anal canal.

The caecum and appendix

The caecum is the first part of the large intestine. It is situated in the right iliac fossa and is completely covered by peritoneum. Like the remainder of the colon, the caecum has three longitudinal bands of muscle on its surface knows as the taeniae coli. These converge on the base of the appendix.

Anteriorly, the caecum is related to the greater omentum and anterior abdominal wall. Its posterior relations include the psoas and iliacus muscles and the femoral nerve. The blood supply is from the anterior and posterior caecal arteries, which are terminal branches of the ileocolic artery.

The appendix

This arises from the posteromedial surface of the caecum below the level of the ileocaecal valve. It is covered by peritoneum and is attached to a short mesentery known as the mesoappendix. The anterior relation of the base of the appendix is the anterior abdominal wall at a point one third of the way along a line joining the anterior superior iliac spine and the umbilicus (McBurney's point). The blood supply is from the appendicular artery, which is a branch of the posterior caecal artery.

> **The tip of the appendix can be found in various positions,** including hanging down into the pelvis, behind the caecum and in front of or behind the terminal ileum. As a result, the clinical features of acute appendicitis can vary and the diagnosis can sometimes be difficult to make.

The colon and rectum

The colon is classified into the ascending, transverse, descending and sigmoid colon.

The blood supply of the colon is shown in **Figure 6.7**. The ileocolic, right and middle colic arteries are branches of the superior mesenteric artery. The superior and inferior left colic arteries are branches of the inferior mesenteric artery. The venous and lymphatic drainage follows the blood supply and enters the portal system.

The rectum

The rectum is about 15 cm long and passes through the levator ani muscles to join the anal canal. The anterior and lateral surfaces of the upper third of the rectum are covered by peritoneum. However, in the middle third of the rectum, only the anterior surface is covered. The lower third of the rectum has no peritoneal covering.

The blood supply of the rectum is from the superior, middle and inferior rectal arteries. The venous drainage is into the inferior mesenteric, internal iliac and internal pudendal veins. The lymphatic drainage is to the pararectal nodes. The lymphatics then follow the superior rectal artery to reach the inferior mesenteric nodes.

The anal canal

The levator ani muscles are sheets of muscle that arise from the side walls of the pelvis and join in the midline to form the floor of the pelvic cavity known as the pelvic diaphragm. The pelvic diaphragm supports the viscera in

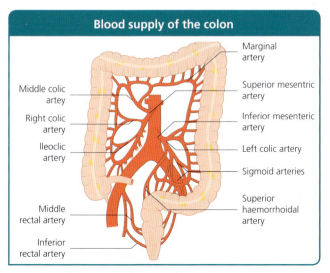

Figure 6.7 Blood supply of the colon.

the pelvic cavity, as well as the structures that pass through it. In combination with the coccygeus muscle, it forms the pelvic diaphragm.

The anus has two muscular sphincters – the internal and external sphincters (**Figure 6.8**). The internal anal sphincter is made up of smooth muscle. The external anal sphincter is striated muscle.

The mucosa of the upper third of anal canal has no somatic sensation. The mucosa of the lower two thirds of the anal canal has a somatic innervation from the inferior rectal nerves. The blood supply to the anal canal is from the superior middle and inferior rectal arteries. The external haemorrhoidal plexus of veins lies deep to the skin of the anal canal and drains via the middle and inferior rectal veins into the systemic venous system. The internal haemorrhoidal plexus of veins lies above the dentate line (**Figure 6.8**) and drains via the superior rectal veins into the portal venous system. The anorectum is therefore the site of an important potential portosystemic anastomosis.

The lymphatics from the anal canal drain into the superficial inguinal group of lymph nodes.

> **The anal canal has cutaneous sensation below the dentate line.** Lesions arising below the dentate line are therefore often painful. Lesions arising above the dentate line are often pain free.

Physiology of the large intestine

The colon has two functions: the absorption of water and electrolytes, and propulsion of the faeces for evacuation. Approximately 1 L of small bowel contents enters the caecum each day, but due to absorption of water, only about 100 g of faeces are evacuated.

Colonic motility is increased by parasympathetic nervous impulses via the vagus and sacral nerves. Motility is decreased by sympathetic nervous impulses via the superior mesenteric plexus, inferior mesenteric plexus and hypogastric plexus. The major control of motility is via the intrinsic (Auerbach's and Meissner's) plexuses in the wall of the colon.

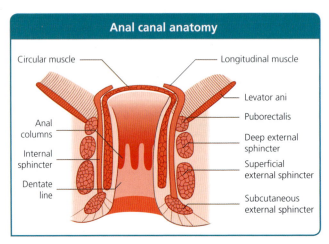

Anal canal anatomy

Circular muscle — Longitudinal muscle

Anal columns

Internal sphincter

Dentate line

Levator ani

Puborectalis

Deep external sphincter

Superficial external sphincter

Subcutaneous external sphincter

Figure 6.8 Anatomy of the anal canal.

History, examination and investigation

Colorectal disease can present as either a surgical emergency from primary care or the emergency department, with a rapid onset of symptoms or to an outpatient clinic with symptoms that have been present for a variable duration of time. The common symptoms and signs of colorectal disease are shown in **Table 6.2**.

Symptoms and signs of colorectal disease	
Symptoms	Signs
Abdominal pain	Abdominal mass
Change in bowel habit	Abdominal tenderness
Rectal bleeding	Abdominal distension
Perianal pain	Rectal mass
Perianal lump	

Table 6.2 Common symptoms and signs of colorectal disease

History

Common symptoms of colorectal disease include abdominal pain, abdominal distension, a change in bowel habit and rectal bleeding.

Abdominal pain

Abdominal pain is a common presentation of colorectal disease. A thorough history is necessary to determine the underlying cause.

Pain arising from the colon is usually located in the lower abdomen and is either constant or colicky. The pain is often relieved by opening the bowels. It is often associated with abdominal distension or a change in bowel habit.

Change in bowel habit

The normal bowel habit varies between individuals. Some people pass a stool several times each day, while other healthy individuals can go several days without passing one. Therefore enquire about a change from the patient's normal pattern rather than absolute frequencies.

Constipation and diarrhoea mean different things to different people. When taking a history, get patients to describe accurately what they mean by these symptoms.

Constipation is common symptom and frequently occurs in the absence of colorectal disease. It may result from dehydration, from systemic illnesses (e.g. hypothyroidism) or as a side effect of medication (e.g. opiate analgesia). Bear in mind that it is also a symptom of intestinal obstruction.

Diarrhoea is also a common symptom. It is often the result of a short-lived bacterial or viral infection. Chronic diarrhoea with or without rectal bleeding is often a feature of inflammatory bowel disease.

Tenesmus is a feeling of an incomplete emptying of the rectum or the constant need to pass stool, despite the rectum being empty. It is a symptom of a mass lesion within the rectum.

Not all constipation is due to mechanical obstruction. Assessment should include the presence of other systemic diseases and possible side effects of medication.

Rectal bleeding

Bleeding per rectum is an embarrassing symptom, and clinical presentation is often delayed as a result. Rectal bleeding is never normal. The amount of blood passed can vary from a few spots, either coating or mixed with the stool, to a large volume passed on its own.

The site of the bleeding determines whether the blood is bright red or dark red. Bleeding from proximal sites in the colon is invariably dark red and is passed either spontaneously or mixed with the stool. Bleeding from the rectum or anal canal is usually bright red and often coats the stool.

Examination

The examination of a patient with potential colorectal disease should begin with an assessment of nutritional status. The patient is also examined for complications of disease such as anaemia. Examination of all patients with potential colorectal disease should involve both an abdominal and a rectal examination.

Abdominal examination

The patient's abdomen, groin and genitalia should be adequately exposed for the examination, but the patient's dignity should be maintained.

The abdomen is inspected for distension and surgical scars. It is then palpated both superficially and deeply, starting away from the site of any potential pathology. Superficial palpation allows tenderness and guarding to be detected. Guarding is involuntary contraction of the abdominal wall musculature arising from irritation of the underlying peritoneum. Deep palpation may reveal abdominal masses.

Percussion may detect shifting dullness due to ascites, or dullness to percussion as a result of hepatomegaly, splenomegaly or abdominal masses. If small bowel obstruction is present, there is often tinkling bowel sounds on auscultation.

Next, examine the groins for hernias. If a lump is detected, define its site clearly. An uncomplicated hernia is both reducible and has a cough impulse. If a hernia is irreducible and tender and has no cough impulse, strangulation should be suspected.

Examination of the abdomen is completed by a digital rectal examination. This begins with inspection of the anus. Digital examination assesses the presence of anal or rectal lesions, the size, shape and contour of the prostate in men, and the presence or absence of any blood on the gloved finger.

Investigation

The investigation of colorectal disease has two aims: to confirm the presence of the disease that has been clinically suspected, and to assess the extent of the disease and the presence of any local or systemic complications.

Blood tests

Blood tests are important in the investigation of colorectal disease, in particular to identify the systemic effects from complications of the disease. Chronic blood loss often results in a hypochromic microcytic anaemia that is detectable on a full blood count. Serum total protein and albumin values provide a measure of nutritional status. Inflammatory markers (e.g. white cell count, C-reactive protein and erythrocyte sedimentation rate) can be useful in assessing patients with infective or inflammatory diseases. Any change in these markers can provide evidence of disease progression or resolution.

Plain radiographs

These are of limited use in the investigation of elective patients with colorectal symptoms but have a role in assessing emergency patients. The indications for a plain abdominal radiograph are a suspicion of:

- Intestinal obstruction
- Intestinal perforation
- Intussusception
- Ingested or inserted foreign body

Plain abdominal radiographs are taken with the patient lying down. An additional erect abdominal radiograph subjects the patient to unnecessary radiation exposure and adds no further information.

In intestinal obstruction, the small bowel, the large bowel or both are dilated. Dilated small bowel is recognised by its position in the centre of the abdomen and by the fact that its markings (representing the plicae circulares) cross the whole width of the bowel. The large bowel is situation at the periphery of the abdomen and is characterised by haustra (small pouches which give the colon its segmented appearance and that do not cross the whole diameter of the bowel).

An erect chest radiograph is useful for looking for free gas under the diaphragm in patients with suspected intestinal perforation.

Abdominal CT and MRI

Contrast-enhanced abdominal CT scanning and MRI have replaced other more invasive radiological investigations (e.g. barium enema) in the investigation of colorectal disease. CT scanning helps to confirm the presence of colorectal lesions, identify their complications and stage colorectal cancer. MRI is particularly useful for assessing rectal and anal pathology as it allows the relationship of lesions to the bowel musculature and other pelvic organs to be clearly defined.

Colonoscopy

Colonoscopy is endoscopic examination of the large bowel and terminal ileum using a fibreoptic endoscope that is passed through the anus. It provides a visual diagnosis and allows biopsies to be taken. Small polyps can also be removed. Sigmoidoscopy is a more limited investigation that allows examination of the rectum and distal colon.

Colonoscopy is used in the assessment of patients with rectal bleeding, a change in bowel habit, unexplained anaemia and suspected colonic malignancy. It is used in screening for colorectal cancer. Bowel preparation is required to obtain an adequate view. Therefore, for 2 days prior to the investigation, the patient is maintained on clear fluid and given strong laxatives. The investigation is performed under sedation. Complications are rare, but major complications include bleeding and bowel perforation.

> A photographic record of the ileocaecal valve should be kept to document that a complete colonoscopy has been achieved.

Abdominal wall hernias

A hernia is a congenital or acquired protrusion of an organ through the wall that normally contains it. Depending on the site of the hernia the wall is the abdomen, muscle fascia or the diaphragm. The hernia consists of a sac, its coverings and its contents. Abdominal wall hernias are common and account for approximately 10% of the general surgical workload.

Hernias are classified as:

- Reducible
- Irreducible
- Obstructed
- Strangulated

With irreducible hernias, there is either a narrow neck or the contents of the hernia are adherent to the sac wall. Obstructed hernias cause intestinal obstruction but the bowel within the hernia remains viable. Strangulation occurs when the venous drainage from the contents of the sac is compromised.

Inguinal hernia

About 3% of adults require surgery for an inguinal hernia at some stage, and 80,000 operations are performed each year in the UK. The male-to-female ratio is 12:1, and the ratio of elective to emergency operation is also about 12:1. The peak incidence is in the sixth decade.

Direct inguinal hernia

A direct inguinal hernia is caused by weakness of the abdominal wall musculature. The hernial sac is located medial to the inferior epigastric artery. In adult males, 35% of inguinal hernias are direct, and they are more common in older patients. Predisposing factors include smoking, ilioinguinal nerve damage and abdominal straining. Complications are unlikely due to the wide neck of the hernial sac.

Indirect inguinal hernia

Indirect inguinal hernias pass through the inguinal canal. The hernial sac is located lateral to the inferior epigastric artery. In adult males, 65% of inguinal hernias are indirect. They are more common on the right side, especially in children. Complications are more common than with direct inguinal hernias.

Clinical features

The lump of an inguinal hernia is often located above and medial to the pubic tubercle.

A reducible hernia usually presents with a lump that increases in size on coughing or straining, and reduces in size or disappears when the patient is relaxed or supine. Examination often shows a cough impulse.

Irreducible but non-obstructed hernias usually cause little pain. If obstruction occurs, colicky abdominal pain, distension and vomiting often occurs. The hernia may be tense, tender and irreducible. If strangulation occurs, the lump becomes red and tender, and the patient will rapidly become systemically unwell.

The features that help to differentiate indirect and direct inguinal hernias are shown in **Table 6.3**.

Investigations

The diagnosis of a hernia is usually based on the clinical features alone. The differential diagnosis is shown in **Table 6.4**. A herniogram where radiological contrast is injected into the peritoneal cavity and the presence of a hernia sought, may help in the investigation of chronic groin pain that may be due to an occult hernia. Ultrasound, CT or MRI scanning can also be useful if a clinically occult hernia is suspected.

Management

- In some patients with painless, easily reducible hernias, surgery should be avoided. However, symptomatic hernias invariably require surgery: Herniotomy involves removal of the sac and closure of the neck of the hernia. This is the treatment of choice in children and adolescents
- Herniorrhaphy involves some form of reconstruction to restore the disturbed anatomy, increase the strength of the abdominal wall and construct a barrier to recurrence. It usually involves the placement of a prosthetic mesh via either an open or a laparoscopic technique
- An open Lichtenstein mesh repair is now regarded as the gold standard technique for inguinal hernia repair as it is associated with a low risk of recurrence

Laparoscopic hernia repair is possible but should be reserved for bilateral or recurrent hernias.

Features of inguinal hernias	
Indirect	Direct
Often descend into the scrotum	Rarely descend into the scrotum
Reduce laterally	Reduced backwards
Controlled by pressure over the deep inguinal ring	Not controlled by pressure over the deep inguinal ring
Defect results in a hernia that is not palpable	Defect results in a hernia that is sometimes palpable
Hernia reappears in the mid-inguinal region	Hernia reappears in the medial part of the inguinal canal

Table 6.3 Features of inguinal hernia

Differential diagnosis of inguinal hernia	
System	Example
Other hernias	Femoral hernia
Lymphoreticular	Inguinal lymph node
	Femoral lymph node
Vascular	Saphena varix
	Femoral artery aneurysm
Genitourinary	Hydrocele of the cord
	Undescended testis
Other	Lipoma of the cord

Table 6.4 Differential diagnosis of inguinal hernia

Femoral hernia

Femoral hernias account for 7% of all abdominal wall hernias. The female-to-male ratio is 4:1. They are more common in middle-aged and elderly women and are rare in children. Despite this, the most common hernia in women is an inguinal hernia.

> All patients presenting with small bowel obstruction should be examined for a possible femoral hernia. Failure to do so risks missing an easily correctable cause of intestinal obstruction.

Clinical features

Femoral hernias present with a groin lump below and lateral to the public tubercle. Unlike inguinal hernias, the lump is often irreducible. Due to their tight neck, femoral hernias are more likely than inguinal hernias to present with complications such as obstruction and strangulation.

> **When a hernia is reduced during a clinical examination, the point at which it disappears will indicate the type of hernia.** A femoral hernia will reduce to a point below and lateral to the public tubercle. An indirect inguinal hernia will reduce to a point above and medial to the public tubercle.

Management

Uncomplicated femoral hernias should be repaired as an urgent elective procedure. Surgery involves dissecting the sac, reducing its contents, ligating the sac and suturing the inguinal and pectineal ligaments. It is important to avoid compromising the femoral vein, which forms the lateral border of the femoral canal.

Umbilical hernia

There are two types of umbilical hernia in adults: true umbilical and paraumbilical hernias. True hernias are rare and occur with abdominal distension (e.g. ascites). The more common paraumbilical hernias occur through the superior aspect of the umbilical scar.

Clinical features

Paraumbilical hernias are more common in women. They usually contain omentum and only rarely contain bowel. As the neck of the hernia is often tight, the hernia is often irreducible. The differential diagnosis of a paraumbilical hernia includes a cyst of the vitellointestinal duct, a urachal cyst and a metastatic tumour deposit (Sister Mary Joseph nodule).

Management

The management of true and paraumbilical hernias is similar. Surgery is usually performed through an infraumbilical incision. Occasionally, particularly during surgery for large

hernias, the umbilicus needs to be excised. The contents of the hernia are reduced. The defect in the linea alba is repaired using an overlapping Mayo repair or a prosthetic mesh.

Incisional hernia

Incisional hernias occur through the scar from a previous operation. Approximately 1% of all abdominal incisions result in incisional hernias. They occur when there is dehiscence of the deep fascial layers but the overlying skin remains intact. Preoperative, operative and postoperative factors (**Table 6.5**) contribute to their aetiology.

The symptoms are often minimal, the cosmetic appearance often being the main concern. As most incisional hernias are wide-necked, strangulation rarely occurs.

Management

A CT or ultrasound scan helps to clarify the site of the muscular defect, the hernial sac and its contents. Surgical repair is challenging and may not always be appropriate. For example, an abdominal wall support can be better for elderly or infirm patients. Surgery is via either an open or a laparoscopic approach. The results of surgery are variable, and recurrence rates of 20% have been reported.

Spigelian hernia

Spigelian hernias occur at the lateral edge of the rectus sheath, usually at the level of the arcuate line.

Risk factors for incisional hernias		
Preoperative	**Operative**	**Postoperative**
Increasing age	Type of incision	Wound infection
Malnutrition	Technique and materials used	Abdominal distension
Sepsis		
Uraemia	Type of operation	Chest infection or cough
Jaundice	Use of abdominal drains	
Obesity		
Diabetes		
Steroids		

Table 6.5 Risk factors for incisional hernias

Obturator hernia

An obturator hernia occurs in the obturator canal. It is usually asymptomatic until strangulation occurs. Patients presents with small bowel obstruction and occasionally complain of pain on the medial aspect of the thigh. In women, a vaginal examination may identify a lump in the region of the obturator foramen.

Intestinal stomas

A stoma is a surgically created communication between a hollow viscus and the skin. The most common types are colostomies (to the colon) and ileostomies (to the small intestine).

Functionally, stomas are end, loop or continent. A loop stoma is usually required to divert the bowel contents away from a distal anastomosis or to rest distal bowel affected by disease.

So that the stoma bag can be applied securely, it is best to position the stoma away from the umbilicus, costal margin and anterior superior iliac spine and away from any scars. The positioning should also be compatible with the patient's usual clothing.

Table 6.6 shows the potential complications of stomas .

Complications of stomas	
Physical	Functional
Necrosis	Excess action
Detachment	Reduced action
Recession	
Stenosis	
Prolapse	
Ulceration	
Parastomal herniation	
Fistula formation	

Table 6.6 Complications of gastrointestinal stomas

Ileostomy

The output of an ileostomy is the contents of the small bowel. The volume is usually 500–1000 mL per day. An output greater than this can result in electrolyte imbalance. If the output of an ileostomy is excessive, consider the presence of inflammatory bowel disease, paraintestinal sepsis or subacute obstruction.

The high bile content of the output can damage the skin, so ileostomies are fashioned with a spout ensuring the opening of the stoma is a few centimetres proud to the skin and is directed into a stoma bag.

Colostomy

The output of a colostomy is normal stool, usually with a volume of less than 500 mL per day. The output is not corrosive to the skin.

Ileostomies and colostomies can be distinguished on examination. An ileostomy is usually situated in the right iliac fossa, has a spout and has a bag that contains liquid small bowel contents. A colostomy is usually situated in the left iliac fossa, is flush with the skin and has a bag that contains firm stool.

Enterocutaneous fistulae

A fistula is an abnormal connection between a hollow viscus and an adjacent organ or the skin. A simple fistula is a direct communication between the gut and the skin. A complex fistula has multiple tracks and is associated with an abscess cavity.

Epidemiology

Enterocutaneous fistulae are rare. Patients who develop one often have prolonged hospital stays and require nutritional support. This presents a large financial burden.

Aetiology

Fistulae result from a leaking anastomosis, inflammatory bowel disease or malignancy.

Clinical features

The first sign of fistula is often a purulent discharge through the skin or an abdominal wound. Small or large bowel contents begin to discharge from the wound.

> The output from a small bowel fistula is bile stained and large in volume. A large bowel fistula usually presents with a faecal discharge.

Fistulae, particularly if they have a high output (more than 500 mL per day) leads to dehydration, electrolyte and acid–base imbalance, malnutrition and sepsis.

Diagnostic approach

The presence and cause of an enterocutaneous fistula will quite rapidly become clinically apparent. The diagnostic approach is to confirm the presence of the fistula and identify any local or systemic complications.

Investigations

When investigating a fistula, determine the anatomy of the tract and whether it is associated with an abscess cavity. A CT or MRI scan will define these and often identifies the underlying cause if it is not clinically apparent. Blood tests are essential to monitor for renal function, sepsis and nutritional status.

Management

The initial management of a fistula is conservative. Surgery is reserved for patients with complex fistulae and those in whom conservative management fails.

Conservative management

This involves protecting the skin from the corrosive gastrointestinal contents. Fluid balance must be carefully maintained and acid–base imbalances corrected. Nutritional support is important and malnutrition should be avoided by parenteral or enteral nutrition.

Somatostatin analogues (e.g. octreotide) may be considered to reduce gastrointestinal and pancreatic secretions in patients with high-output small bowel fistulae.

Surgery

An enterocutaneous fistula will not close if there is separation of two parts of the bowel by either disease or the result of a surgical complication, there is intestinal obstruction beyond the fistula, or there is a chronic abscess cavity. A fistula will also not heal if there is continuity of the epithelium of the bowel and skin. Surgery may be necessary to drain an abscess or remove diseased bowel.

Prognosis

Large bowel fistulae are more likely than small bowel fistulae to close spontaneously. Once sepsis has been controlled, about 60% of small bowel fistulae close with conservative treatment within 1 month. Fistula surgery is associated with a mortality of at least 10%.

Inflammatory bowel disease

Inflammation of the bowel mucosa has several different causes. It can be confined to the colon or affect other parts of the gastrointestinal tract. There may also be extraintestinal clinical features.

Types

Colonic inflammation is common. Its causes are infection, inflammatory bowel disease, ischaemia and radiation.

Epidemiology

Inflammatory bowel disease has a bimodal age distribution with peaks in adolescence and the elderly. Ulcerative colitis is more common than Crohn's disease. Ulcerative colitis is slightly more common in men, and Crohn's disease in women. Both diseases tend to occur in higher socioeconomic groups.

Aetiology

The role of genetic factors is shown by the variable prevalence in different populations and the increased incidence in first-degree relatives. There is also an increased concordance in monozygotic twins and in the site and type of disease in affected families. Possible environmental factors include smoking and use of anti-inflammatory drugs.

The pathological features of ulcerative colitis and Crohn's disease are summarised in **Table 6.7**.

Pathogenesis

Crohn's disease and ulcerative colitis share some pathophysiological features. Both result

from inappropriate activation of the mucosal immune system. The inflammation is driven by the normal bacteria flora in the bowel lumen. The pathological processes result from a defective barrier function of the intestinal epithelium.

Clinical features

Ulcerative colitis

The clinical presentation and progression of ulcerative colitis are variable. The clinical features of mild disease include minimal diarrhoea, intermittent rectal bleeding and little abdominal pain. More extensive disease is invariably associated with an increased stool frequency, significant rectal bleeding and weight loss. Complications result in an acute presentation with abdominal pain.

In 30% of patients with ulcerative colitis, the disease is confined to the rectum. However, 15% of patients develop more extensive disease over a 10-year period. About 20% of patients have total colonic involvement from the outset.

All patients with ulcerative colitis generally fall into the following categories:

- Severe acute colitis
- Intermittent relapsing colitis
- Chronic persistent colitis
- Asymptomatic disease

Assessment of disease severity depends on measuring the frequency of stools and observing the systemic features (**Table 6.8**). These include tachycardia, fever, anaemia and hypoalbuminaemia.

Pathological features of inflammatory bowel disease	
Ulcerative colitis	Crohn's disease
Lesions continuous – superficial	Lesions patchy – penetrating
Rectum always involved	Rectum normal in 50%
Terminal ileum involved in 10%	Terminal ileum involved in 30%
Granulated ulcerated mucosa	Discretely ulcerated mucosa
No fissuring	Cobblestone appearance with fissuring
Normal serosa	
Muscular shortening of the colon	Serositis common
	Fibrous shortening
Fibrous strictures rare	Strictures common
Fistulae rare	Enterocutaneous or intestinal fistulae in 10%
Malignant change well recognised	Malignant change rare
Anal lesions in <20%	Anal lesions in 75%

Table 6.7 Pathological features of inflammatory bowel disease

Assessment of disease severity in ulcerative colitis	
Severity	Features
Mild	Fewer than four stools per day. Systemically well
Moderate	More than four stools per day. Systemically well
Severe	More than six stools per day. Systemically unwell

Table 6.8 Assessment of disease severity in ulcerative colitis

Crohn's disease

The clinical features of Crohn's disease depend on the site of disease. About 50% of patients have ileocaecal disease, producing pain in the right iliac fossa and sometimes a palpable mass. About 25% of patients present with colitis. Extraintestinal manifestations are more common in Crohn's disease than ulcerative colitis (**Table 6.9**).

Diagnostic approach

The diagnostic approach to a patient with inflammatory bowel disease has two aims: to confirm the presence and extent of the disease, and to identify extraintestinal manifestations and complications.

Investigations

In patients presenting with acute colitis, lower gastrointestinal endoscopy:

- Confirms the presence of colitis
- Allows an assessment of the extent of the disease
- Enables biopsies can be taken to differentiate ulcerative colitis from Crohn's disease

On colonoscopy, ulcerative colitis is usually seen as a confluent area extending proximally from the rectum. Crohn's disease may be patchy with 'skip lesions', which are areas of inflamed mucosa interspersed with segments that appear normal. Caution should be exercised when performing a colonoscopy in those with severe disease, as there is an increased risk of colonic perforation, particularly if a biopsy is taken.

If severe colitis is present, the degree of systemic inflammation must be investigated. Useful markers are haemoglobin, white cell count, serum albumin and C-reactive protein. A plain abdominal radiograph is useful if toxic megacolon (**Figure 6.9**) or perforation is clinically suspected.

Management

The management of inflammatory bowel disease depends on the type and site of disease and its severity.

Extraintestinal manifestations of inflammatory bowel disease	
System	Features
Skin	Erythema nodosum, pyoderma gangrenosum
Joints	Asymmetrical non-deforming arthropathy, sacroiliitis, ankylosing spondylitis
Eyes	Anterior uveitis, episcleritis, conjunctivitis
Liver	Primary sclerosing cholangitis, cholangiocarcinoma, chronic active hepatitis
Renal	Nephrolithiasis, amyloidosis

Table 6.9 Extraintestinal manifestations of inflammatory bowel disease

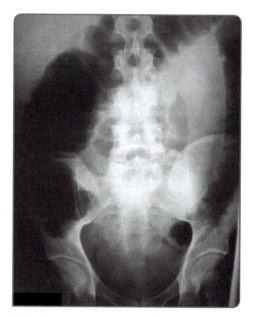

Figure 6.9 Plain abdominal radiograph showing a toxic megacolon in a patient with ulcerative colitis.

Medication

Different drugs may be used for those with active disease and those in remission.

5-Aminosalicylic acid

Drugs that are metaboilised to 5-aminosalicyclic acid (5-ASA) are used in mild to moderate ulcerative colitis and Crohn's disease. They block the production of prostaglandins and leukotrienes. Sulfasalazine was the first agent described. Newer compounds release 5-aminosalicylic acid (5-ASA) at the site of disease activity. Mesalazine is 5-ASA conjugated to prevent absorption in the small intestine and allow delivery of 5-ASA to the colon. Topical agents inserted per rectum can be used in those with left-sided colonic disease. Maintenance therapy is of proven benefit for ulcerative colitis but of unproven benefit in those with Crohn's disease.

Corticosteroids

These are often used when 5-ASA therapy is inadequate and for patients presenting with acute severe disease. They are given orally, topically or parenterally. Their use should be limited to acute exacerbations of the disease. They are of no proven value as maintenance therapy in either ulcerative colitis or Crohn's disease. The benefits of their use in acute exacerbations of the disease must be balanced against their side effects.

Immunosuppressive agents

Immunomodulatory and immunosuppressive agents are often used when steroids cannot be tapered or discontinued due to prolonged disease activity. They include azathioprine, methotrexate and infliximab.

Surgery

Surgery has an important role in both the elective and emergency management of patients with inflammatory bowel disease.

Ulcerative colitis

Approximately 20% of patients with ulcerative colitis require surgery at some point. The indications for elective and emergency surgery are shown in **Table 6.10**. In an emergency, the only appropriate option is often a total colectomy with ileostomy and mucus fistula, a surgically created join between the distal colon and skin designed to allow the release of mucus from the remaining rectum. For elective surgery, the options include:

- Panproctocolectomy (total removal of the colon and rectum) and ileostomy
- Total colectomy and ileorectal anastomosis
- Restorative proctocolectomy with an ileal pouch (a reservoir formed from the small bowel constructed to store small bowel contents and avoid an ileostomy)

A total colectomy and ileorectal anastomosis maintains continence but proctitis (inflammation of the mucosa) often persists within the rectal stump.

The patient needs adequate anal musculature to undergo a restorative proctocolectomy. It is not clear whether a defunctioning ileostomy is necessary after a proctocolectomy.

The functional results of restorative proctocolectomy are often good but morbidity can be high. The mean stool frequency is high at six times per day. Perfect continence is achieved during the day in 90% of patients and at night in 60% of patients. Gross incontinence occurs in 5%. About 50% of patients develop significant complications including small bowel obstruction, pouchitis, genitourinary dysfunction, pelvic sepsis, pouch failure and anal stenosis.

Crohn's disease

The indications for surgery in Crohn's disease are shown in **Table 6.11**. If possible, the patient's nutritional state should be improved preoperatively.

Resection should remove as little small bowel as possible as there is no evidence that having increased resection margins reduces

Indications for surgery in ulcerative colitis	
Emergency	Elective
Toxic megacolon	Chronic symptoms despite medical therapy
Perforation	
Haemorrhage	Carcinoma or high-grade dysplasia
Severe colitis failing to respond to medical treatment	

Table 6.10 Indications for surgery in ulcerative colitis

Indications for surgery in Crohn's disease	
Absolute	Relative
Perforation	Chronic obstructive symptoms
Haemorrhage	Chronic ill-health or debilitating diarrhoea
Carcinoma	
Fulminant or unresponsive acute severe colitis	Intra-abdominal abscess or fistula
	Complications of perianal disease

Table 6.11 Indications for surgery in Crohn's disease

the risk of recurrence. About 30% of patients who undergo ileocaecal resection require further surgery. Strictureplasty (where a stricture is opened longitudinally and closed laterally) is often successful for short strictures, and bypass procedures are rarely required.

Diverticular disease

Colonic diverticulae are outpouchings of the colonic wall. They result from herniation of the gastrointestinal mucosa through the muscular wall at sites where the mesenteric vessels penetrate the bowel wall (**Figure 6.10**). They are most commonly seen in the sigmoid colon.

Epidemiology

The prevalence of diverticular disease increases with age. It affects 10% and 60% of the population, respectively, at 40 and 80 years of age. Diverticular disease is more common in developed countries.

Aetiology and pathogenesis

Diverticular disease is caused by a lack of dietary fibre, which is common in diets in developed countries. The low dietary fibre results in a low stool bulk. This causes increased segmental contraction of the colonic

musculature, which in turn results in colonic muscle hypertrophy. Increased intraluminal pressure as a result of more forceful colonic contractions causes herniation of the mucosa where the colonic musculature is weak.

Inflammation of a segment of diverticular disease results in acute diverticulitis. The intraperitoneal rupture of an inflamed diverticulum, allowing a direct communication between the lumen and peritoneal cavity, resulting in faecal peritonitis. A diverticular fistula forms if the rupture is into an adjacent organ such as the bladder or vagina.

If the lumen of an inflamed diverticulum becomes obstructed due to swelling of the mucosa, a pericolic abscess may form. The intraperitoneal rupture of a pericolic abscess results in purulent peritonitis.

Clinical features

Uncomplicated diverticular disease is often asymptomatic or at worse causes intermittent left iliac fossa pain. There is a tendency towards constipation. Complicated diverticular disease shows several clinical patterns:

- Acute diverticulitis usually presents with more severe and persistent pain in the left iliac fossa. The patient may be pyrexial and tachycardic. An examination often shows tenderness in the left iliac fossa
- A diverticular abscess often causes prolonged left iliac fossa pain associated with signs of systemic sepsis and a swinging pyrexia
- Both purulent and faecal peritonitis cause generalised abdominal pain and signs of generalised peritonitis. Features of severe sepsis are more likely with faecal peritonitis
- A colovesical fistula usually presents with recurrent urinary tract infections and pneumaturia – the passage of air through

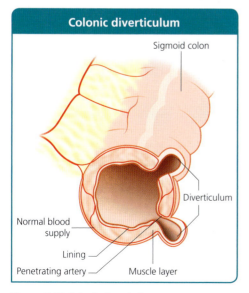

Colonic diverticulum

Sigmoid colon

Diverticulum

Normal blood supply

Lining

Penetrating artery

Muscle layer

Figure 6.10 Colonic diverticulum.

the urethra. A colovaginal fistula results in the passage of faeces through the vagina.

■ A colonic stricture presents with features of large bowel obstruction, often with a background of repeated episodes of acute diverticulitis.

Diagnostic approach

If diverticular disease is suspected, the assessment aims to confirm the diagnosis and exclude other more sinister pathology. It also assesses whether complications are present or may develop.

Complications of diverticular disease include:

■ Diverticulitis
■ Pericolic abscess
■ Purulent peritonitis
■ Faecal peritonitis
■ Fistula – to the vagina, bladder or skin
■ Colonic stricture

Investigations

A plain abdominal radiograph with positive diagnostic features (e.g. free intraperitoneal gas or gas in the bladder) helps in the diagnosis. However, a normal abdominal radiograph cannot exclude the presence of complications of diverticular disease. An abdominal CT with intravenous contrast can image abscesses or fistulae and identify sites of perforation. Flexible sigmoidoscopy is essential to differentiate a benign from a malignant colonic stricture, and allow a histological diagnosis to be obtained in patients with the latter.

Management

Most patients with uncomplicated diverticular disease are managed conservatively with dietary adjustments and occasional use of antispasmotics (e.g. buscopan) and laxatives.

Surgery is only required for those who develop complications.

Medication

Diverticular disease that has few symptoms is managed by dietary modification, stool-bulking agents and the cautious use of laxatives. In patients with acute diverticulitis, the bowel should be 'rested' by restricting oral intake and the administration of intravenous fluids. Intravenous antibiotics are administered, and the patient is observed for the development of complications.

Surgery

If a pericolic abscess forms, percutaneous drainage under radiological guidance is the treatment of choice provided the abscess can be accessed. Patients who develop generalised peritonitis need emergency surgery. This is usually sigmoid resection and left iliac fossa end colostomy (Hartmann's procedure) (**Figure 6.11**). Postoperative mortality is high, especially (about 40%) in patients with faecal peritonitis.

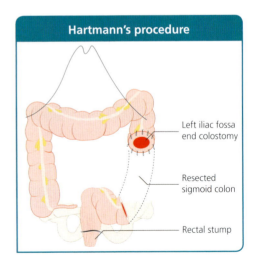

Hartmann's procedure

Left iliac fossa end colostomy

Resected sigmoid colon

Rectal stump

Figure 6.11 Hartmann's procedure.

Colorectal polyps

A polyp is a pedunculated lesion with a base, a stalk and a head. Large bowel polyps are classified as epithelial, mesodermal or hamartomatous (**Table 6.12**).

Not all polyps are tumours. Not all polypoid tumours are benign. Not all benign tumours are polypoid.

Classification of large bowel polyps		
Epithelial	**Mesodermal**	**Hamartomatous**
Adenoma – tubular, villous, tubulovillous	Lipoma	Juvenile
	Leiomyoma	Peutz–Jegher's syndrome
Metaplastic	Haemangioma	

Table 6.12 Classification of large bowel polyps

Juvenile polyps

Juvenile polyps are the most common form of polyp in children. They occur throughout large bowel but are more common in the rectum. They usually present before the age of 12 years with a prolapsing perianal lump or rectal bleeding. They are not premalignant and are treated by local endoscopic resection.

Peutz–Jegher's syndrome

Peutz–Jegher's syndrome is a rare familial condition inherited as an autosomal dominant disorder. It is characterized by circumoral pigmentation and intestinal polyps. Although polyps are found throughout gastrointestinal tract, they are more common in the small intestine.

The disorder presents in childhood with bleeding, anaemia or intussusception. The polyps can become malignant.

Metaplastic polyps

Metaplastic polyps are small plaques approximately 2 mm in diameter. The pathogenesis is unknown and they are not premalignant.

Adenomatous polyps

Adenomas are benign epithelial neoplasms. They are premalignant, and the risk of malignancy increases with their size. Malignancy is more common in villous than tubular lesions.

Most adenomas are asymptomatic. If they become symptomatic, they usually present with bleeding, a mucous discharge or a prolapsing perianal lump. They are usually diagnosed by colonoscopy. Treatment is by transanal excision or colonoscopic snaring. Patients require regular colonoscopic surveillance.

Colorectal cancer

Colorectal cancer can present either electively or as an emergency because of complications. Emergency presentations have a worse prognosis.

Epidemiology

Colorectal cancer is the second most common cause of cancer death. In the UK, there are 20,000 new cases per year, 40% of which are rectal tumours and 60% of which are colonic tumours. About 3% of patients present with more than one tumour (synchronous tumours). A previous colonic cancer increases the risk of a second tumour (a metachronous tumour).

Aetiology

Risk factors for colorectal cancer include age, male sex, a diet rich in meat and fat, inflammatory bowel disease and a personal or family history of colorectal polyps or previous cancer. Most cancers are believed to arise within pre-existing adenomas. The risk of cancer is greatest with villous adenomas.

Familial colorectal cancer (20% of all colorectal cancers) describes cancer in first- or second-degree relatives that does not fulfil the criteria for hereditary non-polyposis colorectal cancer. Hereditary colorectal cancer (5% of all colorectal cancers) is seen in polyposis syndromes (e.g. familial adenomatous polyposis) and hamartomatous polyposis syndromes.

Prevention

The UK NHS Bowel Cancer Screening Programme began in July 2006. If offers screening by faecal occult blood testing every 2 years to all men and women aged 60–69 years. Patients with a positive result are invited for a colonoscopy.

Pathogenesis

Colorectal carcinogenesis is a multistep process involving the progressive accumulation of genetic mutations. These inactivate a variety of tumour suppressor and DNA repair genes, and the activate several oncogenes. This produces changes in the normal epithelium that leads to dysplasia and then invasive cancer.

Clinical features

Colorectal cancer presents via the outpatient clinic or as an emergency. About 40% of cases present as a surgical emergency with either obstruction or perforation. Presentation as an emergency is associated with a poorer outcome.

Caecal or ascending colonic lesions present with iron deficiency anaemia due to occult blood loss, weight loss or a mass in the right iliac fossa. Left-sided colonic lesions often present with abdominal pain and an alteration in bowel habit or rectal bleeding.

> **The emergency presentation of colorectal carcinoma is associated with an increased risk of complications and poorer long-term survival.** This is because the disease is more advanced and there is a greater risk of sepsis and tumour spread associated with perforation.

Diagnostic approach

With potential colorectal cancer, the diagnostic approach is to confirm the disease by endoscopy and biopsy. In patients shown to have a colorectal cancer, the disease should be staged using further radiological investigations.

Investigations

In patients presenting as outpatients, the diagnosis can be confirmed by a combination of flexible sigmoidoscopy, colonoscopy and CT scanning. A CT scan is the investigation of choice for patients presenting with large bowel obstruction. CT scanning also allows staging of the disease.

Management

Surgery is the main mode of treatment for colorectal carcinoma. Some patients with rectal carcinomas may benefit from radiotherapy before surgery. Depending on the postoperative histology results, other patients may need chemotherapy after surgery.

Surgery

The extent of surgical resection is based on the blood supply to the colon and rectum. Depending on site of the tumour, the surgical options are:

- Caecum, ascending colon, hepatic flexure – right hemicolectomy
- Transverse colon – extended right hemicolectomy
- Splenic flexure, descending colon – left hemicolectomy
- Sigmoid colon – high anterior resection
- Upper rectum – anterior resection
- Lower rectum – abdominoperineal resection

Local excision with transanal microsurgery is an option for small lower rectal cancers.

In the surgical resection of colonic lesions, the tumour is excised with a 5 cm proximal clearance and 2 cm distal clearance (**Figure 6.12**). For rectal lesions, a 1 cm distal clearance is adequate. The radial margin should if

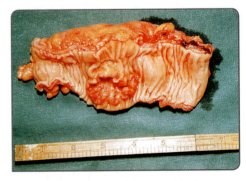

Figure 6.12 Carcinoma of the sigmoid colon.

possible be free of tumour. Lymph nodes are resected up to the origin of the feeding vessel. This should include an 'en bloc' resection of other pelvic organs to which the tumour is adherent.

Laparoscopic surgery is increasingly used for colorectal cancers and is associated with a shorter postoperative recovery and a reduced hospital stay. A defunctioning loop ileostomy is considered if the anastomosis is less than 12 cm from the anal margin.

Prognosis

The simplest staging system for colorectal carcinoma is Duke's classification. This is based on the extent of tumour spread through the bowel wall and the involvement of the lymph nodes (**Figure 6.13**). The 5-year survival is 90%, 70% and 30% for Duke's stages A, B and C, respectively.

> **Neoadjuvant therapy** is chemotherapy or radiotherapy, administered prior to surgery in order to improve the resectability of the tumour. **Adjuvant therapy** is chemotherapy or radiotherapy given after surgery to reduce the risk of recurrence and improve survival.

Chemotherapy

Adjuvant chemotherapy improves the survival of patients with Duke's stage C tumours. It is of no benefit for Duke's stage A tumours, which already have a good prognosis. Its role in Duke's stage B tumours has not been defined.

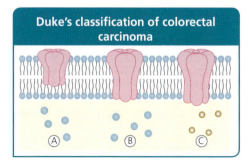

Duke's classification of colorectal carcinoma

Figure 6.13 Duke's classification of colorectal carcinoma. (A) Invasion into muscle. (B) Invasion through muscle. (C) Lymph nodes involved.

Radiotherapy

Local recurrence occurs in 50% of patients with rectal cancer who undergo resection that aims to be curative. The median survival with local recurrence is less than 1 year. Risk factors for local recurrence include:

- The local extent of the tumour
- Nodal involvement
- The presence or absence of a tumour at the circumferential margin

The risk of local recurrence is reduced by radiotherapy. This can be given either preoperatively or postoperatively. Neoadjuvant radiotherapy is given as short course immediately before surgery and has been shown to:

- Reduce local recurrence
- Increase the time to recurrence
- Increase 5-year survival

A combination of chemotherapy and radiotherapy may produce a better outcome.

Anal carcinoma

Anal carcinoma is relatively uncommon but its incidence appears to be increasing. It is more common in homosexual individuals, especially those with genital warts. Patients with genital warts often develop intraepithelial neoplasia, which is a premalignant condition. Human papillomavirus (type 16, 18, 31 or 33) is an important aetiological factor, and approximately 50% of anal tumours contain papillomavirus DNA.

Pathogenesis

Approximately 80% of anal cancers are squamous cell carcinomas. Other rare tumour types include melanoma, lymphoma and adenocarcinoma.

The behaviour of the tumour depends on its anatomical site. Anal margin tumours are usually well-differentiated, keratinising lesions. They are more common in men and have a good prognosis. Anal canal tumours arise above the dentate line. They are usually poorly differentiated, non-keratinising lesions. They are more common in women and have a worse prognosis.

Anal tumours that arise above the dentate line spread to the pelvic lymph nodes. Tumours that arise below the dentate line spread to the inguinal nodes.

Clinical features

The diagnosis of anal carcinoma can be difficult, and about 75% of tumours are initially misdiagnosed as benign lesions.

About 50% of patients present with perianal pain and bleeding. A palpable lesion is identified in only 25% of patients. The anal sphincter is involved in about 70% of patients, which often results in faecal incontinence. Tumours neglected by female patients can cause a rectovaginal fistula. The inguinal lymph nodes are often enlarged, but only 50% of patients with palpable inguinal nodes have metastatic disease.

Investigations

Rectal examination under anaesthetic and biopsy is the most useful 'staging' investigation. Endoanal ultrasound is often impossible due to pain. Abdominal and pelvic CT scanning or MRI are used to assess pelvic spread.

Management

The management of anal carcinoma has changed significantly over the last few years. It was once considered a 'surgical' disease requiring radical abdominoperineal resection. Now most patients are managed with radiotherapy. Radiotherapy is given to both the primary tumour and the inguinal nodes. About 50% of patients respond to treatment, and the overall 5-year survival is 50%. Surgery should be considered for tumours that fail to respond to radiotherapy, large tumours causing gastrointestinal obstruction and small anal margin tumours that do not involve the sphincter.

Perianal conditions

Perianal conditions are common and often painful. They should be easily diagnosed from a complete history and thorough rectal examination.

Anorectal sepsis

Anorectal fistulae occur between the anal or rectal mucosa and the perianal skin. Most anorectal abscesses and fistulae are believe to arise from infections of the anal glands, which lie in the intersphinteric space at the level of the dentate line.

An abscess is a localised collection of pus. A fistula is an abnormal communication between two epithelial surfaces.

Clinical features

An anorectal abscess usually presents as a painful perianal lump. Patients give a history of a previous lump at the same site that often

has discharged spontaneously. Examination may show a fluctuant lump close to the anal margin. Some patients, particularly those with an intersphinteric abscess, present with severe anal pain with no visible signs of an abscess.

An anorectal fistula usually presents with a recurrent purulent perianal discharge. The site of the external opening gives an indication of the site of the internal opening (**Figure 6.14**).

Goodsall's rule states than an external opening situated behind the transverse anal line will open into the anal canal in the midline posteriorly. An anterior opening is usually associated with a radial tract. The rule is not absolute, and the path of the fistula is sometimes complex.

Management

The initial surgery for an anorectal abscess requires only incision and drainage in order

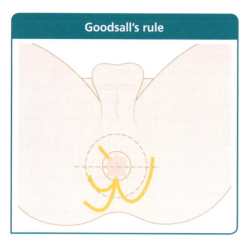

Goodsall's rule

Figure 6.14 Goodsall's rule.

to relieve the sepsis. If there is clinical suspicion of an underlying fistula, this can be further assessed by an outpatient MRI or by a subsequent elective admission for examination under anaesthetic. About 80% of recurrent abscesses are associated with a fistula.

In the opening up of an anorectal fistula, the puborectalis muscle is the key to future continence. However, damage to the other sphincter muscles should also be avoided. A low fistula (an internal opening below the puborectalis) should simply be laid open with a fistulotomy. A high fistula (an internal opening above the puborectalis) requires two-stage surgery, often with the initial placement of a seton followed by its subsequent tightening and removal.

> **A seton is a non-absorbable suture** passed along the fistula tract and tied loosely to encourage drainage. The seton can be sequentially tightened to 'cut through' the tissue and allow healing of the tract.

Haemorrhoids

Haemorrhoids are dilated veins in the lower rectum and anal canal. They affect 50% of the population over the age of 50 years. Dilation of the lower rectal venous plexus appears to be an important aetiological factor.

Clinical features

Haemorrhoids usually present with painless, bright red rectal bleeding, a prolapsing perianal lump or acute pain due to thrombosis. Faecal soiling or pruritus ani also occur.

Haemorrhoids are often classified as internal or external. Internal haemorrhoids arise above the dentate line. The classification of internal haemorrhoids is shown in **Table 6.13**. External haemorrhoids occur below the dentate line and usually present as perianal lumps that occasionally become painful if the tissue becomes thrombosed.

Management

Most patients with haemorrhoids can be managed without surgery.

Medication

All patients should be advised to follow a high-residue diet. Local preparations and creams rarely produce long-term clinical benefit. Outpatient treatment options for first- and second degree internal haemorrhoids include injection with 5% phenol in arachis oil and rubber band ligation. The use of the latter results in better long-term outcome.

Surgery

Haemorrhoidectomy is the treatment of choice for third-degree haemorrhoids. The haemorrhoidal tissue is excised with skin bridges maintained between each wound. Postoperative pain can be reduced with oral metronidazole or the injection of botulinum toxin at the time of surgery. The recently described procedure of stapled haemorrhoidectomy is associated with a reduced operating time, less

Classification of internal haemorrhoids	
Degree	**Clinical features**
First	Bleeding only
Second	Prolapse but reduce spontaneously
Third	Prolapse but can be pushed back
Fourth	Permanently prolapsed

Table 6.13 Classification of internal haemorrhoids

postoperative pain, a shortened hospital stay and a more rapid return to normal activity.

Complications of haemorrhoidectomy include bleeding and anal narrowing.

Anal fissure

An anal fissure is a break in the skin of the anal canal that often results from mucosal ischaemia secondary to muscle spasm of the external anal sphincter. Anal fissures are no longer regarded as a 'tear' in the skin due to the passage of a hard stool. They are associated with increased intra-anal pressure, and treatment aims to reduce the pressure in the anal sphincter.

Clinical features

Anal fissures usually present with pain on defaecation, bright red bleeding and pruritus ani. They are most often seen in patients between 30 and 50 years of age. About 90% lie in the posterior midline; the remaining 10% are in the anterior midline. The fissure is often visible when the buttocks are parted and are seen above a 'sentinel pile' – a small skin tag. Most acute fissures heal spontaneously.

Management

The initial management of anal fissures is usually conservative. Surgery should be considered if the symptoms persist and the fissure fails to heal.

Medication

Stool-bulking agents and topical local anaesthesia produce symptomatic improvement, and about 50% of acute fissures heal with this treatment. The topical use of 0.2% glyceryl trinitrate ointment heals more than 70% of fissures. The most common side effect of glyceryl trinitrate use is headache. A single injection of botulinum toxin can also be used to relax the anal sphincter.

> **Glyceryl trinitrate is a nitric oxide donor that relaxes the internal anal sphincter.** It induces a reversible chemical sphincterotomy and reduces anal resting the pressure by 30–40%.

Surgery

Surgery is the last resort in the management of anal fissures as it is associated with a high risk of faecal incontinence. After surgery, 95% of patients achieve prolonged symptomatic improvement, but 20% have some degree of incontinence (faecal soiling or incontinence of flatus).

The two most common procedures are anal dilatation and internal sphincterotomy. Sphincterotomy is more effective and has a reduced risk of incontinence.

Pilonidal sinus

A pilonidal sinus is a subcutaneous sinus containing hair (**Figure 6.15**). It is lined by granulation tissue and most commonly occurs in the natal cleft between the buttocks. Pilonidal sinuses are occasionally seen in the interdigital clefts on barbers' hands. In all pilonodal sinuses, hair becomes trapped in the sinus resulting in a foreign body reaction that perpetuates the sinus.

Clinical features

Pilonidal sinuses are usually seen in young adults and are rare after the age of 40 years.

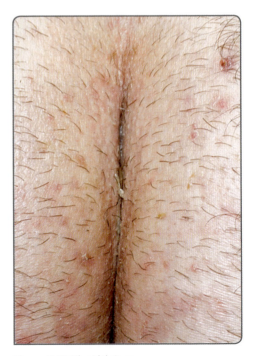

Figure 6.15 Pilonidal sinus.

The male-to-female ratio is 4:1. About 80% of patients present with recurrent pain, and 80% present with a purulent discharge from the natal cleft.

Management

The treatment of choice is surgery. There are three surgical options. The first is excision and leaving the wound open to heal by secondary intention. The second is excision and primary closure. The third is the use of a skin flap to cover the wound (e.g. the Karydakis procedure). Skin flap procedures aim to excise the sinus, flatten the natal cleft and keep the resulting scar away from the midline.

Rectal prolapse

A complete rectal prolapse is a full-thickness prolapse of the rectum through the anus (**Figure 6.16**). It contains two layers of rectal wall with a peritoneal sac between them. It usually occurs in elderly adults. The female-to-male ratio is approximately 6:1. It is invariably associated with weak pelvic and anal musculature. The sigmoid colon and rectum are often floppy and mobile, predisposing to prolapse.

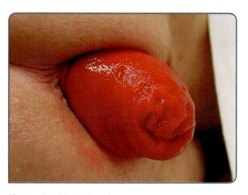

Figure 6.16 Rectal prolapse.

An incomplete rectal prolapse is limited to the rectal mucosa. It occurs in children and adults and is often associated with excessive straining, constipation and haemorrhoids. In children, it is sometimes associated with cystic fibrosis.

Clinical features

Rectal prolapse occurs at the extreme ages of life. A rectal prolapse in a child is usually noted by the parents and must be differentiated from colonic intussusception and a juvenile rectal polyp. In adults, it usually presents with a prolapsing anal mass after defaecation. In both children and adults it may be reduced spontaneously or with gentle manual pressure. Bleeding, mucus discharge or incontinence may be troublesome particularly in adults. Examination usually shows poor anal tone and the prolapse may be visible on straining. The differential diagnosis in an adult is haemorrhoids, a prolapsing rectal tumour and an anal polyp.

Management

Many patients with a complete prolapse are elderly and too frail to undergo surgery. They should be given bulk laxatives and their carers taught how to reduce the prolapse. In children, improvement is often seen with dietary advice and the treatment of constipation.

Surgery

Surgery is rarely required in children. In adults, urgent treatment is required if the prolapse is irreducible or ischaemic. If the patient is fit for surgery, the operation can be performed via a perineal or an abdominal approach. Abdominal procedures can be performed laparoscopically.

Answers to starter questions

1. A hernia is an abnormal protrusion of a tissue or organ from its normal anatomical site. It usually involves a weakness in the retaining structure, a sac and the contents of the hernia. The commonest site for hernias is the abdominal wall and the commonest types of hernia are inguinal and femoral. Inguinal hernias can be either direct or indirect. Direct hernias result from a weakness in the transversalis fascia and present as a direct protrusion through the posterior wall of the inguinal canal. Indirect hernias occur as a result of persistence of the processus vaginalis.

2. An enterocutaneous fistula is an abnormal connection between the gastrointestinal tract and the overlying skin. A simple fistula is a direct communication, whereas a complex fistula is associated with an abscess cavity. Many enterocutaneous fistulae are complex. They are difficult to manage as the underlying cause may not be directly amenable to surgical correction. The patients are at risk of both local and systemic complications. Local complications include infection, skin corrosion and systemic complications such as nutritional and metabolic dysfunction. Treatment often requires parenteral nutritional support over a long period.

3. Colonic diverticulae are outpouchings of the colonic wall. They result from herniation of the gastrointestinal mucosa through the muscular wall at sites where mesenteric vessels penetrate the bowel wall. These sites display potential weakness and increased intraluminal pressure, resulting from a low residue diet and colonic muscular hypertrophy, both of which predispose to their formation.

4. In terms of the clinical presentation of colorectal cancers, the colon can be divided into right and left sides. Small bowel contents entering the right colon are liquid and the stool becomes increasingly solid as it transits the colon. Accordingly, right-sided colon cancers (apart from those occurring close to the ileocaecal calve) can grow to a large size before they cause obstruction. As a result, they often present with anaemia due to occult blood loss and abdominal mass. Left-sided colon cancers may present with rectal bleeding due to more overt blood loss, a change in bowel habit or intestinal obstruction.

5. When colorectal cancers present as an emergency they do so with either intestinal obstruction or colonic perforation. To present with obstruction, they have will have grown to a larger size and present with more advanced disease. There is a higher risk of lymph node involvement or distant metastases. If perforation occurs, the tumour must have penetrated the bowel wall with a higher risk of locally advanced disease or direct contamination of the peritoneal cavity with tumour cells.

6. Perianal sepsis presents as either an acute abscess or a perianal fistula. Both often arise as result of infection of the anal glands found between the internal and external anal sphincter at the level of the dentate line. Depending on the direction of spread of the sepsis, the anal sphincter may be involved and inadvertent surgical damage can result in faecal incontinence. In the surgical management of a perianal abscess, it is most prudent to simply drain the infection and to try and identify a fistula tract once the infection has settled.

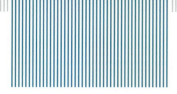
Chapter 7
Hepatobiliary surgery

Introduction	139	Gallstone disease	150
Case 6 Jaundice	140	Pancreatic cancer	152
Core science	141	Liver and biliary cancer	155
History and examination	145	Portal hypertension and ascites	157
Obstructive jaundice	148	Splenic disorders	160

Starter questions

Answers to the following questions are on page 161.

1. Why do pale stools and dark urine occur in obstructive jaundice?
2. How do pathological conditions of the gallbladder relate to their clinical presentation?
3. Why is liver cancer more common in Africa and South East Asia?
4. Why is the prognosis for pancreatic cancer so poor?
5. Why can removal of the spleen lead to sepsis?

Introduction

Hepatobiliary surgery encompasses surgery of the liver, gallbladder and pancreas. It commonly deals with gallstones and their complications.

Hepatobiliary disease often presents with either abdominal pain or jaundice. Its complications result in sepsis and physiological derangement, and are potentially life-threatening. When these occur, they need to be corrected before surgical or interventional radiological procedures are performed.

The incidence of various conditions (e.g. hepatocellular carcinoma) differs markedly in different continents and has to be considered when formulating a differential diagnosis. Hepatobiliary malignancy is rare in the western world.

Case 6 Jaundice

Presentation

A 70-year-old woman, Mrs Marjorie Taylor, presents to her general practitioner with a 2-week history of gradually increasing jaundice. Her urine has become darker and her stools have become pale. She is referred to the jaundice clinic in the local hospital for further investigation and assessment.

Initial interpretation

Painless jaundice, dark stools and pale urine suggest that Mrs Taylor has developed obstructive jaundice. A normal appearance of the stools and urine would suggest a prehepatic or hepatic cause.

History

For the past 2 weeks, Mrs Taylor has noticed that the whites of her eyes have become increasingly yellow. Her skin is also yellow and she has started to itch. She has noticed a gradual worsening of her symptoms. She has no abdominal pain and her general health remains good. Her urine has become brown. Her stools are creamy in colour.

Interpretation of history

Obstructive jaundice results from blockage of the common bile duct and is most commonly due to either gallstones or a pancreatic tumour. This causes a rise in serum conjugated bilirubin and jaundice,

Further history

Mrs Taylor is otherwise well with no significant past medical history. She has no abdominal pain. Her weight has remained steady. She is taking no medication, has never received a blood transfusion and

Jaundice: investigation

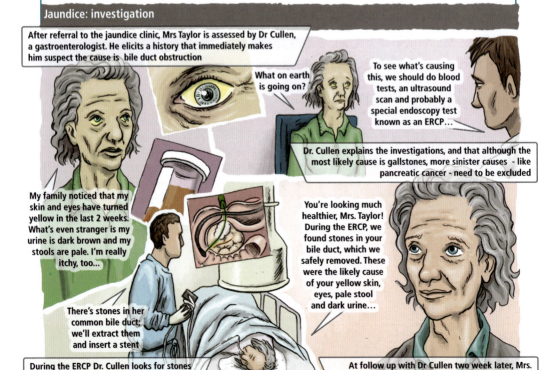

After referral to the jaundice clinic, Mrs Taylor is assessed by Dr Cullen, a gastroenterologist. He elicits a history that immediately makes him suspect the cause is bile duct obstruction

What on earth is going on?

To see what's causing this, we should do blood tests, an ultrasound scan and probably a special endoscopy test known as an ERCP...

Dr. Cullen explains the investigations, and that although the most likely cause is gallstones, more sinister causes - like pancreatic cancer - need to be excluded

My family noticed that my skin and eyes have turned yellow in the last 2 weeks. What's even stranger is my urine is dark brown and my stools are pale. I'm really itchy, too...

You're looking much healthier, Mrs. Taylor! During the ERCP, we found stones in your bile duct, which we safely removed. These were the likely cause of your yellow skin, eyes, pale stool and dark urine...

There's stones in her common bile duct; we'll extract them and insert a stent

During the ERCP Dr. Cullen looks for stones or stricture in the common bile duct and is prepared to insert a stent, if required

At follow up with Dr Cullen two week later, Mrs. Taylor is feeling back to normal and is glad to hear no sinister cause of her symptoms was found

Case 6 *continued*

has not recently travelled abroad. Her alcohol intake is minimal and she has had no previous abdominal surgery.

Examination

On examination, Mrs Taylor appears comfortable and is obviously jaundiced. The abdominal examination is normal with no masses or tenderness. There is no hepatomegaly and the gallbladder is not palpable. There are no signs of chronic liver disease such as clubbing, ascites or spider naevi.

Interpretation of findings

In a women of this age, the differential diagnosis of painless obstructive jaundice is either common bile duct stones or a pancreatic carcinoma obstructing the common bile duct.

Investigations

In the jaundice clinic, blood samples are taken to carry out liver function tests. A raised bilirubin confirms the clinical impression of jaundice. The serum alkaline phosphatase is raised and the liver transaminases (alanine transaminase and aspartate transaminase) are normal. This suggests an obstructive jaundice. Clotting factor and urea and electrolyte levels are normal. An abdominal ultrasound shows multiple stones within the gallbladder (**Figure 7.1**) and the common bile duct is dilated to 20 mm. No obvious stones are seen within the common bile

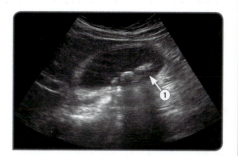

Figure 7.1 Ultrasound showing gall stones ① within the gallbladder.

duct. The pancreas is not clearly visualised due to overlying bowel gas.

Diagnosis

Mrs Taylor probably has obstructive jaundice and, in view of her excellent health, this is most likely to be due to gallstones within the common bile duct. She is admitted the following week for endoscopic retrograde pancreatography (ERCP), which is performed under sedation as both a diagnostic and a therapeutic investigation. This shows three small stone within the distal common bile duct.

A sphincterotomy (incision of the sphincter of Oddi) is performed and a balloon catheter is passed into the bile duct. This allows the stones to be extracted. A stent is placed in the bile duct. Mrs Taylor makes an uncomplicated recovery from the procedure and her jaundice improves over the next 2 days. She is then readmitted 2 weeks later for a laparoscopic cholecystectomy, from which she makes an uncomplicated recovery.

Core science

Anatomy

The hepatobiliary tree consists of the liver, hepatic and common bile ducts, gallbladder and pancreas.

Liver

The liver (**Figure 7.2**) is the largest organ in the body. It lies in the right hypochondrium and extends into the epigastrium. It is related to

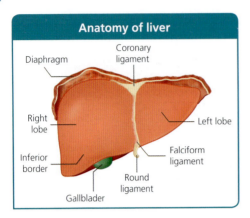

Anatomy of liver

Diaphragm

Coronary ligament

Right lobe

Left lobe

Inferior border

Falciform ligament

Round ligament

Gallbladder

Figure 7.2 Gross anatomy of the liver.

the abdominal section of the oesophagus, the stomach, the duodenum, the hepatic flexure of the colon and the right kidney and adrenal gland.

Lobes of the liver

Anatomically, the falciform ligament divides the liver into the right and left hepatic lobes. The right lobe is further divided into the quadrate and caudate lobes, although these are both functionally part of the left lobe. The liver is surrounded by a strong fibrous capsule.

> **Functionally, the liver is divided into eight segments with defined blood supplies and biliary drainage.** When planning liver resections for malignant disease, it is more important to take into account the functional anatomy than the lobar anatomy.

Porta hepatis

The porta hepatis is on the posterior–inferior surface of the liver and contains the:

- Right and left hepatic ducts
- Right and left branches of the hepatic artery
- Portal vein
- Hepatic lymph nodes

Blood supply

The liver's blood supply is from the hepatic artery and portal vein, and it drains via three hepatic veins into the vena cava.

Ligaments

The falciform ligament, which ascends from the umbilicus, contains the ligamentum teres, which is the remains of the umbilical vein. The falciform ligament splits into two on the surface of the liver. The right-hand portion forms the upper layer of the coronary ligament, whereas the left side forms the upper layer of left triangular ligament. The extreme edge of the coronary ligament forms the right triangular ligament. The coronary and triangular ligaments connect the liver to the inferior surface of the diaphragm. An area of the superior surface of the liver that is devoid of peritoneum is known as the bare area.

Extrahepatic biliary apparatus

The extrahepatic biliary apparatus (**Figure 7.3**) is made up of the:

- Right and left hepatic ducts
- Common hepatic duct
- Common bile duct
- Gallbladder
- Cystic duct

The right and left hepatic ducts leave the right and left lobes of the liver in the porta hepatis and join to form the common hepatic duct. This descends in the free edge of the lesser omentum and is joined by cystic duct to form the common bile duct. This in turn passes behind the first part of duodenum and across the posterior surface of the pancreas. It drains into the second part of the duodenum at the ampulla of Vater. The terminal part of the common bile duct is surrounded by smooth muscle and is known as the sphincter of Oddi.

Gallbladder

The gallbladder, which lies on the visceral surface of the liver, comprises the fundus, body and neck. The neck is continuous with cystic duct. The gallbladder is closely related to the anterior abdominal wall, the visceral surface of the liver, the transverse colon and the first and second parts of the duodenum. It

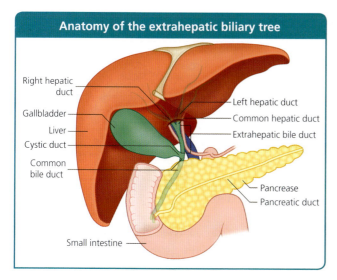

Figure 7.3 Anatomy of the extrahepatic biliary tree.

receives blood via the cystic artery, a branch of the right hepatic artery, and drains directly into the portal vein.

> **The fundus of the gallbladder** projects beyond the inferior margin of the liver and comes into contact with the abdominal wall at the tip of the 9th costal cartilage. This is the point of maximal tenderness in patients with acute cholecystitis.

Pancreas

The pancreas lies retroperitoneally and is both an endocrine and an exocrine gland. It is made up of the head, neck, body and tail. The head lies within the curve of the duodenum. The uncinate process projects from the head, and the superior mesenteric artery and vein separate the head from the body. The tail, along with the splenic artery and vein, extends into the lienorenal ligament.

The pancreas is closely related to the following (**Figure 7.4**):

- The transverse mesocolon and stomach anteriorly
- The inferior vena cava, aorta, portal vein, common bile duct and left kidney posteriorly
- The first part of duodenum and splenic artery superiorly

Pancreatic ducts

There are two pancreatic ducts – the main

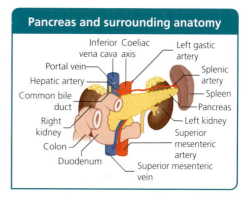

Figure 7.4 Anatomical relations of the pancreas.

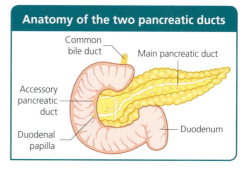

Figure 7.5 Anatomy of the two pancreatic ducts.

duct and the accessory duct (**Figure 7.5**). The main pancreatic duct is also known as the duct of Wirsung. It begins in the tail and, together with the common bile duct, drains into the second part of the duodenum. The accessory duct, or duct of Santorini, begins in the head of the pancreas. It usually drains into the main duct but occasionally opens separately into the duodenum.

Blood supply

The pancreas is supplied by the superior and inferior pancreaticoduodenal arteries. The superior pancreaticoduodenal artery is an indirect branch of the hepatic artery, whereas the inferior pancreaticoduodenal artery arises from the superior mesenteric artery. The splenic artery, which supplies the body and tail, branches directly off the coeliac trunk. The veins correspond to the arteries and drain into the portal system.

Pancreatic cell types

About 80% of the pancreas is composed of acinar cells, which form the exocrine portion of the gland. The endocrine tissue is contained in the islets of Langerhans dispersed within the gland. The islets consist of type A (20%), B (70%) and D (10%) cells, which produce glucagon, insulin and somatostatin, respectively.

The spleen

The normal spleen weighs about 150 g. It lies within the anterior leaf of the dorsal mesogastrium parallel to the 9th to 11th ribs. It is closely related to the tail of pancreas, the greater curvature of stomach, the left kidney, the lienorenal ligament and the greater omentum. The blood supply is from splenic artery and short gastric arteries. The splenic artery divides within the hilum to form four or five end-arteries.

Physiology

Approximately 75% of the blood entering the liver is venous blood from the portal vein; the rest is arterial blood from the hepatic artery. The terminal branches of the hepatic portal vein and hepatic artery enter the hepatic sinusoids (**Figure 7.6**). The sinusoids are distensible vascular channels lined with endothelial cells and bounded circumferentially by hepatocytes (liver cells). As the blood flows through the sinusoids, plasma is filtered into the space between the endothelium and the hepatocytes. The blood leaving

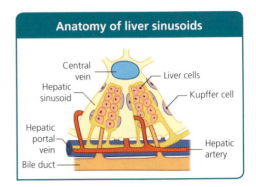

Figure 7.6 Anatomy of the liver sinusoids.

the sinusoids empties into the central vein of each lobule. These central veins join to form the hepatic veins, which leave the liver and drain into the inferior vena cava.

The intrahepatic biliary apparatus

The biliary system is a series of ducts conveying bile from the liver into the lumen of the small intestine. The hepatocytes are arranged in 'plates' with their apical surfaces surrounding the hepatic sinusoids (Figure 7.6). The basal surfaces of adjoining hepatocytes join to enclose dilated intercellular spaces called bile canaliculi, into which the hepatocytes secrete bile. The bile then flows in the canaliculi in parallel to the sinusoids but in the opposite direction to the blood flow. At the ends of the canaliculi, the bile enters into the bile ducts, which are lined by epithelial cells. The bile ducts are in close proximity to the terminal branches of the portal vein and hepatic artery, and with them form a portal triad.

Bile

Bile is a fluid containing water, electrolytes, bile acids, cholesterol, phospholipids and bilirubin. Adults produce approximately 500 mL of bile each day. Bile acids are formed from cholesterol in the hepatocytes. Cholesterol is converted into bile acids (cholic and chenodeoxycholic acids), which are then conjugated to amino acids (glycine or taurine) and actively secreted into the canaliculi. Bile acids are important for the digestion and absorption of fats and fat-soluble vitamins from the small intestine.

Waste products

Waste products, including bilirubin, are secreted into the bile for removal from the body. Bilirubin is a tetrapyrrole and is a normal product of haem catabolism. Unconjugated bilirubin is formed in the reticuloendothelial system of the spleen. It is not water soluble so is transported to the liver bound to albumin. In the liver it is conjugated with glucuronic acid, rendering it water soluble and allowing its excretion in bile.

The spleen

The spleen is an important component of the lymphoreticular system, which is involved in regulating immunity. It is a site of haemopoesis in the fetus and in patients with bone marrow pathology. It also has an important role in the maturation and destruction of red blood cells. In addition, it is a component of both the humoral and cell-mediated immune systems. Antigens are trapped in the spleen and IgM is produced in the germinal centres. The spleen also produces molecules (opsonins) that facilitate the phagocytosis of encapsulated bacteria.

History and examination

Patients with hepatobiliary disease often present with jaundice, with or without abdominal pain. They also present with symptoms related to the complications of liver disease, such as ascites or bleeding disorders. Common symptoms and signs of hepatobiliary disease are shown in **Table 7.1**.

History

Jaundice is yellow discoloration of the sclerae and skin due to the deposition of bilirubin within the tissues. It results from hyperbilirubinaemia and is classified according to where in the physiological metabolic pathway the pathology occurs. The three categories (**Table 7.2**) are:

- Pre-hepatic – pathology occurring before the liver
- Hepatic – pathology occurring within the liver
- Post-hepatic – due to obstruction of the biliary tree

In assessing a patient with jaundice, the history seeks to define the underlying cause. The rate of onset and progression of the symptoms may give a clue to the likely aetiology. Deeply jaundiced patients often itch due to the deposition of bilirubin in the skin. Those with a post-hepatic cause may have pale stools and dark urine. Other features that should be obtained from the history include drug ingestion, blood transfusion, foreign travel, family history, alcohol intake and potential contact with infectious diseases. The presence or absence of abdominal pain may also give an indication of the underlying cause.

Hepatobiliary disease	
Symptoms	Signs
Jaundice	Jaundice
Epigastric and right upper quadrant pain	Abdominal mass
	Abdominal tenderness
Pale stools and dark urine	Hepatosplenomegaly
Itch	Ascites

Table 7.1 Common symptoms and signs of hepatobiliary disease

Classification of jaundice		
Pre-hepatic	Hepatic	Post-hepatic
Haemolytic disorders	Alcoholic liver disease	Common bile duct stones
Congenital hyperbilirubinaemia	Viral hepatitis	Pancreatic carcinoma
	Drug-induced hepatitis	Cholangiocarcinoma
	Metastatic disease	Biliary strictures
		Mirizzi's syndrome

Table 7.2 Classification of jaundice

Examination

The examination of a patient with hepatobiliary disease starts with a general examination for systemic signs, followed by an abdominal examination to identify the underplaying pathology.

General examination

The general examination of patients with hepatobiliary disease may show jaundice or other stigmata of liver disease such as clubbing, palmar erythema, spider naevi and gynaecomastia.

Abdominal examination

Palpation of the liver for size and surface characteristics should be part of every abdominal examination (**Figure 7.7**). A two-handed technique is used. With the left hand in the right renal angle, the right hand should is aligned parallel to the right costal margin, initially in the right iliac fossa. The patient is asked to breathe slowly in and out. With each expiration, the right hand is advanced towards the costal margin, and pressure is applied to potentially palpate the edge of the liver as it descends during the next inspiration.

If the liver is palpable, the surface is assessed for tenderness, firmness and irregularity. A measurement is made of how far the

liver descends beyond the costal margin in the mid-clavicular line. Percussion of the liver (see page 30) may also give an estimate of its size.

The gallbladder may also occasionally be palpable below the costal margin and may be tender or non-tender, with or without the presence of jaundice (**Table 7.3**).

> To test for Murphy's sign, place a hand on the patient's gallbladder and ask them to breathe in deeply. If the gallbladder is tender, the patient catches their breath on inspiration.

Palpation for the spleen is very similar to that for the liver (**Figure 7.8**). The diseased spleen enlarges medially and inferiorly. A two-handed technique is used, with the left hand in the left renal angle and the right parallel to the left costal margin.

Causes of gallbladder enlargement	
With jaundice	Without jaundice
Carcinoma of the head of the pancreas	Acute cholecystitis
	Carcinoma of the gallbladder
Carcinoma of the ampulla of Vater	Mucocele of the gallbladder
	Empyema of the gallbladder

Table 7.3 Causes of gallbladder enlargement

Palpation of the liver

Figure 7.7 Palpation of the liver.

Palpation of the spleen

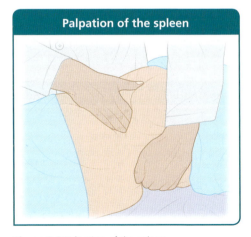

Figure 7.8 Palpation of the spleen.

Ascites

Ascites is free fluid within the abdomen. It results from a range of conditions but large volumes lead to abdominal distension irrespective of the underlying aetiology. Ascites has two diagnostic physical features: shifting dullness and a fluid thrill (see page 30).

Shifting dullness is dullness to percussion that occurs in the flanks and moves when the patient changes position, such as rolling onto their side.

A fluid thrill is elicited by tapping one side of abdomen and feeling the vibration when it reaches the other side. The patient or an assistant places the edge of their hand in the midline of the abdomen to prevent the percussion wave being transmitted through the abdominal wall.

Investigation

Liver function tests

Liver function tests are a series of biochemical assays (**Table 7.4**) used in combination to assess the function of the liver. They are used to detect the presence of liver damage and to distinguish between different liver disorders. They are also used to assess changes in the patient's clinical condition.

> **Interpreting liver function tests in combination gives a more accurate picture of liver function than relying on individual test results in isolation.**

Abdominal ultrasound

Abdominal ultrasound is used to image the liver, spleen, kidneys, pancreas and aorta. It is also used to assess the structure of the gallbladder, the thickness of the gallbladder wall and the presence of gallstones. The diameter of the common bile duct is also measured. Ultrasound is mainly used in the assessment of patients with abdominal pain, jaundice and pancreatitis.

Endoscopic retrograde cholangiopancreatography

ERCP combines endoscopy and fluoroscopy to assess the biliary and pancreatic duct systems.

Liver function tests		
Liver function test	Significance	Normal range
Albumin	Marker of hepatic protein synthesis	35–50 g/L
Total protein	Marker of hepatic protein synthesis	60–85 g/L
Prothrombin time	Hepatic protein synthesis (clotting factors I, II, V, VII and X)	0.9–1.2 s
Alanine transaminase)	Cytoplasmic, mitochondrial and serum enzymes Blood level increases with hepatocyte damage The most specific marker of hepatocyte damage	3–35 IU/L
Aspartate transaminase	Cytoplasmic, mitochondrial and serum enzymes Found in liver, kidneys, heart, skeletal muscle, red blood cells and brain A marker of hepatocyte damage	3–35 IU/L
Alkaline phosphatase	Systemic hydrolase enzyme in the liver, bile duct, kidney, bone and placenta Marker of bile duct blockage and inflammation	20–140 IU/L
Total bilirubin	Marker of haemoglobin catabolism and bilirubin liver conjugation	3–17 µmol/L
Conjugated bilirubin	Marker of liver bilirubin conjugation	1.5–6.0 µmol/L
Gamma-glutamyl transferase	Hepatocyte and biliary epithelium enzyme Marker of hepatobiliary damage and a sensitive indicator of biliary outflow obstruction	Men 11–50 IU/L Women 7–32 IU/L

Table 7.4 Liver function testshepatobiliary disease

The stomach and duodenum are visualised through a side-viewing endoscope. The ampulla of Vater is identified and cannulated, and radiological contrast is injected into the biliary and pancreatic ducts. Therapeutic interventions can be performed at the same time, such as:

- Endoscopic sphincterotomy – division of the sphincter of Oddi
- Stone extraction
- Insertion of a biliary stent

The principle indications for ERCP are the assessment and management of obstructive jaundice, suspected common bile duct stones and pancreatic and biliary cancers.

The major risks of ERCP are bleeding and pancreatitis. The latter occurs after about 2% of all procedures.

Magnetic resonance cholangiopancreatography

Magnetic resonance cholangiopancreatography (MRCP) is the use of MRI to image the biliary and pancreatic ducts. Unlike ERCP, it is a non-invasive technique with few risks. Unfortunately, it does not allow therapeutic procedures to be performed. Many patients with an abnormality detected on MRCP will need to proceed to ERCP.

Obstructive jaundice

If there is obstruction of the extrahepatic biliary tract, the serum levels of conjugated bilirubin increase, resulting in its accumulation in the tissues and its excretion in the urine. Obstructive jaundice then follows.

Epidemiology

Biliary obstruction occurs in about 5 per 1000 patients per year.

Aetiology

Obstructive jaundice results from both benign and malignant processes (**Table 7.5**), with the most common cause being gallstones.

Causes of obstructive jaundice		
Common	**Infrequent**	**Rare**
Common bile duct stones	Ampullary carcinoma	Benign strictures
Carcinoma of the pancreas	Pancreatitis	Recurrent cholangitis
Malignant nodes in porta hepatis	Liver secondaries	Mirizzi's syndrome
		Sclerosing cholangitis
		Cholangiocarcinoma
		Biliary atresia
		Choledochal cysts

Table 7.5 Causes of obstructive jaundice

Clinical features

The accumulation of bilirubin in the skin and sclera produces jaundice. Patients also often complain of itch and notice pale stools and dark urine. Other clinical features depend on the underlying cause and include fever, abdominal pain and weight loss. The duration and clinical course are variable and are further influenced by the development of complications. A deranged production of clotting factors results in a bleeding tendency.

Diagnostic approach

The assessment of any patient with jaundice requires an initial confirmation that the patient is jaundiced. Further investigation is used to differentiate pre-hepatic, hepatic and post-hepatic causes, leading to identification of the underlying cause (**Figure 7.9**).

Investigations

Investigation of a jaundiced patient allows the differentiation of pre-hepatic, hepatic and post-hepatic causes in about 90% cases. In obstructive jaundice, the levels of serum and urine conjugated bilirubin are increased and liver function tests are deranged. The increase

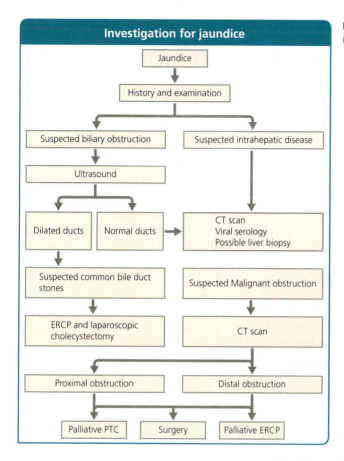

Figure 7.9 Algorithm for the investigation of jaundice.

in serum alkaline phosphatase is relatively more than that of the aspartate aminotransferase and alanine aminotransferase. The converse is seen in patients with hepatocellular causes of jaundice (**Table 7.6**). The serum albumin level may be reduced and clotting studies deranged.

The normal common bile duct (CBD) is less than 8 mm in diameter. The diameter increases with age and after previous biliary surgery. It also increases in patients with bile duct obstruction. Transabdominal ultrasound has a high sensitivity and specificity for detecting dilatation of the CBD, and may also allow identification of the underlying cause (e.g. a stone in the CBD, pancreatic carcinoma).

Abdominal CT or MRCP scanning is useful in obese individuals or if there is excessive bowel gas. Both imaging modalities are better at imaging the lower end of the common bile duct and the pancreas. In those with obstructive jaundice due to a pancreatic tumour, it allows

Differential diagnosis of jaundice			
	Pre-hepatic	Hepatic	Post-hepatic
Conjugated bilirubin	Absent	Increased	Increased
Aspartate aminotransferase and alanine aminotransferase	Normal	Increased	Normal
Alkaline phosphatase	Normal	Normal	Increased
Urine bilirubin	Absent	Present	Present
Urine urobilinogen	Present	Present	Absent

Table 7.6 Differential diagnosis of jaundice

staging and the assessment of operability. ERCP allows biopsies or brush cytology specimens to be taken, stone extraction to occur or the insertion of a biliary stent (**Figure 7.10**).

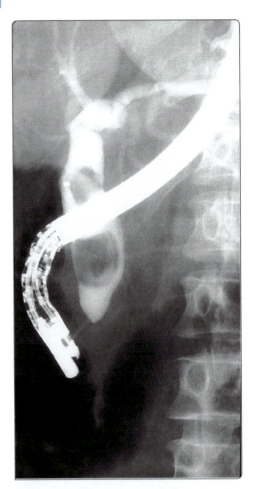

Figure 7.10 Endoscopic retrograde cholangiopancreatography showing stones in the common bile duct.

Management

The management of obstructive jaundice involves the correction of any complications, decompression of the biliary tree and treatment of the underlying cause. Broad-spectrum antibiotic prophylaxis should be given. Parenteral vitamin K and fresh frozen plasma can be administered to correct the clotting disorder. Fluid expansion will reduce the risk of the hepatorenal syndrome.

> **Hepatorenal syndrome is renal failure after intervention in a patient with obstructive jaundice** but its pathophysiology is poorly understood. It is caused by Gram-negative endotoxin absorption from the gut.

Gallstone disease

Gallstones are small stones composed of a combination of cholesterol and bile salts. They are one of the most common causes of morbidity in the developed world and have a varied clinical presentation.

Epidemiology

Gallstones are found in about 12% and 24% of adult men and women, respectively. The prevalence of gallstones increases with age. Only about 20% of gallstones ever become symptomatic. About 10% of patients with stones in their gallbladder will also have stones in their common bile duct.

Aetiology

There are three types of gallstone:

- Cholesterol stones (15%)
- Mixed stones (80%)
- Pigment stones (5%)

Cholesterol stones are caused by a change in the solubility of the bile constituents. Bile acids act as a detergent that keeps the cholesterol in

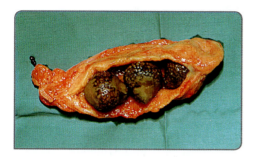

Figure 7.11 Multiple pigment stones in the gallbladder.

solution. However, if the bile becomes supersaturated with cholesterol, microcrystals form, predisposing to stone formation. Biliary infection, bile stasis and changes in gallbladder function are also contributory factors. Mixed stones are a variant of cholesterol stones. Pigment stones are made of bilirubin and calcium salts and occur in haemolytic conditions (**Figure 7.11**).

Biliary colic and acute cholecystitis

Biliary colic arises as a result of intermittent obstruction of the cystic duct due to the presence of a gallstone within Hartmann's pouch. Acute cholecystitis results from persistent obstruction of the cystic duct. Increased pressure and dilatation of the gallbladder results in an acute inflammatory response. Secondary bacterial infections occur in about 20% of cases, most commonly involving *Escherichia coli, Klebsiella* and *Streptococcus faecalis.*

Clinical features

Biliary colic typically presents with intermittent right upper quadrant abdominal pain precipitated by food. The pain radiates to the back and scapula and usually resolves spontaneously after 30 minutes to a few hours. The systemic upset is mild and the abdominal signs are usually minimal.

Acute cholecystitis presents with constant right upper quadrant abdominal pain of longer duration. This is often associated with fever, tachycardia and localised tenderness in the right upper quadrant. Murphy's sign – guarding in right upper quadrant on deep inspiration – may be present. Jaundice is uncommon in uncomplicated acute cholecystitis.

Complications of acute cholecystitis include:

- Gangrenous cholecystitis
- Perforation of the gallbladder
- Cholecystoenteric fistula (a communication between the gallbladder and duodenum)
- Gallstone ileus (small bowel obstruction due to a stone within the lumen)

Diagnostic approach

The various clinical presentations of gallstones can often be differentiated by an accurate history and through clinical examination. Investigations should then be selected to confirm the diagnosis, monitor the clinical course and plan appropriate treatment.

Investigations

Liver function tests are often normal in both biliary colic and acute cholecystitis. In acute cholecystitis, the white cell count is usually raised.

Abdominal ultrasound is the initial radiological investigation of choice. In patients with biliary colic, stones are usually seen within a normal gallbladder. In acute cholecystitis, the diagnostic features include the presence of gallstones in a distended, thickwalled gallbladder. Fluid may be noticed around the gallbladder. The CBD should also be visualised, its diameter assessed and the possibly of stones within the CBD considered. A dilated common bile duct and deranged liver function tests indicate the need for further assessment for the presence of biliary obstruction.

Management

The initial management of biliary colic or acute cholecystitis invariably involves symptom control with analgesia and/or antibiotics. A large proportion of patients will proceed to surgery.

Conservative management

The initial management of acute cholecystitis is with intravenous fluids and opiate analgesia. Intravenous antibiotics should be given to prevent secondary infection. Overall, about 80% of patients improve with conservative treatment.

Surgery

Laparoscopic cholecystectomy should be considered for fit patients. The timing of the surgery is, however, controversial. Evidence suggests that it is safe to carry out early surgery, i.e. less than 72 hours after the onset of symptoms.

Empyema of the gallbladder

If acute cholecystitis fails to resolve, an empyema of the gallbladder can form in which the gallbladder becomes grossly distended with pus. Patients present with features of severe sepsis and have a tender palpable gallbladder. Management is with intravenous antibiotics, urgent decompression using a percutaneous drain or an emergency cholecystectomy.

Mucocele of the gallbladder

A mucocele of the gallbladder refers to gross distension of the gallbladder with mucus; it results from prolonged obstruction of the cystic duct. Patients present with right upper quadrant abdominal pain, and abdominal examination will show a mass in the right hypochondrium. The diagnosis is confirmed by abdominal ultrasound, and treatment is by laparoscopic cholecystectomy.

Mirizzi's syndrome

Mirizzi's syndrome is hepatic or common bile duct obstruction resulting from extrinsic compression from an impacted stone in the cystic duct or Hartmann's pouch. The obstruction is either mechanical or from inflammation around the common hepatic duct. Patients present with right upper quadrant abdominal pain and jaundice.

Acute cholangitis

Acute cholangitis results from infection in an obstructed biliary tree, usually as a result of gallstones. Patients often have features of severe sepsis, and if untreated it can lead to hepatic abscess formation. Management is with intravenous antibiotics and an ERCP to decompress the biliary tree. If the treatment is delayed, the mortality is high.

> **Charcot's triad is the classical clinical presentation of acute cholangitis,** with intermittent right upper quadrant abdominal pain, jaundice and fever.

Gallstone ileus

Gallstone ileus is rare cause of small bowel obstruction. It usually follows an episode of acute cholecystitis when a fistula develops between the gallbladder and small bowel. Large gallstones are able to pass directly into the small intestine and can cause obstruction when they arrest at the ileocaecal valve. A plain abdominal radiograph may show both dilated small bowel and air in the biliary tree. Management consists of removal of the obstructing stone and cholecystectomy.

Pancreatic cancer

Pancreatic tumours can arise from either the exocrine or endocrine areas of the pancreas. The underlying pathology, clinical presentations, management and outcomes are very different for the two types of tumour.

Pancreatic adenocarcinoma

Pancreatic adenocarcinoma arises from the exocrine pancreas and accounts for 95% of all pancreatic tumours.

Epidemiology

Pancreatic adenocarcinoma is the second most common digestive system tumour. Its incidence is increasing in the developed world and it is more common in men. It is uncommon below the age of 50 years: 80% of patients are 60–80 years of age. Most tumours present late and the prognosis, even after potentially curative surgery, is poor. Approximately 75% of patients have metastases at presentation.

Aetiology

The aetiology of pancreatic adenocarcinoma is unknown. Risk factors include family history of pancreatic cancer, alcohol intake and smoking.

Clinical features

About 30% of patients present with obstructive jaundice. Although this is classically described as 'painless jaundice', most patients develop pain at some stage. About 50% of patients present with epigastric pain, which radiates through to the back. Approximately 90% of patients develop anorexia and weight loss. The clinical presentation depends on where in the pancreas the tumour develops. Tumours in the body or tail usually present with pain and weight loss, and those in the head with weight loss and jaundice. The gallbladder is sometimes palpable on abdominal examination.

> **If the gallbladder is palpable in the presence of jaundice, gallstones are unlikely to be present and a pancreatic carcinoma should be suspected.** The gallbladder is palpable because, if gallstones are not present, it is not inflamed and can dilate when biliary obstruction occurs.

Investigation

The diagnosis of pancreatic adenocarcinoma is usually made during the investigation of obstructive jaundice or abdominal pain.

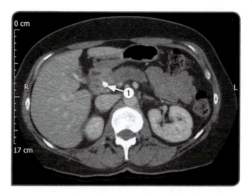

Figure 7.12 Abdominal CT scan showing a pancreatic carcinoma ① with a biliary stent in situ.

Abdominal ultrasound will detected about 80% of pancreatic cancers. It can show the level of biliary obstruction, exclude the presence of gallstones and identify a pancreatic mass. Abdominal CT is more than 95% sensitive in detecting pancreatic tumours and was until recently the most useful of the staging investigations (**Figure 7.12**). MRCP is increasingly used to image the pancreas and liver as both ultrasound and CT often fail to detect small hepatic metastases. Serum CA 19.9, a tumour marker relatively specific for pancreatic cancer, may also be raised.

Management

Pancreatic resection is the only hope of curing the disease. The possibility of surgical resection is assessed by measuring the tumour size (<4 cm), the absence of invasion of the superior mesenteric artery or portal vein and the absence of ascites, nodal, peritoneal or liver metastases.

Surgery

Whipple's procedure is the surgical treatment of choice and involves a pancreaticoduodenal resection. The head of the pancreas and duodenum are excised, and a pancreaticojejunostomy, hepaticojejunostomy and duodenojejunostomy are then formed (**Figure 7.13**). Octreotide is given by some surgeons for 1 week after surgery to reduce pancreatic secretions.

Postoperative complications are common. About 10% of patients develop diabetes and

Postoperative anatomy of Whipple's procedure

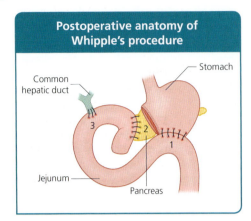

Figure 7.13 Postoperative anatomy following a Whipple's procedure. ① Gastrojejunostomy. ② Pancreaticoduodenostomy. ③ Choledochoduodenostomy.

30% of patients require digestive enzyme supplements to treat malabsorption. Complications of a Whipple's procedure include:

- Delayed gastric emptying
- Gastrointestinal haemorrhage
- Intra-abdominal fluid collections
- Pancreatic fistula

Because pancreatic adenocarcinoma presents late, only 15% of tumours are suitable for surgical resection. Even after apparently curative resection, the prognosis is poor.

Palliative treatment

About 85% of patients with pancreatic cancer are not suitable for curative resection. In these patients palliation of symptoms can be achieved either surgically or endoscopically. Palliative treatment aims to relieve the bile duct obstruction and jaundice, prevent duodenal intestinal obstruction and relieve the pain. Surgical palliation has a higher complication rate at first but produces better symptom control in the long term.

Endoscopic stenting of the common bile duct, performed at ERCP, is possible in over 95% of patients. Complications include bleeding, perforation and pancreatitis. Biliary drainage can also be achieved surgically by choledochojejunostomy or cholecystojejunostomy.

A 'triple bypass' involves a choledochojejunostomy, gastrojejunostomy and enteroenterostomy. This prevents duodenal obstruction and often avoids recurrent jaundice.

Prognosis

The operative mortality after a Whipple's procedure is less than 5% in centres where surgeons are experienced in the technique. However, even in patients suitable for resectional surgery, the 5-year survival is only 30%.

Pancreatic neuroendocrine tumours

Neuroendocrine tumours arise from the islets of Langerhans in the exocrine pancreas, and often produce hormones. In a small number of patients, exocrine tumours of the pancreas are associated with a series of genetic disorders known as multiple endocrine neoplasia (MEN) syndrome (**Table 7.7**). These are inherited in an autosomal dominant fashion.

Insulinomas

Insulinomas are rare, are usually solitary and occur at any age. They are slightly more common in women. Approximately 90% are benign and 10% are associated with MEN type 1 syndrome. They often present with hypoglycaemia that is induced by exercise. To confirm the diagnosis, it is necessary to show hypoglycaemia when symptoms are present. Insulin levels are usually normal or raised. The diagnosis confirmed by CT.

Resection is the only way to cure MEN and has a 10-year survival rate of over 90%. Hepat-

Multiple endocrine neoplasia syndrome	
	Features
Type 1	Parathyroid adenoma, pituitary adenoma, pancreatic islet cell tumour
Type 2A	Phaeochromocytoma, medullary carcinoma of the thyroid, parathyroid hyperplasia
Type 2B	Phaeochromocytoma, medullary carcinoma of the thyroid, Marfanoid features, visceral ganglioneuromas

Table 7.7 Multiple endocrine neoplasia syndrome

ic artery embolisation and chemotherapy are useful adjuncts in metastatic disease.

Gastrinomas

Gastrinomas occur in the duodenum and pancreas. Their overproduction of gastrin results in Zollinger–Ellison syndrome and about 20% of patients with gastrinomas have MEN type 1 disease. Patients present with severe peptic ulcer disease and diarrhoea. The hypersecretion of gastric acid is controlled by either a proton pump inhibitor or surgery. The tumour is removed by distal pancreatectomy or a Whipple's procedure. Metastatic disease is managed with chemotherapy or α-interferon.

Glucagonomas

Glucagonomas are rare and occur as part of MEN type 1 syndrome. Patients present with rashes and mucositis, and the disease has often also metastasised. The diagnosis is confirmed by raised serum glucagon levels. Surgery is beneficial even if the disease has metastasised, and octreotide may help to control the symptoms.

Liver and biliary cancer

Two types of malignant tumour occur within the liver: tumours arising from the liver parenchyma (hepatocellular carcinoma) or from the biliary tree (cholangiocarcinoma).

- Alcohol
- Anabolic steroids
- Primary liver diseases, e.g. primary biliary cirrhosis and haemochromatosis

Hepatocellular carcinoma

Hepatocellular carcinoma (HCC) is a primary malignant tumour of the liver that can present as either a solitary lesion or multiple tumours. As most tumours present late, screening of high-risk patients has been introduced in those countries with a high prevalence.

Epidemiology

HCC is one of the most common malignant tumours in Africa and south-east Asia. Its incidence mirrors the population prevalence of chronic hepatitis B and C. It is more common in men. The peak age at presentation is 40 years in Africa and Asia, and 80 years in Europe. In Europe, secondaries tumours of the liver (e.g. colon, lung and breast) are 30 times more common than HCC.

Aetiology

Important aetiological factors in HCC include:

- Cirrhosis of the liver
- Viral hepatitis, particularly hepatitis B and C
- Mycotoxins such as aflatoxin, produced by *Aspergillus flavus*

Clinical features

The most common clinical features are right hypochondrial pain and the presence of a mass. Malaise, weight loss and low-grade pyrexia often occur, and jaundice is a late feature. Haemobilia (bleeding in the biliary tree) or haemoperitoneum (bleeding into the peritoneum) are often the immediate cause of death.

Diagnostic approach

The possibility of an HCC should be suspected in any patient with cirrhosis who shows evidence of clinical deterioration.

Investigations

HCCs can be imaged by ultrasound or CT scanning (**Figure 7.14**).

Progressive increases in serum alpha-fetoprotein, a normal fetal serum protein produced by the yolk sac and liver, are seen in many patients with HCC. Slightly increased and often fluctuating serum alpha-fetoprotein levels are also seen in hepatitis and cirrhosis. In patients with HCC, serum levels correlate with the size of the tumour. The rate of increase in serum HCC levels correlates with the growth of the

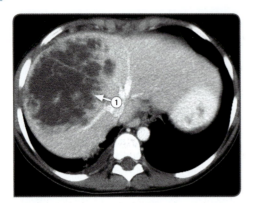

Figure 7.14 CT scan showing hepatocellular carcinoma ①.

tumour. Tumour resection usually causes a fall in serum alpha-fetoprotein that is measured serially to assess the response to treatment.

Management

Only about 25% patients who present with an HCC are suitable for surgery. Most patients are only suitable for palliative treatment.

Surgery

The surgical options are surgical resection of the tumour and liver transplantation. Surgical resection involves either hemi-hepatectomy (i.e. removal of a lobe of the liver) or segmental resection (i.e. removal of the affected segment or segments of the liver). Many tumours cannot be resected as they are too large, involve major vessels or are associated with advanced cirrhosis or metastatic disease. Cirrhosis increases the operative mortality from about 5% to more than 20%. Liver transplantation should be considered for irresectable disease confined to the liver, but metastases occur after transplantation in 30–40% of patients.

Palliative treatment

Palliative interventions include chemotherapy, cryotherapy (i.e. freezing of tumour deposits) and chemoembolisation (i.e. local delivery of chemotherapy into a blood vessel feeding a tumour). The median survival in those with irresectable disease is 6 months.

Prognosis

After surgical resection, the 5-year survival is typically 30–60%. The 5-year recurrence rate

is over 80%, and only a small proportion of patients are cured. After transplantation, the 5-year survival is less than 20%.

Cholangiocarcinoma

Cholangiocarcinoma is a rare biliary tree tumour that accounts for about 1000 deaths a year in the UK. It arises from the epithelium of the biliary tract and about 25% of lesions are intrahepatic. It often presents late with inoperable disease. Risk factors for cholangiocarcinoma include:

- Increasing age
- Primary sclerosing cholangitis
- Choledocholithiasis
- Biliary papillomatosis
- Choledochal cysts
- Liver flukes (*Clonorchis sinensis*)

Clinical features

Most patients present with obstructive jaundice, and pain and fever are uncommon. Late presentation is associated with fatigue, malaise and weight loss.

Investigation

Liver function tests usually show an obstructive jaundice (Table 7.6). Serum CA19.9 a tumour marker for pancreatic cancer, may be raised. The diagnosis is confirmed by CT, MRI or ERCP, the latter also being used for treatment. Specimens can be obtained for cytology or histology and a biliary stent can be inserted.

Management

Cholangiocarcinoma can only be cured by resection of the tumour followed by biliary reconstruction. Liver transplantation is occasionally performed for cholangiocarcinoma but is controversial due to high recurrence rates. Cure rates are low and the median survival is less than 12 months.

Liver metastases

As a result of its rich blood supply from the systemic and portal circulations, the liver is one of the most common site for metastatic spread.

About half of liver metastases arise from tumours of the gastrointestinal tract. Other tumours that spread to the liver include those of lung, breast, ovary and kidney.

> In the developed world, metastatic tumours in the liver are 20 times more common than hepatocellular carcinomas.

Clinical features

Patients presenting with liver metastases may or may not be known to have had a primary tumour. The presence of liver metastases is often a sign of extensive malignant disease, and patients often present with weight loss and cachexia. Symptoms directly related to the liver disease include jaundice and right upper quadrant abdominal pain. Examination often shows tender hepatomegaly, with the liver having an irregular surface.

Investigations

The presence of liver metastases is confirmed by an abdominal ultrasound or CT scan (**Figure 7.15**). If a histological diagnosis is required to guide future treatment, an image-guided core biopsy should be performed.

Management

Solitary or a limited number of liver metastases, particularly those of colorectal origin, may be suitable for liver resection or radiofrequency ablation. However, the vast majority of patients have multiple metastases, and these, especially when they are in both lobes, are only suitable for palliative treatment. Chemotherapy can be delivered systemically or via the hepatic artery.

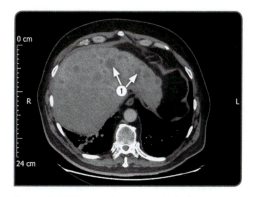

Figure 7.15 CT scan showing multiple liver metastases ①.

Portal hypertension and ascites

Increased pressure in the portal vein is one of the commonest causes of ascites. Investigation of ascites is aimed at assessing the portal circulation or identifying another cause.

Portal hypertension

Portal hypertension is due to raised pressure in the portal vein and its tributaries. It is associated with many conditions, cirrhosis being the most common.

The normal pressure in the portal vein is 5–10 mmHg. Portal hypertension is defined as a portal pressure of more than 12 mmHg. Above this pressure, complications are more likely to occur.

Epidemiology

The prevalence of portal hypertension mirrors that of cirrhosis of the liver. It is more common in men. In Western Europe it is associated with alcohol intake, and in Africa and south-east Asia it is associated with hepatitis B and C.

Aetiology

Portal hypertension is classified as pre-hepatic, intrahepatic or post-hepatic and the causes are shown in **Table 7.8**. Portal hypertension results from an increase in vascular resistance, usually within the liver. The portal venous pressure rises and portal venous flow

Causes of portal hypertension		
Pre-hepatic	Intrahepatic	Post-hepatic
Portal vein thrombosis	Schistosomiasis	Caval abnormality
Splenic vein thrombosis	Primary biliary cirrhosis	Constructive pericarditis
Tropical splenomegaly	Chronic active hepatitis	
Arteriovenous fistula	Sarcoidosis	
	Cirrhosis	
	Budd–Chiari syndrome	
	Veno-occlusive disease	

Table 7.8 Causes of portal hypertension

is reduced. Raised pressure encourages the development of portosystemic anastomoses – vascular communications between the portal and systemic circulations. These develop at several sites:

- Gastro-oesophageal junction
- Lower rectum
- Periumbilical veins
- Retroperitoneal veins (of Retzius)
- Perihepatic veins (of Sappey)

Clinical features

Cirrhosis produces features of hepatocellular disease, portal hypertension, variceal bleeding and ascites. Liver disease presents with right upper quadrant abdominal pain, jaundice, anorexia, nausea and vomiting. When obtaining a history, it is important to evaluate alcohol intake, blood transfusions, previous hepatitis, family history of liver disease and high-risk sexual activity.

Examination may show stigmata of liver disease – jaundice, spider naevi, palmar erythema, clubbing, gynaecomastia, a change in mental state, encephalopathy, bruising and peripheral oedema. Caput Medusae describes the appearance of distended umbilical veins radiating from the umbilicus to join the systemic veins.

About 90% patients with portal hypertension develop oesophageal varices and an upper gastrointestinal bleed occurs in 30% of these patients. The bleeding is often massive and torrential.

Diagnostic approach

The diagnostic approach to a patient with portal hypertension should be to determine the underlying cause, assess the severity of the liver disease and detect the presence of potential complications.

Investigations

To detect and assess the extent of liver disease, liver function tests and clotting studies should be performed. Serum samples should also be taken for hepatitis serology.

Abdominal ultrasound is used to assess both the size and the architecture of the liver and spleen and the possible presence of ascites. Doppler ultrasound will assess flow in the portal vein and to assess the collateral circulation. A direct measurement of portal venous pressure is rarely performed due to the invasive nature of the investigations and the risk of complications. In patients who present with an upper gastrointestinal bleed, an urgent upper gastrointestinal endoscopy should be performed. This can be both a diagnostic and a therapeutic procedure.

Management

The management of patients with portal hypertension requires a close collaboration between gastroenterologists, radiologists and surgeons. Portal pressure can be reduced by the use of drugs or radiologically or surgically created shunts between the portal and systemic circulations. Surgery is often the last resort.

Medical

In patients with known oesophageal varices, the portal pressure and the risk of oesophageal bleeding can be reduced by using beta-blockers. Transjugular intrahepatic portosystemic shunting (TIPSS) is a radiological procedure that involves creating an intrahepatic portosystemic shunt. First, the hepatic vein is cannulated via the internal jugular vein. Next, the intrahepatic portal vein is punctured percutaneously. A guidewire is then passed from the portal vein into the hepatic vein, and a stent is passed along the guidewire. Complications of TIPSS include encephalopathy and liver failure.

Surgery

Surgical portocaval shunts are less common since the introduction of TIPSS and liver transplantation for end-stage liver disease. Shunts are total, partial or selective.

Total shunts are wide and decompress all the portal circulation. After a total shunt, there is no portal venous flow to the liver. Over 90% long-term patency is achieved but 30–40% of patients will develop encephalopathy.

Partial shunts are narrow and only partially decompress the portal circulation; some portal vein flow is maintained. About 20% of partial shunts will either stenose or occlude but only 10% of patients will develop encephalopathy.

Selective shunts decompress part of portal circulation. With these, flow through the portal vein is maintained.

Ascites

Ascites is free fluid within the abdominal cavity. Over 70% of cases are due to liver disease.

Aetiology

Peritoneal fluid is produced by the visceral capillaries and drains via the diaphragmatic lymphatics. The normal peritoneal cavity contains approximately 100 mL of fluid that is a transudate. Ascites is either a transudate (low protein levels) or an exudate (high protein levels). The causes of ascites are shown in **Table 7.9**.

Clinical features

Ascites usually presents with abdominal distension. The patient may give a history of alcohol excess, suggestive of portal hypertension as the underlying cause. There may also be a known history of malignancy, cardiac or renal failure. Examination invariably confirms abdominal distension and shifting dullness, or a fluid thrill may be elicited.

Causes of ascites	
Exudate (high protein content)	Transudate (low protein content)
Malignancy – ovarian, gastric and colorectal carcinomas	Cardiac – right ventricular failure, constrictive pericarditis
Infection – tuberculosis	Liver – cirrhosis, veno-occlusive disease
Renal – nephrotic syndrome, renal failure	Myxoedema
Pancreatitis	Malnutrition

Table 7.9 Causes of ascites

Diagnostic approach

The diagnostic approach to a patient with ascites is to identify the underlying cause and assess the severity of the underlying disease process

Investigation

A diagnostic peritoneal tap with a needle and syringe allows peritoneal fluid to be sent for analysis. This includes protein estimation, cytology, bacteriology and biochemistry. A transudate has a total protein level of less than 30 g/L. Causes of a transudate include cirrhosis and heart failure. An exudate has a total protein of more than 30 g/L. Causes of an exudate include carcinomatosis and infection.

Management

It is hard to treat ascites in cirrhosis effectively. Medical measures include sodium restriction and diuretics. Spironolactone (a potassium-sparing diuretic) is usually the drug of choice. In those with ascites refractory to medical therapy, options include:

- Repeated paracentesis (drainage of ascites) of large volumes of fluid
- Peritoneovenous shunting
- Portocaval shunting
- TIPPS
- Liver transplantation

Splenic disorders

The spleen is an important component of the lymphoreticular system but it is possible to live without it, provided certain precautions are taken to reduce the risk of infection. It enlarges, sometimes massively, in various disease states. Causes of splenomegaly are shown in **Table 7.10**.

> **In splenomegaly, the size of the spleen is variable.** In the UK, massive splenomegaly is usually due to chronic myeloid leukaemia or myelofibrosis.

Surgical removal of the spleen (splenectomy) is necessary in some patients. Indications for splenectomy are:

- Trauma
- Spontaneous rupture
- Hypersplenism
- Neoplasia
- Hydatid cysts
- Splenic abscesses

Splenic trauma

Splenic rupture should be suspected in any patient with abdominal trauma and shock, especially if there are shoulder tip pain and lower rib fractures. Patients require prompt resuscitation. An abdominal CT will confirm the diagnosis and identify the extent of the injury.

Management

Non-operative management of splenic trauma is acceptable if the injury is isolated and the patient is stable. Patients should be closely monitored. Splenectomy is required if the patient remains cardiovascularly unstable despite adequate fluid resuscitation. Repair of the spleen with sutures or tissue adhesives with preservation of the spleen should be considered if possible. This maintains the splenic tissue and prevents postoperative infection.

Overwhelming post-splenectomy infection

Overwhelming post-splenectomy infection (OPSI) is systemic infection due to encapsulated bacteria. It occurs when the spleen is no longer present to phagocytose certain bacteria. About 50% of cases are due to *Streptococcus pneumoniae*, but other organisms, including *Haemophilus influenzae* and *Neisseria meningitidis*, also cause it. OPSI occurs in about 4% of post-splenectomy patients who have not received prophylaxis. The mortality is approximately 50%. The greatest risk of OPSI is in the first 2 years after surgery.

Prevention

Penicillin is the antibiotic prophylaxis of choice in all patients undergoing splenectomy. However, little consensus exists over the duration of prophylaxis. Immunisation against pneumococcus and Haemophilus should also be given. Immunisation should be given 2 weeks prior to a planned splenectomy and given immediately postoperatively following emergency surgery. Antibiotic prophylaxis should be started within days of surgery.

Causes of splenomegaly	
System	Examples
Haematological	Chronic myeloid leukaemia, myelofibrosis, lymphoma, polycythaemia rubra vera, haemolytic anaemia
Metabolic	Glycogen storage disease, connective tissue disease
Infectious	Infectious mononucleosis, malaria
Autoimmune	Amyloidosis, sarcoidosis
Other	Portal hypertension

Table 7.10 Causes of splenomegaly

Answers to starter questions

1. Jaundice is yellow discolouration of the sclerae and the skin due to the deposition of bilirubin within the tissues. It results from hyperbilirubinaemia and can be classified according to where in the physiological metabolic pathway the pathology occurs. In obstructive jaundice the outflow of conjugated bilirubin from the liver is impaired. Conjugated bilirubin is water soluble and is excreted by the kidney, resulting in dark urine. Failure of its excretion into the gastrointestinal tract causes pale stools.

2. Gallstones are common and most remain asymptomatic. The symptomatic presentation of gallstones can be explained in relation to the pathology they cause. Biliary colic occurs when a stone lodges in Hartmann's pouch and the pressure within the gallbladder rises. Acute cholecystitis occurs when the obstructed gallbladder becomes inflamed. Mirizzi syndrome results from obstruction of the hepatic ducts by the inflamed gallbladder. Gallstone ileus occurs when the inflamed gallbladder fistulates in to the small bowel and intestinal obstruction occurs as a result of stone within its lumen.

3. HCC is one of the commonest malignant tumours in Africa and south-east Asia. Important aetiological factors in HCC include cirrhosis, viral hepatitis (particularly Hepatitis B and C, mycotoxins) aflatoxin produced by *Aspergillus flavus*, alcohol and primary liver diseases – primary biliary cirrhosis, haemochromatosis.

4. The commonest site for tumours to arise within the pancreas gland is within its head. They usually present with obstructive jaundice. They can grow to a large size before they cause symptoms. The head of the pancreas is related to a number of major vascular structures. As a result tumours may have metastasised before they present and local invasion may preclude surgical resection.

5. The spleen is an important component of both the humoral and cell mediated immune systems. Antigens are trapped and IgM is produced in germinal centres. It produces opsonins for the phagocytosis of encapsulated bacteria. Overwhelming post splenectomy infection (OPSI) is systemic, and most often due to encapsulated bacteria such as *Streptococcus pneumoniae*. Other organisms that can lead to OPSI include *Haemophilus influenzae* and *Neisseria meningitidis*.

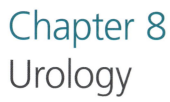

Chapter 8
Urology

Introduction. 163
Case 7 Abdominal pain and
    microscopic haematuria . . . 164
Case 8 Urinary frequency 165
Case 9 Painless haematuria
    and a loin mass 166
Core science 167
History and examination 172

Urinary tract infection 176
Ureteric and bladder calculi 178
Renal cancer 180
Bladder cancer 182
Bladder outflow obstruction 183
Prostate cancer 185
Testicular disorders 186
Penile disorders 189

Starter questions

Answers to the following questions are on page 191.

1. Why is benign prostatic hyperplasia so common?
2. Why is passing a kidney stone so painful?
3. What is the transurethral resection syndrome and why does it occur?
4. Why do renal cell carcinomas sometimes present with systemic features?
5. Why has the prognosis of testicular tumours improved dramatically?
6. Why is testicular torsion a surgical emergency?

Introduction

Urology is a surgical speciality that deals with diseases of the urinary tract – the kidneys, ureter, bladder and urethra – in both men and women, and with diseases of the male reproductive system. Urinary symptoms are a common reason for general practice consul-tations, and a complete history may suggest the underlying cause. With the increasing use of urinalysis in assessing patients in other medical fields, significant urinary pathology is often identified in patients who are other-wise asymptomatic.

Case 7 Abdominal pain and microscopic haematuria

Presentation

A 30-year-old man, Martin Green developed a sudden onset of right loin pain while in his office at work. It was the most severe pain he had ever experienced. His colleagues called an ambulance and he was taken to the local accident and emergency department.

Initial interpretation

A sudden onset of severe loin pain in a young previously fit and healthy man suggests a renal or ureteric problem. Further clinical assessment and investigation should aim to identify the site and cause of the pathology.

History

Martin developed the pain sitting at his desk and can recall the exact moment it began. The intensity of the pain increased and decreased every few seconds. It radiated from his loin down into his groin. He felt cold and clammy and wanted to pass urine. He went to the bathroom but was able to pass only a small volume, which he noticed contained some blood. Over the next few minutes, the pain seemed to move further down into his groin and eventually reduced in intensity.

Interpretation of history

Severe colicky loin-to-groin pain associated with blood in the urine in an otherwise fit and healthy young man is highly suggestive of ureteric colic.

Further history

Martin has no pain on passing urine (dysuria), does not need to pass urine quickly when the sensation occurs (urgency) and is not passing urine more often than normal (frequency). He has no significant past medical history. There is no family history of kidney stones. He has not previously had similar symptoms and says he never wants to experience this again!

Examination

On examination, Martin appears uncomfortable. His temperature and pulse rate are in the normal range. There is tenderness in the right loin, but no other findings from the remainder of the abdominal examination. Examination of the groins shows no evidence of a hernia, and both testicles are normal.

Interpretation of findings

The clinical presentation is highly suggestive of ureteric colic due to the passage of a stone down the ureter. As the stone moves progressively downwards, the symptoms migrate with it . The pain resolves when either migration ceases or the stone is passed into the bladder.

The differential diagnosis of ureteric colic includes appendicitis and pyelonephritis. In women, it is important to consider an ectopic pregnancy and salpingitis. In elderly men, a leaking abdominal aortic aneurysm can present with similar symptoms.

Investigations

In the emergency department the urine appears normal to the naked eye, but dipstick testing (urinalysis) shows blood in it. This is known as microscopic haematuria. There is no evidence of nitrites from the breakdown of urinary nitrates by bacteria, to suggest a urinary tract infection (UTI).

A urine sample is sent to the microbiology laboratory. Microscopy shows the presence of red blood cells. The results of microbiological culture, available 48 hours later, are negative. Blood tests indicate normal values for the full blood count and urea and electrolytes.

A plain kidney–ureter–bladder (KUB) radiograph of the abdomen demonstrates a tiny calcified abnormality in the pelvis along the line of the right ureter. A CT-KUB – a CT scan performed to assess the kidneys, ureters and bladder – identifies a 4 mm stone at the right vesicoureteric junction.

Diagnosis

The investigations have confirmed a small right ureteric calculus at the junction

between the ureter and bladder. Martin remains symptom free and is discharged from hospital 12 hours later.

> **Most ureteric calculi less than 5 mm in diameter will pass spontaneously, so surgical intervention can be avoided.** Initial conservative management is to ensure adequate hydration with oral or intravenous fluids and giving analgesia. Urgent intervention is required only if there is evidence of infection or renal failure. Large stones over 5 mm in diameter that lie in the lower ureter and fail to pass spontaneously can usually be broken up by shock-wave lithotripsy.

Case 8 Urinary frequency

Presentation

A 20-year-old woman, Emma Smith, presents to her general practitioner with a 24-hour history of pain on passing urine and passing urine more frequently than normal.

Initial interpretation

Urinary frequency is a common symptom, particularly in women, and is suggestive of a UTI.

History

Emma describes to her doctor a burning sensation when she passes urine. She is also passing urine more often than normal and has to go quickly when she feels she needs to pass urine. Her urine is foul smelling.

Interpretation of history

Frequency, urgency and dysuria are the key symptoms of a UTI.

Further history

Emma is sexually active and had a similar episode 6 months previously that improved with a course of antibiotics.

Examination

On examination, Emma looks well. Her temperature and pulse rate are normal. Examination of her abdomen reveals some suprapubic tenderness but no loin tenderness.

Interpretation of findings

The findings suggest that Emma has an uncomplicated UTI. If there was a high fever and loin tenderness. This would suggest a diagnosis of pyelonephritis.

Investigations

A midstream specimen of urine (MSU) provided in the general practice surgery reveals cloudy urine. Urinalysis demonstrates the presence of red blood cells,

Case 8 *continued*

white blood cells and nitrites, suggestive of a UTI.

The urine sample is sent to the microbiology laboratory at the local hospital for microscopy, culture and sensitivity analysis. Microscopy confirms the presence of red and white cells in the urine. Urine culture shows a pure growth of *Escherichia coli* that is sensitive to the antibiotic trimethoprim.

Diagnosis

The clinical picture and urinalysis suggest an uncomplicated lower UTI.

Knowing the likely aetiological bacteria, the general practitioner prescribes oral trimethoprim and Emma's symptoms improve with treatment. The appropriateness of treatment is confirmed by microscopy, culture and sensitivity analysis of a repeat urine specimen 1 week later, which shows that the infection has cleared.

Uncomplicated UTIs in women do not require extensive investigation as the incidence of an underlying renal or bladder abnormality is extremely low.

Case 9 Painless haematuria and a loin mass

Presentation

A 75-year-old man, William Blythe, is referred to the urology clinic at his local hospital with a 3-month history of painless haematuria.

Initial interpretation

Painless haematuria at any age is never normal and carries a high risk of underlying urological disease. Urgent referral to a urology clinic for further assessment and investigation is therefore necessary. Common causes of macroscopic painless haematuria include:

- UTI
- Bladder carcinoma
- Benign prostatic hyperplasia
- Ureteric calculi
- Renal cell carcinoma

History

For the past 3 months, William has noticed blood in his urine on most days.

It is not associated with pain, and he has no other urinary symptoms.

Interpretation of history

Haematuria is never normal. In an elderly man, an underlying urological malignancy is the most likely cause.

Further history

William is generally fit and healthy. His only other chronic medical problem is hypertension, for which has been taking medication for 5 years.

Examination

Examination shows William to be healthy. His blood pressure is 140/100 mmHg. Abdominal examination demonstrates a non-tender mass in his right loin. The bladder is not palpable.

Interpretation of findings

Painless haematuria and the presence of a loin mass suggest a renal neoplasm.

Case 9 *continued*

Subsequent investigation aims to confirm the diagnosis.

Investigations

Urinalysis confirms the presence of haematuria, and urine microscopy shows red blood cells in the urine. The haemoglobin level is normal, and renal function as assessed by serum sodium, potassium, urea and creatinine, is normal.

On ultrasound scanning, there is a 6 cm mass in the lower pole of the right kidney. A CT scan confirms the presence of a solid lesion within the right kidney (**Figure 8.1**). The radiological appearances are those of a renal cell carcinoma. There is no evidence of tumour spread to the perinephric fat, renal vein or vena cava. The liver and lungs appear normal with no suggestion of metastatic disease. There are no findings of note in the contralateral kidney.

Diagnosis

The findings suggest a diagnosis of renal cell carcinoma that is confined to the kidney with no evidence of metastatic disease.

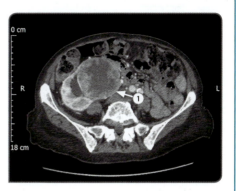

Figure 8.1 Abdominal CT scan showing a right renal cell carcinoma ①.

This is regarded as being operable and William undergoes a laparoscopic nephrectomy without complication. Postoperative histology of the lesion confirms a renal cell carcinoma. No adjuvant treatment is required.

> **In patients being considered for a nephrectomy, it is vital first to prove that the other kidney has normal function** in order to prevent removal of the only functioning kidney.

Core science

Anatomy of the upper renal tract

The upper renal tract comprises the kidney and ureters and extends to the vesicoureteric junction.

The kidneys

The kidneys lie in a retroperitoneal position on the posterior abdominal wall and are largely covered by the costal margins. The right kidney lies slightly lower than the left. The relations of the kidneys are shown in **Table 8.1**.

Each kidney is surrounded by a fibrous capsule (**Figure 8.2**), outside which are the perinephric fat and fascia. The renal hilum is found on the medial border of each kidney and transmits the ureter, renal vein and branches of the renal artery. The arterial supply is from the renal artery, which arises directly from the aorta. The venous drainage is to the renal vein and inferior vena cava.

Structure

The substance, or parenchyma, of the kidney is classified into two major areas: the

Anatomical relations of the kidney

Position	Right kidney	Left kidney
Anterior	Suprarenal gland	Suprarenal gland
	Liver	Spleen
	Second part of duodenum	Stomach
		Pancreas
	Hepatic flexure of colon	Splenic flexure of colon
Posterior	Diaphragm	Diaphragm
	Costodiaphragmatic recess	Costodiaphragmatic recess
	Twelfth rib	Twelfth rib
	Psoas muscle	Psoas muscle

Table 8.1 Anatomical relations of the kidney

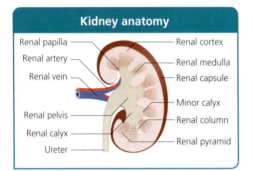

Figure 8.2 Anatomy of the kidney.

renal cortex lies superficially, and the renal medulla lies more deeply (**Figure 8.2**). These are formed into about 15 cone-shaped renal lobes, each containing renal cortex surrounding a portion of medulla called a renal pyramid. Between the renal pyramids are projections of cortex called renal columns.

The nephrons, which are the functional urine-producing structures of the kidney, span both the cortex and the medulla (**Figure 8.3**). The initial region of the nephron that filters the blood is the glomerulus, which is located in the cortex. The glomerulus is a network of capillaries surrounded by Bowman's capsule. This leads into a renal tubule, which passes from the cortex deep into the medullary pyramids. Each renal tubule is made up of a proximal tubule, a loop of Henle and a distal convoluted tubule and collecting duct. Collections of renal tubules that drain into a single collecting duct are known as medullary rays. These lie in the renal cortex.

The ureters

The ureters are also located retroperitoneally. They run downwards over the psoas muscles along the line formed by the tip of the transverse processes of the lumbar vertebrae. The ureters cross the bifurcation of the common iliac artery and continue on the lateral wall of

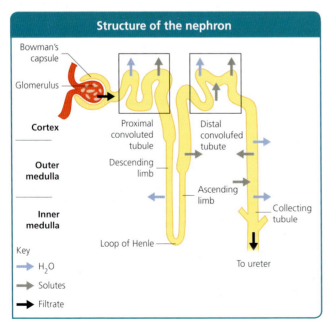

Figure 8.3 Structure of the nephron.

Anatomical relations of the ureter

Position	Right ureter	Left ureter
Anterior	Duodenum	Pelvic colon
	Terminal ileum	Left colic and ileocolic vessels
	Right colic and ileocolic vessels	Left testicular or ovarian vessels
	Right testicular or ovarian vessels	
Posterior	Psoas muscle	Psoas muscle
	Bifurcation of right common iliac artery	Bifurcation of left common iliac artery

Table 8.2 Anatomical relations of the ureter

the pelvis to the region of ischial spine. The anatomical relations of the ureters are shown in **Table 8.2**.

The ureters are lined by transitional epithelium.

> **Three natural constrictions are found along the course of the ureters:** where they join the renal pelvis, cross the brim of the pelvis and enter the bladder. These constrictions are points where ureteric calculi may be held up when they are passed.

Anatomy of the lower renal tract

The lower urinary tract includes the bladder and urethra, along with the prostate gland in men.

The bladder

When empty, the pyramidal urinary bladder is an extraperitoneal structure. Distension of the bladder causes the peritoneum to be stripped off the anterior abdominal wall.

The superior surface of the bladder is covered by the pelvic peritoneum. Anteriorly, it lies behind the pubis. The apex is attached to the umbilicus by the median umbilical ligament (**Figure 8.4**), which represents the remnant of the fetal urachus. The inferolateral surfaces are related to the levator ani and obturator internus muscles. In men, the bladder

Anatomy of the bladder

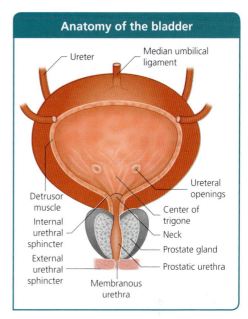

Figure 8.4 Anatomy of the bladder.

neck fuses with the prostate and the base is related to the rectum, vas deferens and seminal vesicles. In women, the posterosuperior surface of the bladder is related to the uterus, and the base is related to the vagina and cervix.

The ureters join the bladder at its upper lateral angles. Inside the bladder, the ureteric orifices are joined by the interureteric ridge. The triangular area outlined by the interureteric ridge and the urethral orifice is known as the trigone. The bladder wall is made of smooth muscle and lined by transitional epithelium.

Sphincters

The bladder has two sphincters. The internal sphincter is made up of smooth muscle and is found at the bladder neck. The external sphincter lies distal to the internal sphincter and is formed of voluntary muscle. The blood supply to the bladder is from the superior and inferior vesical arteries, which are branches of the internal iliac artery. The lymphatic drainage is to the iliac and para-aortic nodes.

Nerve supply

The bladder has both a motor and a sensory nerve supply. The motor supply is autonomic.

The sympathetic supply arises from L1 and L2 and inhibits bladder contraction. The parasympathetic supply arises from S2 to S4 and is the motor supply to the detrusor muscle (the smooth muscle of the bladder that causes urination). The sensory supply of the bladder is parasympathetic.

The prostate

The prostate is a fibromuscular and glandular organ that surrounds the proximal urethra in men (**Figure 8.5**). It has five lobes: the anterior, posterior, middle and two lateral lobes. Above, it is continuous with the base of the bladder. Below, the apex sits on the sphincter urethrae in the deep perineal pouch. Posteriorly, the prostate is separated from the rectum by Denonvillier's fascia. Anteriorly, it is separated from the pubis by extraperitoneal fat. The prostate is surrounded by the prostatic venous plexus.

The ejaculatory ducts, formed by fusion of the vas deferens transmitting sperm from the testes and the seminal vesicles secreting fluid to form semen, enter the upper posterior part of the prostate and open into the urethra. The blood supply of the prostate is from the inferior vesical artery.

The male urethra

The male urethra is about 20 cm long and is divided into three anatomically discrete sections.

The prostatic urethra This is about 4 cm long. It has a longitudinal elevation on its posterior wall that is known as the urethral crest. The prostatic sinus lies along each side of this. In the middle of the urethral crest is an elevation known as the verumontanum. The ejaculatory ducts open on each side of the utricle (a small indentation in the prostatic urethra).

The membranous urethra This is about 2 cm long and is the narrowest part of the urethra. It passes through the external urethral sphincter in the deep perineal pouch.

The spongy urethra This passes through the corpus spongiosum of the penis. The external urethral orifice is the narrowest part of the urethra. As soon as the urethra enters the meatus, it dilates into a terminal fossa.

The testis

The testes (**Figure 8.6**) lie within the scrotum and are surrounded by a capsule, the tunica albuginea. The epididymis can be classified into the head, body and tail.

The testicular tissue is composed of about 250 lobules, which are separated by septae. The lobules consist of one or more seminiferous tubules, which start and end at the rete testis. Efferent ducts then transport the sperm from the rete testis into the epididymis. This extends from the upper pole of the testis to the caudal pole. The vas deferens connects the epididymis to the urethra.

Renal physiology

The primary functions of the kidney are to regulate the volume and chemical composition

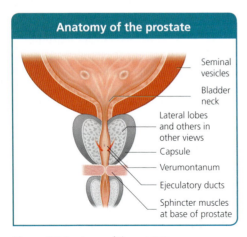

Anatomy of the prostate

- Seminal vesicles
- Bladder neck
- Lateral lobes and others in other views
- Capsule
- Verumontanum
- Ejaculatory ducts
- Sphincter muscles at base of prostate

Figure 8.5 Anatomy of the prostate.

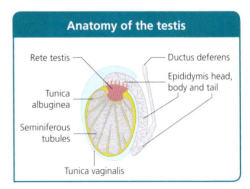

Anatomy of the testis

- Rete testis
- Ductus deferens
- Tunica albuginea
- Epididymis head, body and tail
- Seminiferous tubules
- Tunica vaginalis

Figure 8.6 Anatomy of the testis.

of the blood. Its secondary functions are the metabolism of vitamin D and the production of renin, an enzyme that activates the renin-angiotensin system, and erythropoietin, a glycoprotein hormone that increases erythropoiesis.

The nephron

Each kidney contains about 1 million nephrons, of two types. Cortical nephrons regulate the chemical composition of the urine. Juxtamedullary nephrons concentrate the urine.

The glomerular endothelium is fenestrated (i.e. has holes within it) so solute-rich but protein-free fluid passes from the blood vessels into the Bowman's capsules. The composition of this filtrate is modified as it passes through the renal tubule by resorption into and secretion from the peritubular capillaries. This occurs mainly in the proximal convoluted tubule. The loop of Henle has an important role in water balance.

Blood supply of the nephron

The glomerular capillaries receive blood from the afferent arterioles and then drain into the efferent arterioles. The high capillary pressure in the glomerulus facilitates filtration. The peritubular capillaries receive blood from the efferent arterioles. The resorption that occurs here is assisted by the low capillary pressure.

> Over 99% of the fluid filtered in the glomerulus is resorbed in the peritubular capillaries.

Juxtaglomerular apparatus

The juxtaglomerular apparatus abuts the afferent arteriole and distal convoluted tubule and has a role in regulating the content of the filtrate. At this point, the cells of the distal convoluted tubule are known as the macula densa. These monitor the sodium content of the filtrate. The juxtaglomerular cells are specialised smooth muscle cells in the arteriole that act as baroreceptors and secrete renin.

Control of renal function

Normal renal function is maintained in the nephrons by a control of filtration from the glomerular capillaries and resorption from the nephrons into the peritubular capillaries.

Filtration

About 20% of the blood that enters the glomerulus is filtered. The rate of filtration is known as the glomerular filtration rate and is controlled by intrinsic and extrinsic mechanisms. Intrinsic mechanisms includes myogenic regulation by changes in constriction of the arteriolar smooth muscle, and tubuloglomerular feedback, with changes in response to the sodium concentration in the distal convoluted tubule. Extrinsic mechanisms include sympathetic neural stimulation and the renin–angiotensin system that controls sodium and water resorption.

Resorption

In the proximal convoluted tubules, resorption is primarily driven by sodium. Sodium passively diffuses out of the proximal convoluted tubule and is actively transported into the peritubular capillaries. This movement of sodium has three important effects:

- It creates an osmotic gradient for water resorption
- It creates an electrical gradient for negatively charged ions, such as chloride
- It allows secondary active transport of potassium in the proximal convoluted tubule

Regulation of urine concentration and volume

Maintaining the concentration of the body fluids is integral to homeostasis. Concentration is measured in osmolarity, such that a concentrated solution has a high osmolarity and a dilute solution a low one. If the osmolarity of the blood rises, water reabsorption increases and urinary volume decreases. If blood osmolarity falls, the opposite response occurs.

Antidiuretic hormone

Blood osmolarity is measured by specialised neurones in the hypothalamus that are known as osmoreceptors. These determine how much antidiuretic hormone (ADH) is secreted by the posterior pituitary gland. ADH increases the permeability of the collecting ducts to water, which increases water reabsorption in the collecting duct and decreases urinary volume. When the osmolarity of the blood rises, ADH release is increased. When blood osmolarity falls, ADH release is decreased.

Aldosterone

Aldosterone is produced in the renal cortex. It increases sodium resorption and potassium excretion in the distal convoluted tubule. The release of aldosterone is stimulated by:

- Low plasma sodium levels
- High plasma potassium levels
- Low blood volume and pressure

History and examination

Urinary disease can present with changes in the appearance of the urine, abnormalities of micturition, abdominal pain or systematic symptoms of renal failure, such as weakness and lethargy. The common symptoms and signs of urinary disease are shown in **Table 8.3**.

History

The most common symptoms of urinary disease are haematuria, loin pain, urinary frequency and dysuria.

Haematuria

Haematuria is the passage of blood in the urine. The amount passed can cause minimal discolouration or be what appears to be frank blood. If the blood is coming from the lower urinary tract, it may appear only at the end of micturition. The causes of haematuria are shown in **Table 8.4**.

Haematuria can be painless or associated with variable degrees of pain. Painless haematuria always requires complete investigation as it is often the presenting symptom of tumours of the upper or lower renal tract. Certain drugs (e.g. rifampicin) or vegetables (e.g. beetroot) can discolour the urine.

> In women, it is important to differentiate a possible haematuria from menstrual bleeding.

Loin pain

Pain from the kidney is felt in the loin, in the angle between the 12th rib and the edge of the erector spinae muscle. Depending on the pathology, it can range from a constant dull ache to severe, colicky pain. Pain from the bladder usually occurs in the suprapubic region. Pain from the prostate gland may be felt in the perineum.

Common symptoms and signs of urinary disease	
Symptoms	Signs
Haematuria	Loin tenderness
Loin pain	Loin mass
Urinary frequency, urgency, dysuria	Prostatic enlargement or irregularity
Urinary hesitancy, poor stream, dribbling	Testicular lump or tenderness
Testicular pain or lump	

Table 8.3 Common symptoms and signs of urinary disease

Causes of haematuria	
Site	Pathology
Kidney	Renal calculus, transitional cell carcinoma, renal cell carcinoma, pyelonephritis, trauma
Ureter	Ureteric calculus, transitional cell carcinoma
Bladder	Transitional cell carcinoma, bladder calculus, acute cystitis
Prostate	Prostatitis, urethral trauma

Table 8.4 Causes of haematuriametastasis

Lower urinary tract symptoms	
Filling or irritative	Voiding or obstructive
Frequency	Poor stream
Urgency	Hesitancy
Dysuria	Terminal dribbling
Nocturia	Incomplete emptying
	Incontinence

Table 8.5 Lower urinary tract symptoms

Lower urinary tract symptoms

Lower urinary tract symptoms can be categorised as shown in **Table 8.5**.

Filling or irrative symptoms

Irritative urinary tract symptoms are more common in women:

- Dysuria is pain on passing urine rather than difficulty passing urine
- Frequency is the passage of urine more often than normal, usually in small volumes
- Urgency is the strong desire to pass urine and the urgent need to void

The triad of dysuria, frequency and urgency is highly suggestive of a UTI.

Pneumaturia is a bizarre and rare symptom usually described as the sensation of passing bubbles in the urine. It is almost always caused by a vesicocolic fistula.

Obstructive urinary symptoms

Obstructive urinary tract symptoms are more common in men and are a feature of obstruction of bladder outflow. Hesitancy is difficulty in initiating the urinary stream. This is often followed by a decrease in strength of the urinary flow that finishes with terminal dribbling. It is often associated with a sensation of incomplete emptying of the bladder. Patients may also need to get up from sleep and void several times overnight – nocturia.

If the obstruction is nearly complete, an overflow of urine can occur resulting in incontinence. Acute urinary retention usually presents with severe lower abdominal pain and a complete inability to pass urine. The symptoms can be instantly relieved by the passage of a urethral catheter.

Examination

The examination of the urinary system in both sexes requires an abdominal examination. In men, the scrotum should be assessed and a rectal examination performed.

Abdominal and prostate

Assessment of the kidneys and bladder should form part of every abdominal examination. The normal empty bladder should be impalpable. Enlargement of the bladder, usually as a result of outflow obstruction, results in a smooth lower midline mass extending towards the umbilicus. The abdominal swelling caused by a chronically obstructed bladder is not tender. In contrast, the bladder in acute urinary retention is usually exquisitely tender.

The kidneys should be palpated using a bimanual technique (**Figure 8.7**). The anterior hand is placed lateral to the rectus muscle and immediately over the posterior hand in the renal angle. If the patient is asked to breathe deeply, the lower poles of the kidney descend. When the two hands are firmly pushed together as the patient breathes out, the kidney may be felt to move between them. The lower pole of the normal right kidney is often palpable. The left kidney is usually impalpable. If the

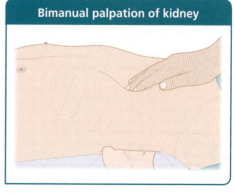

Bimanual palpation of kidney

Figure 8.7 Bimanual palpation of the kidney.

kidney can be felt, its size and surface consistency should be described.

When assessed on digital rectal examination, the normal prostate is smooth and has a firm consistency. It has two lateral lobes with a median groove. Its size should be assessed and the presence of any nodules evaluated. The clinical features of a normal, hyperplastic and malignant prostate are shown in **Table 8.6**.

Scrotum

The scrotum should be examined from the front with the examiner sitting beside the patient or kneeling on the floor. Inspect the scrotum to observe any obvious swelling and any changes in the overlying skin such as redness and oedema. The testis, epididymis and spermatic cord are palpated on each side between the thumb and index and middle fingers (**Figure 8.8**). The size, surface and consistency of the testes should be assessed. If a lump is identified, its relation to the testis and epididymis should be recorded.

Clinical assessment of the prostate gland	
State	**Features**
Normal	Smooth, symmetrical, rubbery, mobile, median grove
Hyperplastic	Large, smooth, rubbery, asymmetrical, mobile, median groove
Malignant	Hard, irregular, asymmetrical, fixed, loss of median groove

Table 8.6 Clinical assessment of the prostate gland

Examination of the scrotum

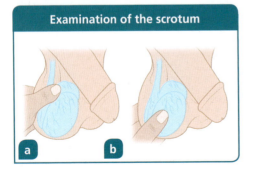

a   b

Figure 8.8 Examination of the scrotum. (a) Palpation of the epididymis. (b) Palpation of the testis.

> The scrotum should be examined as part of all abdominal examinations in men. Scrotal pathology can cause abdominal symptoms, and failure to examine the scrotum can lead to diagnostic errors.

Investigation

Investigation of the urinary tract invariably involves an assessment of the urine. It also includes radiological assessment of the upper urinary tract or direct visualisation of the lower urinary tract.

Urinalysis

Urinalysis is a simple, cost-effective procedure that provides a chemical evaluation of the urine. It is usually performed by the bedside using test strips that evaluate the presence or absence of key factors (**Table 8.7**).

Urine microscopy and culture

Microscopy of the urine is a simple and informative test that should be performed on all patients suspected of having renal disease. To avoid contamination, a midstream specimen is collected. Microscopy shows the presence of red blood cells, while blood cells, epithelial cells, bacteria and casts. It is now usually performed using automated methods. If bacteria are present, the urine should be cultured to determine the antibiotic sensitivities of the organisms present. Culture results are usually available within 2–3 days.

Interpretation of urinalysis results	
Test	**Result indicates**
Leukocytes	Urinary tract infection
Nitrites	Gram-negative bacteria
Protein	Renal inflammation
Ketones	Dehydration, diabetic ketoacidosis
Blood	Infection, malignancy, calculi

Table 8.7 Interpretation of urinalysis results

Urine cytology

Urine cytology is the collection and evaluation of epithelial cells shed from the urinary tract. The urine sample is centrifuged and the sediment viewed under a microscope. Urinary cytology is useful in the diagnosis of high-grade tumours but may miss low-grade, non-invasive tumours.

> **CT-KUB is now the investigation of choice for assessing patients with suspected ureteric calculi.** It has a high sensitivity for identifying stones, will detect any complications and sometimes show an alternative pathology if no stones are detected.

Renal ultrasonography

Ultrasonography is the imaging modality of choice for assessing the kidney, bladder and prostate gland. The prostate is imaged using an ultrasound probe inserted into the rectum (transrectal ultrasound).

Ultrasound is indicated in the assessment of:

- Acute renal failure
- Chronic renal failure
- Hydronephrosis
- Congenital anomalies
- Renal cysts and neoplasms

It can be repeated after voiding, providing an indication of the residual volume and thus an indirect assessment of bladder function.

Renal ultrasonography can be combined with Doppler imaging to assess flow in the renal artery and vein.

Kidney–ureter–bladder radiograph

A KUB radiograph is a plain abdominal radiograph to assess the urinary tract. It may identify radiopaque ureteric stones and nephrocalcinosis. Intravenous urography was until recently also used in the assessment of the urinary tract. It has, however, largely been superseded by the use of CT scanning.

Computed tomography

CT of the urinary tract can be performed as either contrast-enhanced or a non-contrast-enhanced scanning. It is used in detecting:

- Renal calculi
- Renal and bladder neoplasms – for detection and staging
- Renal trauma

Radioisotope renography

Conventional radiological imaging techniques are good at assessing the structure of the kidney and detecting any associated pathology. However, it is also important to assess the relative function of the two kidneys.

Radioisotope renography (**Figure 8.9**) is imaging of the kidneys after the injection of a radioisotope. The two most common radiolabelled pharmaceutical agents are technetium-labelled MAG3 (mercaptoacetyltriglycine) and DTPA (diethylene triamine pentacetic acid). MAG3 is excreted by the proximal tubule. DTPA is filtered by the glomerulus and may be used to measure the glomerular filtration rate. DMSA (dimercaptosuccinic acid) can be used to assess the extent of renal scarring in children with vesicoureteric reflux and the risk of future renal impairment.

Urodynamic studies

Urodynamic studies are used to assess the function of the bladder by measuring the pressure and volume of urine within it. From this, they provide information on the storage and voiding of the urine. Uroflowmetry measures the volume of urine passed with time and is used to calculate the flow rate (**Figure 8.10**). Characteristic pressure traces and flow rates are seen in different conditions.

Cystoscopy

Cystoscopy is an endoscopic procedure used to assess the urethra and bladder visually. The camera is inserted via the urethra under either local or general anaesthesia. Lesions within the bladder can then be biopsied or removed. Interventional procedures can also be performed, such as the insertion of a ureteric stent, the resection of a tumour or lithotripsy to break up and remove ureteric stones.

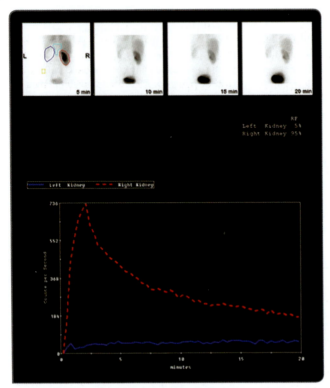

Figure 8.9 MAG3 renogram showing a non-functioning left kidney.

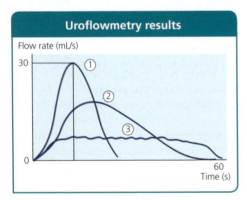

Figure 8.10 Characteristic uroflowmetry results. ① Normal. ② Benign prostatic hyperplasia. ③ Urethral stricture.

Urinary tract infection

Several terms are encountered in relation to UTIs:

- Bacteriuria is the presence of bacteria within the urine
- Significant bacteriuria is defined as more than 105 colony-forming units per millilitre of urine
- Cystitis is infection within the bladder
- Pyelonephritis is infection involving the upper urinary tract

Epidemiology

As women have a shorter urethra than men, they are more likely to develop lower UTIs.

At least 50% of women will develop a UTI as some time, and recurrence is common. Infections are more prevalent in women who are sexually active. Other risk factors include diabetes and pregnancy. UTIs in men are often associated with an abnormality of the urinary tract.

> The term 'honeymoon cystitis' has been applied to the observation that UTIs are more frequent during the early months of a relationship due to more frequent sexual intercourse.

Aetiology

Urine located proximal to the distal urethra is normally sterile. Most UTIs are due to organisms found in the faecal flora and are invariably the result of an ascending infection. They are most commonly caused by *E. coli. Proteus mirabilis* and *Pseudomonas aeruginosa* also cause infection, particularly if there is an underlying abnormality. Rarely, UTIs arise secondary to a bacteraemia (e.g. with *Staphylococcus aureus*).

Pathogenesis

Host defences against urinary infection include the voiding of urine, urinary antibodies, desquamation (i.e. shedding of cells) of the epithelial surface and antibacterial enzymes.

UTIs can be uncomplicated or complicated. Uncomplicated UTIs have no underlying structural abnormality. Complicated UTIs arise secondary to a structural lesion and can result in renal damage. Complications include pyonephrosis, which can occur if there is coexisting upper tract obstruction.

Clinical features

Acute cystitis is usually mild and symptoms include suprapubic pain, frequency, urgency and dysuria. The clinical examination is often normal. Acute pyelonephritis presents with pyrexia, frequency, dysuria and loin pain. Patients are often systemically unwell, and examination invariably shows a high fever and loin tenderness.

Diagnostic approach

Investigation aims to establish the diagnosis of a UTI, identify the organism involved and its antibiotic sensitivity, and exclude a structural or pathological abnormality of the urinary tract.

Investigations

The diagnosis of a UTI can be suggested by urinalysis. The presence of nitrites or leucocyte esterase is highly suggestive of infection with a Gram-negative organism. The diagnosis should be confirmed by microscopy and culture. An MSU will invariably be positive for the infecting organism.

Investigation in adults should involve renal ultrasound and cystoscopy, supplemented by other modalities as guided by the clinical presentation. Investigation in children includes renal ultrasound and DMSA scanning to assess renal damage. A micturating cystogram, an investigation performed by instilling radiological contrast in to the bladder via a catheter and assessing flow and reflux during micturition, can be used to evaluate vesicoureteric reflux.

> All upper and lower UTIs in adult men should be investigated by ultrasound, CT scanning or cystoscopy to identify any predisposing pathology.

Management

Acute cystitis is treated with increased fluid intake and antibiotics. Trimethoprim is the antibiotic of choice. Symptoms can be improved by alkalisation of the urine with potassium citrate. An MSU should be checked at 7 days to confirm that the infection has been cleared.

Acute pyelonephritis is treated more aggressively, using intravenous antibiotics. Obstruction of the upper urinary tract is considered if the symptoms fail to settle within 48 hours.

Pyonephrosis requires urgent decompression, usually by a percutaneous nephrostomy. If inadequately treated, it can result in the development of a perinephric abscess.

Ureteric and bladder calculi

Stones can be found within the kidney, ureter or bladder. Renal stones can migrate to the ureter and cause severe symptoms. Bladder stones form directly within the bladder and can be asymptomatic.

Ureteric calculi

Stones within the renal pelvis can remain asymptomatic for many years. It is only when they start to migrate along the ureter that symptoms occur.

Epidemiology

The lifetime risk of developing a ureteric calculus is about 5%, and the recurrence rate is about 50%. They are more common in men, with most presenting between 30 and 60 years of age.

Aetiology

Urinary tract calculi form from crystalline aggregates of proteins high in glutamic and aspartic acid. Stone formation is more likely with increased urinary concentrations of constituents (e.g. calcium and uric acid), the presence of promoter substances and a reduction in the concentration of inhibitors. The relative proportions of different types of ureteric calculi are:

- Calcium oxalate – 40%
- Calcium phosphate – 15%
- Mixed oxalate and phosphate – 20%
- Struvite – 15%
- Uric acid – 10%

Chronic infection with urease-producing organisms (e.g. Proteus) can precipitate stone formation within the renal pelvis. A magnesium ammonium phosphate or 'staghorn' calculus can result. Large staghorn calculi may be asymptomatic but can lead to a deterioration in renal function.

Clinical features

Ureteric calculi usually present with pain due to migration of the stone and obstruction to urinary flow. Ureteric colic is typically severe, colicky, loin-to-groin pain. It may radiate into the scrotum in men and the labia in women. It may be associated with urinary frequency, urgency and dysuria. The pain may settle if the stone is passed or fails to migrate further.

Abdominal examination is usually normal though there may be some loin tenderness. The different diagnosis of ureteric colic is shown in **Table 8.8**. Complications of ureteric calculi include obstruction, ureteric strictures and infection.

> About 90% of ureteric calculi are idiopathic and about 10% are due to a metabolic derangement, including hyperparathyroidism, vitamin D excess and primary hyperoxaluria.

Diagnostic approach

The clinical presentation of a ureteric calculus is often supported by the history and either macroscopic or microscopic haematuria. Radiological assessment may confirm the presence of a stone.

Investigations

Haematuria is invariably present in patients with ureteric calculi and can be confirmed by urinalysis or urine microscopy. Serum electrolytes and calcium should be checked to ensure normal renal function and exclude hypercalcaemia. An MSU should be obtained for microbiological evaluation to assess the

Differential diagnosis of ureteric colic	
Non-renal causes	Renal causes
Appendicitis	Tumour (known as clot colic)
Diverticulitis	
Ectopic pregnancy	Pyelonephritis
Acute salpingitis	Retroperitoneal fibrosis
Torted ovarian cyst	Ureteric stricture
Abdominal aortic aneurysm	Papillary necrosis

Table 8.8 Differential diagnosis of ureteric colic

presence or absence of infection. Due to the ability to manipulate images, CT-KUB has a higher sensitivity for stone detection than an intravenous urogram (**Figure 8.11**). If no stone is seen, there may be an alternative diagnosis.

More formal metabolic investigation with a 24-hour urinary collection should be considered if there is:

- A family history of stone formation
- Bilateral stone disease
- Inflammatory bowel disease, chronic diarrhoea or malabsorption
- A history of bariatric surgery
- Medical conditions associated with urolithiasis
- Nephrocalcinosis
- Osteoporosis or a pathological fracture
- Stones that are composed of cystine, uric acid or calcium phosphate suggest an underlying metabolic disorder

Management

Most cases of ureteric colic can be managed conservatively with adequate hydration, opiates and anti-inflammatory analgesia until the stone has passed and the symptoms resolve.

Conservative management

Most ureteric calculi less than 5 mm in diameter pass spontaneously. If the calculus is

Treatment of ureteric calculi	
Site in ureter	Treatment
Upper third	Extracorporeal shock-wave lithotripsy
Middle third	Extracorporeal shock-wave lithotripsy or ureteroscopy
Lower third	Ureteroscopy or lithotripsy

Table 8.9 Treatment of ureteric calculi

larger than 5–10 mm and fails to pass spontaneously, intervention is considered, depending on the position of the calculus in the renal tract (**Table 8.9**).

Lithotripsy

Lithotripsy is the use of mechanical shock waves to break the stones. It requires an energy source – a spark-gap electrode or piezoceramic array, which is a coupling device between the patient and the electrode – a water bath, to provide air-free contact with the patient's skin, or cushion and a method of stone localisation – such as fluoroscopy or ultrasound. Lithotripsy is usually performed as an outpatient procedure with the patient sedated.

Surgery

Overall, fewer than 1% patients with stones require open surgery. If large stones are present in the renal pelvis or upper ureter, percutaneous nephrolithotomy is necessary as an elective procedure, particularly if the stone is more than 3 cm in diameter or there is a staghorn calculus (**Figure 8.12**).

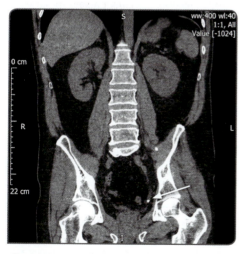

Figure 8.11 Coronal reconstruction of a CT-KUB showing a radiopaque calculus (arrow) in the distal left ureter.

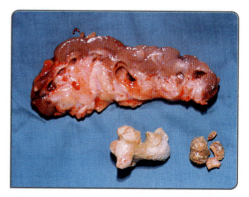

Figure 8.12 A staghorn calculus from the renal pelvis.

Indications for emergency intervention in patients with ureteric calculi include:

- Infection with urinary tract obstruction
- Severe urinary infection
- Intractable pain or vomiting
- Impending acute renal failure
- Obstruction in a solitary or transplanted kidney
- Bilateral obstruction

Acute infection in an obstructed kidney is a urological emergency. The patient is usually unwell with loin pain, swinging pyrexia and dysuria. Rapid renal destruction may occur if drainage via emergency percutaneous nephrostomy is not performed.

Bladder calculi

Bladder calculi are distinct pathological entities from ureteric calculi. There is no recognised association with ureteric stones, and they are not the result of ureteric calculi that migrate to the bladder.

Epidemiology

Bladder calculi are uncommon in the developed world and the incidence is decreasing. They invariably occur in men. In developing countries, they are seen in both children and adults.

Aetiology

Bladder calculi are usually associated with urinary stasis with infection. Foreign bodies (e.g. suture material) can also act as a focus for stone formation. Stones vary in size and can be multiple. Most stones in adults are formed of uric acid.

Long-standing untreated bladder stones are associated with the development of squamous cell carcinoma of the bladder.

Clinical features

Many bladder calculi are asymptomatic. If they do cause symptoms, these include suprapubic pain, dysuria and haematuria. The abdominal examination may be normal. Patients may present in acute urinary retention.

Investigations

Most stones can be seen as radio opaque foreign bodies on a plain abdominal radiograph, filling defects on ultrasound or abdominal CT scan, or directly visualised on cystoscopy. Uric acid stones are radiolucent on plain X-ray, but may have an opaque calcified layer. Underlying bladder abnormalities should be sought.

Management

Bladder stones can be removed by fragmentation, usually using transurethral cystolitholapaxy. Indications for surgery for bladder calculi include recurrent UTIs and frank haematuria. Extracorporeal shock-wave lithotripsy, which is used in the management of ureteric calculi, is relatively ineffective for bladder calculi.

Historically, stones were diagnosed by passing a urethral 'sound' and the surgical approach involved 'cutting for a stone' via either a perineal or a suprapubic approach.

Renal cancer

Benign tumours of the kidney are rare, and all renal neoplasms should be regarded as potentially malignant. Renal cell carcinomas are increasingly identified on radiological investigations performed for unrelated reasons.

Epidemiology

About 80% of all kidney tumours are renal cell carcinomas, also known as hypernephromas, clear cell carcinomas or Grawitz's tumours. They account for over 3% of all new cases of cancer diagnosed in men and around 2% of all cancers in women. The male-to-female ratio is approximately 2:1. The incidence is increased in patients with von Hippel–Lindau syndrome.

> von Hippel–Lindau syndrome is rare autosomal dominant condition that predisposes patients to tumours of the kidney, central nervous syndrome and neuroendocrine system. It results from the mutation of a tumour suppressor gene on chromosome 3.

Pathologically, renal cell cancers may extend into the perinephric fat, renal vein and inferior vena cava. Blood-borne spread can result in isolated 'cannon ball' pulmonary metastases so called because of their large round appearance on a chest X-ray.

Aetiology

Renal cell carcinomas arise from the proximal renal tubule. Risk factors include a positive family history, smoking, obesity and exposure to occupational chemicals (e.g. cadmium).

Clinical features

The most common presentation is painless haematuria. Only about 10% of patients present with the classic triad of haematuria, loin pain and a renal mass, the latter being a sign of advanced disease. Other clinical presentations include a pyrexia of unknown origin and hypertension.

> Renal cell carcinomas occasionally produce hormones that influence the clinical presentation. Polycythaemia can occur due to erythropoietin production. Hypercalcaemia can occur from the production of a parathyroid hormone-like hormone.

Diagnostic approach

Investigation aims to identify the cause of the haematuria and assess the extent of spread and operability of the tumour.

> The appearance of a varicocele, particularly in the left side of the scrotum, in a middle-aged or elderly man should prompt an investigation for renal cell carcinoma.

Investigations

Urinalysis will confirm the presence of blood in the urine. The diagnosis can often be confirmed from an ultrasound scan showing a mass in the kidney. Abdominal CT scanning confirms the diagnosis and allows staging of the disease and an assessment of renal vein and caval spread (see **Figure 8.1**). An echocardiogram should be considered if a thrombus is seen in the inferior vena cava extending above the diaphragm, possibly into the heart and increasing the risk of tumour embolisation.

Management

Unless there is extensive metastatic disease, treatment invariably involves surgery. This is usually radical nephrectomy, with removal of the kidney and perinephric fat. The kidney is approached through either a transabdominal or a loin incision, although laparoscopic surgery may be considered for small localised tumours. The renal vein is ligated early during the surgery to reduce spread of the tumour cells. The kidney and its adjacent tissue (adrenal gland and perinephric fat) are excised. Solitary metastases (e.g. to the lung) can occasionally be resected.

Radiotherapy and chemotherapy have little place in the treatment of renal cell carcinoma. However, recently developed novel targeted therapies (e.g. monoclonal antibodies against vascular endothelial growth factor receptors) have shown promise in those with metastatic disease.

Prognosis

When the tumour is confined to the kidney, the 5-year survival is approximately 70%.

Other renal tumours

Rarer tumours arising in the kidney include renal oncocytomas, angiomyolipomas, cystic nephromas and metanephric adenomas. All are considered benign. Renal oncocytomas arise from the collecting ducts. Angiomyolipomas are composed of blood vessels, smooth muscle and fat, and are associated with tuberous sclerosis. Cystic nephromas are often asymptomatic and are typically discovered incidentally on radiological imaging.

Bladder cancer

Bladder cancers are the most common tumours of the urinary system. Most are transitional cell carcinomas, and they can occur in both the bladder and the ureters. Superficial tumours confined to the epithelium are usually of low grade and are associated with a good prognosis. Tumours that invade the muscle are often of high grade and have a poorer prognosis.

Epidemiology

Bladder cancer accounts for around 1 in 30 new cancers. The male-to-female ratio is 3:1.

Aetiology

Of all bladder carcinomas:

- 90% are transitional cell carcinomas
- 5% are squamous cell carcinomas
- 2% are adenocarcinomas

Transitional cell carcinomas should be regarded as representing a 'field change' throughout the urothelium – the squamous epithelium of the urinary tract. About 80% of transitional cell carcinomas are superficial and well differentiated, and only 20% of all tumours progress to muscle invasion. Aetiological factors for transitional cell carcinoma are occupational chemical exposure (e.g. analine dyes and chlorinated hydrocarbons), cigarette smoking and pelvic irradiation.

> *Schistosoma haematobium* infection, often seen in the developing world, is associated with an increased risk of squamous carcinoma of the bladder.

Clinical features

About 80% of patients present with painless haematuria. Bladder tumours can also present with treatment-resistant urinary infection, bladder irritability and sterile pyuria (white cells in the urine in the absence of infection).

Diagnostic approach

Bladder tumours are usually detected during the investigation of painless haematuria. Once a tumour has been identified, the whole renal tract must be assessed as transitional cell carcinomas have a tendency to be multifocal.

Investigations

Investigation involves cystoscopy and biopsy. Pathological staging requires bladder muscle to be included in the specimen as tumours are divided into superficial or muscle-invading according to the depth of tumour invasion. The grade of the tumour is also important, as high grade tumours are at increased risk of local invasion and metastatic spread. Cytology of the urine may be useful.

> In patients with transitional cell carcinoma of the bladder, urine cytology may show malignant cells. However, the result may be normal, and the absence of malignant cells does not exclude the diagnosis of cancer.

Management

Superficial transitional cell carcinoma is treated by transurethral resection and regular cystoscopic follow-up. Prophylactic chemotherapy should be considered if there are risk factors for recurrence or muscle invasion. Immunotherapy may also be required. *Bacillus Calmette–Guerin* is an attenuated strain of *Mycobacterium bovis* that reduces the risk of recurrence and progression in about 50% of cases.

Carcinoma in situ is an aggressive form of cancer and is often associated with positive cytology. About 50% of patients progress to muscle invasion. Immunotherapy should be considered, to reduce the risk of progression to invasive disease. If this fails, the patient may need radical cystectomy.

For patients with invasive transitional cell carcinoma, the options are radical cystectomy and radiotherapy. After removal of the bladder, urinary diversion can be achieved using an ileal conduit (implantation of the ureters in to an ileal loop used to form a stoma; **Figure 8.13**) or the formation of a neo-bladder from a loop of small bowel. Ureteric transitional cell carcinomas are usually managed by nephro-ureterectomy.

Urinary diversion has the potential to cause local or metabolic complications (**Table 8.10**). The most common metabolic consequence as a result of electrolyte absorption through the bowel mucosa is a hyperchloraemic acidosis, which is often asymptomatic and detected on routine blood tests.

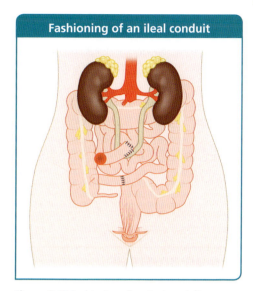

Fashioning of an ileal conduit

Figure 8.13 Fashioning of an ileal conduit.

Early and late complications of urinary diversion

Early	Late
Urinary tract infections	Metabolic derangements
Urinary leakage	Renal stones
Small bowel obstruction	Ureteral strictures
Fluid collections – urinomas, haematomas	Malignant transformation in the reservoir

Table 8.10 Early and late complications of urinary diversion

Bladder outflow obstruction

Over 70% of men with lower urinary tract symptoms have proven bladder outflow obstruction. The causes of this can be structural or functional and are shown in **Table 8.11**.

Urethral strictures

A urethral stricture is a physical narrowing of the urethra resulting in obstruction of the outflow of the bladder. Causes of urethral strictures are shown in **Table 8.12**. The management can be with dilatation, urethrotomy

Causes of bladder outflow obstruction

Structural	Functional
Urethral valves	Bladder neck dyssynergia
Urethral strictures	Neurological disease
Benign prostatic hyperplasia	Drugs
Carcinoma of the prostate	
Bladder neck stenosis	

Table 8.11 Causes of bladder outflow obstruction

Causes of urethral strictures	
Pathology	**Examples**
Trauma	Instrumentation, urethral rupture
infection	Gonorrhoea, non-specific urethritis, syphilis, tuberculosis
Inflammation	Balanitis xerotica obliterans
Neoplasia	Squamous, transitional cell or adenocarcinoma

Table 8.12 Causes of urethral strictures

(surgical division of the stricture) or urethroplasty (refashioning of the urethra).

Benign prostatic hyperplasia

Benign prostatic hyperplasia is an increase in the size of the prostate gland due to an increase in the number of cells. It is a common phenomenon in ageing men.

Epidemiology

It affects 50% of men older than 60 years, and 90% of men older than 90 years.

Aetiology

Benign prostatic hyperplasia is due to hyperplasia of both the stromal and epithelial cells of the prostate. It occurs from a mismatch between the rates of cell proliferation and apoptosis that favours cell proliferation. This is caused by an imbalance between dihydrotestosterone (a metabolite of testosterone) and oestrogens within the prostate gland, with a relative increase in the latter.

Large discrete nodules form around the urethra. These then compress the urethra, causing a partial or sometimes complete obstruction of urinary flow.

Clinical features

Benign prostatic hyperplasia presents with either obstructive and/or irritative bladder symptoms (Table 8.5). In some men, the initial presentation is acute urinary retention.

Diagnostic approach

Acute urinary retention is diagnosis clinically and confirmed by a relief of symptoms after the passage of a urinary catheter. The assessment of chronic bladder outflow obstruction requires urinary flow measurement followed by a clinical, radiological and pathological assessment to identify the underlying cause.

Investigations

Chronic bladder outflow obstruction can be confirmed by uroflowmetry (see **Figure 8.10**). Other investigations include urea and electrolyte measurement to check renal function, an ultrasound scan to exclude hydronephrosis, causing back pressure on the kidneys, and measurement of the post-micturition urine volume, showing possible incomplete voiding. A serum prostate-specific antigen level should be measured to exclude malignancy.

Management

The aims of treatment are to relieve the symptoms, improve quality of life and treat complications resulting from bladder outflow obstruction.

Medication

Drug treatment is often the first line of management, particularly in those with mild symptoms. Effective drugs include α-adrenergic antagonists (e.g. tamsulosin, which relaxes the muscles of bladder neck) and 5α-reductase inhibitors (e.g. finasteride, which reduces dihydrotesterone levels and as a result the size of the prostate).

Surgery

Transurethral resection of the prostate (TURP) is the surgical treatment of choice for bladder outflow obstruction caused by benign prostatic hyperplasia. The bulk of the prostate is reduced endoscopically, the fragments of prostatic tissue are washed from the bladder, and an irrigation catheter is inserted. Obstruction is reduced and urinary symptoms improved in over 90% of patients. Absorption of the bladder irrigation fluid (glycine) can result in acute hyponatraemia and is known as transurethral resection syndrome.

> Transurethral resection syndrome is an uncommon complication of TURP that results when the irrigation fluid is absorbed into the systemic circulation. Clinical features include confusion, hypotension, collapse and bradycardia. Investigation reveals hyponatraemia.

Prognosis

After TURP, urinary retention occurs in about 5% of patients following removal of the catheter in the early postoperative period. Post-prostatectomy incontinence is a transient phenomenon in many men but becomes a persistent problem in fewer than 5%. Retrograde ejaculation occurs in about 80%.

Prostate cancer

With an ageing population the incidence of prostate cancer is increasing. However, many men will die with the disease rather than from the disease.

Epidemiology

Prostate cancer is the most common cancer in men and accounts for nearly a quarter of all new cancers in men. It is more common in Europe and North America and rare in Asia. It is uncommon below the age of 50 years. The incidence is increasing due the discovery of prostate cancers after TURP for apparently benign disease and, more recently, the increased use of serum prostate-specific antigen testing.

> About 5–10% of operations for benign prostatic disease reveal unsuspected prostate cancer.

Aetiology

Prostate cancer is an adenocarcinoma and usually arises in the posterior part of the gland. It spreads through the capsule into the bladder neck, pelvic wall, rectum and perineural spaces. Lymphatic spread is common. Haematogenous spread occurs to the axial skeleton.

The tumours are graded using the Gleason score, which is based on the glandular and cellular pattern of the tumour.

Clinical features

Early tumours are often asymptomatic. About 60% of patients present with symptoms of bladder outflow obstruction. The remainder present with bone pain or cord compression as a result of spinal metastatic disease. Renal failure can occur due to bilateral ureteric obstruction.

With locally advanced tumours, the diagnosis can be confirmed by rectal examination, which shows a hard nodule or a loss of the central sulcus of the prostate gland.

> The clinic presentation of prostate cancer is usually symptoms of bladder outflow obstruction or bone metastases.

Diagnostic approach

The diagnosis of prostate cancer can be suspected on digital rectal examination and confirmed by biopsy and the measurement of prostate-specific antigen. Once the disease has been confirmed, it should be staged by CT or MRI scanning in those in whom surgery is being considered.

Investigations

Transrectal ultrasound is a key investigation. It confirms the diagnosis and allows an ultrasound-guided transrectal biopsy to be performed. Sclerotic secondary deposits may been seen on a radiograph of the lumbar spine and pelvis. Nuclear medicine bone scanning will also detect the presence of metastases.

Prostate-specific antigen

Prostate-specific antigen (PSA) is a protein produced by the epithelial cells of the prostate. A serum level of 4 ng/mL is the upper limit of normal, and a level greater than 10 ng/mL is highly suggestive of prostatic carcinoma. It is a useful marker for monitoring the response to treatment. Serum PSA can, however, also be raised in BPH.

Management

This depends on the stage of the disease, the patient's age and his general fitness. For disease localised to the prostate gland, the options are observation, radiotherapy and radical prostatectomy. Hormonal therapy is the mainstay of treatment for metastatic disease.

Radical prostatectomy

Radical prostatectomy involves removal of the entire prostate gland along with the seminal vesicles. The urethra is anastomosed to the base of the bladder. Radical prostatectomy is associated with an improvement in mean survival over simple observation, and a 50% reduction in the risk of metastatic disease. However, erectile dysfunction occurs in 50% of patients.

Hormonal therapy

In about 80% of prostate cancers, growth is androgen dependent. Hormonal therapy therefore involves androgen depletion. This produces good palliation until tumours 'escape' from hormonal control, which eventually occurs in almost all patients if they live long enough and do not die from other causes. Androgen depletion can be achieved with luteinising hormone releasing hormone agonists (e.g. goserelin), anti-androgenic agents (e.g. cyproterone acetate and flutamide) or complete androgen blockade with a combination of drugs.

Testicular disorders

Testicular disorders are relatively rare. However, the testes are one the most common sites of malignancy in young men. Due to its sudden onset and severity, acute testicular pain is one the dramatic surgical presentations, requiring urgent assessment and intervention.

Testicular tumours

Testicular tumours are one of the most common malignancies seen in young men. With improved chemotherapy regimens, the outcome has significantly improved in the last 20 years. The two main types of testicular tumours are teratomas and seminomas.

Epidemiology

The incidence of testicular tumours has doubled in the past 25 years. Teratomas and seminomas now have an equal incidence, with a peak age of presentation of 25 and 35 years, respectively. The highest incidence is seen in white individuals, with figures five times higher than those for other ethnic groups.

Aetiology

The cause of testicular tumours is unknown but there is almost certainly a genetic predisposition. Risk factors include testicular maldescent, Klinefelter's syndrome and a positive family history of testicular tumours.

> **Klinefelter's syndrome is genetic disorder in which the standard male karyotype is associated with an extra X chromosome.** The principal clinical features are hypogonadism and impaired fertility, with an increased risk of testicular cancer.

Clinical features

Testicular tumours usually present with a testicular swelling or lump. The amount of pain is variable but often minimal. Examination shows a testicular lump that cannot be separated from the underlying testis (**Figure 8.14**). Patients may present with gynaecomastia or symptoms of metastatic disease, usually abdominal or back pain or respiratory symptoms.

Diagnostic approach

The diagnosis can usually be suspected from the clinical assessment, but investigations may help to confirm the diagnosis.

Investigations

The diagnosis can often be confirmed by testicular ultrasonography. A pathological diagnosis is made from an inguinal orchidectomy. There is no place for scrotal exploration and a testicular biopsy as opening up of the tunica vaginalis risks seeding of tumour from the testis to the scrotal skin. The disease can be staged by thoracoabdominal CT scanning.

Unlike with many other tumours, serum tumour markers are useful in both staging the disease and assessing the response to treatment. The tissues from which seminomas and teratomas arise have different embryological origins. Alpha-fetoprotein is produced by yolk sac elements and is not produced by seminomas. Beta-human chorionic gonadotrophin is produced by trophoblastic elements, and elevated levels seen in both teratomas and seminomas.

Management

Treatment for testicular cancer is very effective. Nearly all men are cured by a combination of surgery, chemotherapy and radiotherapy.

Surgery

In most cases, initial surgical treatment is by inguinal orchidectomy. The spermatic cord is divided at the deep inguinal ring before the testis is mobilised. Testis-preserving surgery may be necessary in men with synchronous bilateral tumours or only one testis.

Adjuvant therapy

Seminomas are radiosensitive. Stage I and II disease is managed by inguinal orchidectomy with radiotherapy to the ipsilateral abdominal and pelvic nodes. Stage II and higher disease should be treated with orchidectomy, radiotherapy and chemotherapy.

Teratomas are not radiosensitive. Stage I disease is treated by orchidectomy alone and

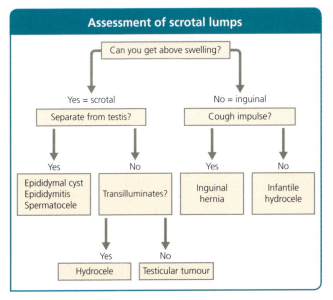

Figure 8.14 Assessment of scrotal lumps.

surveillance. Orchidectomy should be performed and chemotherapy should be given to men with stage II disease, those who relapse and those who have metastatic disease at presentation.

Prognosis

Testicular cancers are very sensitive to chemotherapy and are curable even when they have metastasised. In those with disease localised to the testis, the 5-year survival is more than 95%. Even in those with metastatic disease at presentation, cure rates of 80% have been reported.

Testicular torsion

Testicular torsion is a common surgical emergency in adolescent boys as the peak incidence is in the second decade of life. It results from twisting of the testicle on its blood supply. A high insertion of the tunica vaginalis (known as a bell clapper testis) predisposes to the condition. The underlying abnormality is often bilateral, and the contralateral testis is usually lying horizontally.

Clinical features

Testicular torsion usually presents with acute scrotal pain. About 50% of patients have had a previous episode of pain. However, it may present with acute abdominal pain and no testicular symptoms. It is therefore essential to examine the scrotum in all boys who present with acute abdominal pain. Urinary symptoms are uncommon.

Examination shows an exquisitely tender high-riding testis, often with a small hydrocele.

> Testicular torsion can present with abdominal pain, but no testicular pain. It is therefore important to examine the testes in all boys irrespective of age, presenting with acute abdominal pain.

Management

Testicular torsion is a clinical diagnosis requiring urgent surgical exploration. The diagnosis is usually obvious and investigation wastes time as the viability of the testis is reduced with a delay in surgical intervention. The outcome is best in those operated on less than 6 hours after the onset of symptoms.

If the testis is black and infarcted, it should be removed. If its viability is in doubt, the testis should be wrapped in a warm swab and observed after several minutes. Viability can be assessed by any duskiness of the testis resolving and it returning to its normal pink colour. If the testis is assessed to be viable both testes should be fixed within the scrotum.

Approximately 60% of testes are salvageable and orchidectomy can be avoided. However, if patients are re-examined 6 months after surgery, 10% of testes are found to be atrophic. Long-term subfertility is occasionally a problem and is possibly due to an autoimmune response affecting both testes, due to testicular antigens entering the blood stream at the time of the initial torsion.

> If a diagnosis of testicular torsion is suspected, investigation is not required as testicular torsion is a clinical diagnosis requiring urgent surgical exploration. The diagnosis is usually obvious.

Epididymitis

Epididymitis is a bacterial infection of the epididymis. It usually presents in adult males. As it is uncommon in adolescents, be wary about making the diagnosis in this age group.

Clinical features

Patients usually present with gradual-onset and prolonged testicular pain that may not be severe. Frequency and dysuria may be present. Examination will show a swollen and tender testis with the greatest swelling located over the epididymis. Treatment is with antibiotics.

Varicocele

A varicocele is dilatation of the veins of the pampiniform plexus, the veins that drain the testis. There are several veins in the scrotum but these coalesce to one or two in the inguinal canal. By the deep inguinal ring, there is only one testicular vein. The left testicular vein drains into the left renal vein. The right testicular vein drains directly into the inferior vena cava.

Clinical features

Most varicoceles present in adolescence or early adult life. About 95% occur on the left and are idiopathic. Most are asymptomatic, but vague scrotal discomfort may occur. Examination shows the typical 'bag of worms' (the dilated veins), which reduces in size in the supine position (**Figure 8.15**). Varicoceles are occasionally associated with infertility.

> As the left testicular vein drains into the left renal vein, a varicocele may be the presenting sign of left renal cell carcinoma with a tumour obstructing the renal vein.

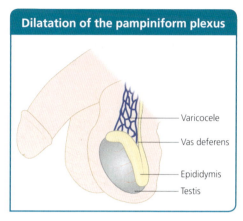

Dilatation of the pampiniform plexus

Varicocele
Vas deferens
Epididymis
Testis

Figure 8.15 Dilatation of the pampiniform plexus forming a varicocele.

Management

Varicoceles need treatment only if they are symptomatic. The veins can be ligated via either a scrotal, an inguinal or a laparoscopic approach. Recurrence can occur due to the collateral drainage via the cremasteric vein.

Penile disorders

Penile disorders are rare and often present late due to the embarrassing nature of the symptoms that they cause.

Penile cancer

Penile cancer is a squamous cell carcinoma that is rare in developed countries. It is most commonly seen in uncircumcised men and is rare under the age of 50 years. The tumour spreads to the inguinal nodes.

Aetiology

Human papillomavirus and poor hygiene are believed to be important aetiological factors. Erythroplasia of Queyrat is squamous cell carcinoma in situ of the glans penis and is a precursor of invasive disease.

Clinical features

Penile cancer usually presents as an ulcerating lesion on the glans penis or the foreskin. Pain

and a foul-smelling discharge may be present. The inguinal lymph nodes may be enlarged.

> The lymphatic drainage of the penis and the skin of the scrotum is to the inguinal lymph nodes. Malignant disease at these sites can present with inguinal lymphadenopathy.

Management

Management depends on the size of the lesion. Surgical treatment can range from circumcision to either partial or complete amputation of the penis. If the inguinal lymph nodes are involved, block dissection of these nodes should be considered. Radiotherapy may be of benefit for small lesions confined to the glans penis.

Urethritis

Urethritis is inflammation of the urethra. It usually results from a sexually transmitted infection. The disease is classified as either gonococcal urethritis, caused by *Neisseria gonorrhoeae*, or non-gonococcal urethritis, most commonly caused by *Chlamydia trachomatis*.

Clinical features

In men, the most common presentation is a purulent urethral discharge. A burning discomfort on micturition may also be present. In women, urethritis may be relatively asymptomatic but dysuria is usually present.

Management

The diagnosis can be confirmed if Gram staining of a urethral smear shows more than five polymorphonuclear cells per high-power field. Both gonococcal and non-gonococcal urethritis are managed with appropriate antibiotics. Patient education is important regarding the nature of sexually transmitted infections. Patients should abstain from sex until the infection has resolved, and sexual partners should be traced.

Priapism

Priapism is a persistent erection of the penis. Priapism can be either high or low flow:

- Low-flow priapism is more common and is due to venous stasis and ischaemia
- High-flow priapism is uncommon and is due to the development of an arteriocavernosal fistula after blunt or penetrating penile trauma

Delayed presentation or treatment results in a loss of erectile function.

Clinical features

Low-flow priapism presents with painful persistent erection. The penile shaft is firm, and the glans penis is usually soft. High-flow priapism is often painless. There is invariably a clear history of trauma. Aspiration of the corpora will distinguish the two types. In high-flow priapism, the blood is arterial. In low-flow priapism, the blood is dark and viscous and is similar to venous blood.

Management

Low-flow priapism requires urgent aspiration, which is successful in only 30% cases if used alone. Additional treatment is the instillation of a vasoconstrictor (e.g. phenylephrine). Detumescence can be achieved in 70% of patients and maintenance of erectile function following resolution of the priapism is present in about 40%.

High-flow priapism requires closure of the arteriocavernosal fistula, which is often performed by an interventional radiologist.

Erectile dysfunction

Erectile dysfunction is sexual dysfunction characterised by the regular or repeated inability to develop or maintain an erection, resulting in poor sexual performance. It can have a significant impact on quality of life. Causes of erectile dysfunction are shown in **Table 8.13**.

Clinical features

It is important to ascertain as to whether full erections are sometimes achieved, for example during asleep. This shows that the physical structures are functioning. Other factors leading to erectile dysfunction should be identified.

Management

The aim is to treat the cause of erectile dysfunction. Modifiable or reversible factors

Causes of erectile dysfunction	
Cause	Examples
Psychological	Performance anxiety, depression
Neurological	Stroke, spinal cord injury, diabetic neuropathy
Vascular	Peripheral vascular disease, hypertension
Endocrine	Hypogonadism, hyperprolactinaemia
Trauma	Cavernosal trauma
Drug-induced	Antidepressants, antihypertensives

Table 8.13 Cause of erectile dysfunction

should be addressed. It usually cannot be cured, but curative therapies should be planned where appropriate. Treatments should be selected according to efficacy, safety, invasiveness and patient preference.

Effective drugs include phosphodiesterase inhibitors (e.g. sildenafil). Vacuum devices and the intracavernosal injection of prostaglandins may be helpful. Semi-rigid, malleable or inflatable penile prostheses can be surgically inserted to produce an erect state.

Answers to starter questions

1. Benign prostatic hyperplasia results from proliferation of the epithelial and stromal cells of the prostate gland. Its prevalence increases with age. It occurs as a result of a mismatch between cell proliferation and apoptosis, favouring cell proliferation. It is caused by an imbalance between dihydrotestosterone (a metabolite of testosterone) and oestrogens within the prostate gland. This is a normal phenomenon of ageing, causing enlargement of the prostate with age, even if it does not cause symptoms.

2. Ureteric colic occurs when a stone passes along the ureter. Stones in the kidney are usually painless. They only cause symptoms when they start to migrate. Once they enter the bladder symptoms usually settle. If migration of the stone arrests along the course of the ureter pain may also settle. The pain occurs due to spasm and dilatation of the ureter as the stone passes through the narrow lumen of the ureter. The site and nature of the pain changes as the stone migrates.

3. During a TURP the bladder is irrigated with glycine to wash away both blood and the prostatic chippings. TUR syndrome is an uncommon complication of TURP due to the absorption of irrigation fluid into the systemic circulation. Clinical features include confusion, hypotension, collapse and bradycardia. Investigations reveal hyponatraemia.

4. Renal cell carcinomas usually present with haematuria and a renal mass. However they occasionally produce hormones that influence the clinical presentation. Polycythaemia can occur due to erythropoietin production. Hypercalcaemia can occur due to production of a PTH-like hormone.

5. Testicular tumours are one of the commonest malignancies in young men. Surgical treatment usually involves an inguinal orchidectomy followed by chemotherapy and radiotherapy dependent on the type and stage of the tumour. Testicular cancers are very sensitive to chemotherapy and are curable even when metastatic. With the improvement in chemotherapy regimens, the prognosis has improved dramatically over the past three decades.

6. Testicular torsion results from a twisting of the testicle on its own blood supply, resulting in ischaemia of the testicle. The presentation is with sudden onset of testicular pain and examination shows a high-riding testicle in the scrotum. The diagnosis is clinical with no need for extensive investigation. If the diagnosis is suspected, urgent surgical exploration of the scrotum is required. The risk of irreversible testicular necrosis increases with time, while investigation simply delays the surgery that is required.

Chapter 9
Vascular surgery

Introduction 193
Case 10 Cold painful foot 194
Core science 195
History, examination and
investigation 198
Intermittent claudication
and chronic limb ischaemia 203
Acute limb ischaemia 205
Diabetic foot 207
Carotid artery disease 208
Abdominal aortic aneurysm 210
Vascular trauma 212
Varicose veins 213
Venous hypertension and leg
ulceration 215
Lymphatic conditions 216
Raynaud's disease 218

Starter questions

Answers to the following questions are on page 220.

1. Why does atheroma kill?
2. Why does embolic acute limb ischaemia result in more dramatic clinical features than that due to thrombosis?
3. How do compartment syndromes occur?
4. Why are diabetics at increased risk of chromic limb ischaemia?
5. What are the potential advantages of endovascular repair of an abdominal aortic aneurysm?
6. How does chronic venous insufficiency cause leg ulceration?

Introduction

Arterial disease is a common cause of morbidity and mortality in the developed world. It affects any part of the arterial system in isolation or in combination, presenting as ischaemic heart disease, cerebrovascular disease or peripheral vascular disease. The underlying risk factors are well understood. The medical management of these risk factors, both radiological investiga- tions and non-surgical interventions are as important as surgical intervention. Indeed, surgery is often the last resort once other less invasive procedures have been tried. Surgery also forms part of the multidisci- plinary approach to venous disease. This is also common and places a huge economic burden on society. It often presents with leg ulceration.

Case 10 Cold painful foot

Presentation

A 90-year-old woman, Mrs Marjory Smith, is awoken from sleep with a sudden onset of pain in her right foot. She wakes her husband, who notices that the foot looks pale and feels cold.

Initial interpretation

The sudden onset of a painful and cold extremity with pallor indicates a failure of circulation to the limb and is indicative of acute limb ischaemia.

History

Marjory is a relatively fit and active 90-year-old. She has no significant past medical history.

Interpretation of history

Acute limb ischaemia arises from either a thrombotic or an embolic cause. Thrombosis often occurs in patients who have an underlying atheroma. These patients usually give a history of intermittent claudication – calf pain on walking. They frequently have had symptoms or signs of arterial disease at other sites, for example ischaemic heart disease or cerebrovascular disease. Emboli usually occur in previously normal arteries.

Further history

Marjory has had no previous limb pain. She has no history of ischaemic heart disease or stroke. She is not taking any regular medication. She has never smoked.

Examination

On examination, Marjory is in severe pain. Her pulse is irregularly irregular and suggests atrial fibrillation. Abdominal examination is unremarkable, with no expansile epigastric mass to suggest an abdominal aortic aneurysm. On examination, the left leg appears normal, with all pulses present. The right leg is pale and feels cooler than the left. The right femoral pulse is present, but all pulses are absent below the groin. Sensation in the right foot is reduced and capillary return is delayed. There is no muscle tenderness.

Interpretation of findings

These findings suggest that Marjory has acute limb ischaemia. As there are no previous symptoms but atrial fibrillation is present, this is probably embolic in origin. The most likely source of the embolus is the left atrium. The embolus is likely to have arisen in the heart and become dislodged as a result of the atrial fibrillation.

Investigations

Acute limb ischaemia is usually a clinical diagnosis. Further investigation aims to differentiate between thrombotic and embolic causes. It is also used to determine the site of the occlusion and assess the state of the collateral circulation. Duplex ultrasonography is used to determine the site of the occlusion. Angiography with a view to balloon angioplasty is considered if acute occlusion in the presence of chronic limb ischaemia is suggested.

The patient undergoes duplex ultrasonography, which shows that the circulation in the left leg is normal, with normal triphasic flow in the dorsalis pedis and posterior tibial arteries. No arterial blood flow is detected below the level of the superficial femoral artery in the right leg.

Diagnosis

Duplex ultrasonography has confirmed an acute embolic occlusion of the right superficial femoral artery. It suggests that the embolus has lodged at the bifurcation

Case 10 *continued*

of the common femoral artery at the origin of the superficial femoral artery. Marjory is given analgesia and then undergoes urgent surgery.

Management

A femoral embolectomy is performed under local anaesthesia (**Figure 9.1**). In this procedure, an incision is made in Marjory's right groin. Vascular clamps are then applied to the common femoral, superficial femoral and profunda femoris arteries to reduce the arterial inflow and backflow into the operative field.

An incision (an arteriotomy) is made in the common femoral artery, and a Fogarty balloon catheter is passed up and down the femoral artery and its branches with the balloon deflated. Next, the balloon is inflated and the catheter slowly withdrawn. Thrombus is extracted from the vessels, and flow is re-established. The vessels are flushed with heparinised saline, and the arteriotomy is closed. When the surgical procedure is complete, the foot is checked to determine that the pallor has resolved, capillary return is present and the peripheral pulses are felt.

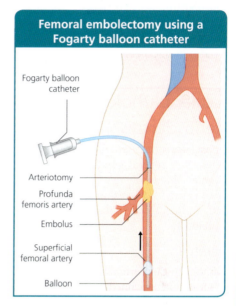

Femoral embolectomy using a Fogarty balloon catheter

Fogarty balloon catheter

Arteriotomy

Profunda femoris artery

Embolus

Superficial femoral artery

Balloon

Figure 9.1 A femoral embolectomy using a Fogarty balloon catheter.

After surgery, the patient is anticoagulated with warfarin. A cardiology opinion on the management of the atrial fibrillation is obtained.

Core science

The arteries carry oxygenated blood away from the heart. The veins return deoxygenated blood to the heart. They are connected by capillaries, which are the site of oxygen and nutrient exchange.

Vascular anatomy

The walls of arteries and veins have three layers (**Figure 9.2**):

The **tunica intima** is the thin inner layer. It includes the vascular endothelium, which is the epithelial layer that lines all the arteries and veins.

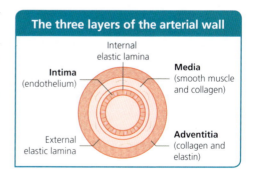

The three layers of the arterial wall

Internal elastic lamina

Intima (endothelium)

Media (smooth muscle and collagen)

External elastic lamina

Adventitia (collagen and elastin)

Figure 9.2 The three layers of the arterial wall.

The **tunica media** is the middle layer. It is made up of smooth muscle cells and sheets of elastin, both arranged circularly.

The **tunica adventitia** is the outer layer. It is mainly made up of fibrous connective tissue and varies in thickness between arteries and veins.

Vascular pathology

Arteriosclerosis

Arteriosclerosis (i.e. hardening of the arteries) describes several conditions including atheroma, Mönckeberg's arteriosclerosis (medial calcific sclerosis) and atherosclerosis, all of which result in narrowing of arteries (**Table 9.1**).

Atheroma

This is the most important cause of morbidity and mortality in developed countries. It results in arterial narrowing, leading to ischaemic heart disease, peripheral vascular disease and cerebrovascular disease. The cause of atheroma is unknown, but many risk factors have been identified (**Table 9.2**). The complications of atheroma are summarised in **Figure 9.3**.

Aetiology

High plasma levels of serum low-density lipoprotein cholesterol lead to the accumulation of cholesterol in the intima of the arteries. First, fatty streaks are produced (**Figure 9.4**), and ultimately there is fibrous plaque formation (**Figure 9.5**).

Atheroma forms at sites of haemodynamic stress, such as a narrowing or division of the arteries. Endothelial injury at these sites is an initiating factor. Inflammation is also a feature of atheromatous plaques and may be involved in progression of the disease. The inflammation is promoted by various factors (e.g. myeloperoxidase) produced by macrophages.

Risk factors for atheroma	
Major	Other
Hypertension	Age
Diabetes mellitus	Obesity
Smoking	Male sex
Hyperlipidaemia	Alcohol
Family history	Lack of exercise
	Low socioeconomic status

Table 9.2 Risk factors for atheroma

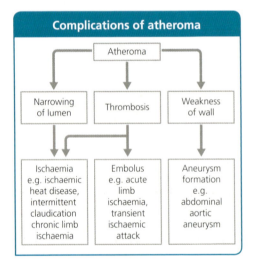

Figure 9.3 Complications of atheroma.

Common arterial diseases	
Disease	Nature
Atheroma	Due to lipid deposition within the tunica intima of the arterial wall
Mönckeberg's arteriosclerosis	Due to calcification of the tunica media of medium-sized arteries
Atherosclerosis	Characterised by thickening of the small arteries and commonly seen in the kidneys secondary to hypertension or diabetes mellitus

Table 9.1 Common arterial diseases

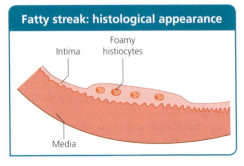

Figure 9.4 Histological appearance of a fatty streak.

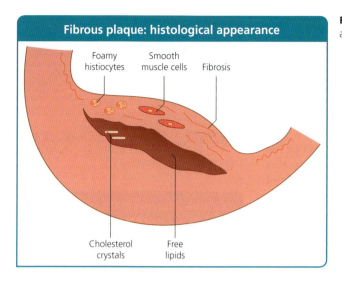

Figure 9.5 Histological appearance of a fibrous plaque.

Inflammation results in lymphocyte accumulation, the proliferation of fibroblasts and collagen production.

Fatty streaks and fibrous plaques

Fatty streaks are seen even in infants as slightly elevated areas of the arterial wall of medium- to large-sized arteries. They are caused by the accumulation of a small number of lipid-laden histiocytes and some free lipid.

Fibrous plaques are usually found in medium-sized to large arteries. They have a classic structure. The lipid is both free and contained within foamy histiocytes, which are lipid-filled macrophages. Fibrosis develops around the lipid. The central core of the plaque consists of cholesterol crystals, foam cells, debris and thrombus. Smooth muscle cells migrate from the media, proliferate and, with connective tissue cells, form a cap over the lesion.

Advanced disease is associated with calcification of the atheroma.

Complicated plaques

Ulceration or fissuring of the fibrous cap exposes the plaque contents to the circulation, resulting in thrombus formation. Inflammation associated with the plaque destroys the media, weakening the vessel wall. The vascular consequences of atheroma are therefore:

- Arterial narrowing causing ischaemia
- Arterial occlusion resulting in infarction
- Arterial wall weakening resulting in aneurysm formation
- Arterial embolism

Thrombosis

A thrombus is a solid mass of blood constituents that forms in both arteries and veins. It consists of fibrin, platelets and entrapped red blood cells. If the thrombus occludes a vessel, it causes infarction. Released fragments of thrombus can travel in the bloodstream to occlude distal vessels.

Contact with damaged endothelium or the contents of an atheromatous plaque triggers the coagulation cascade. This ultimately results in the conversion of fibrinogen monomer to fibrin polymer. On contact with fibrin or collagen, the platelets release their granules, which promotes the aggregation of adjacent platelets. As a result, a mass of fibrin and platelets covers the endothelial defect. Factors that promote thrombus formation include:

- Vessel wall changes
- Changes in blood constituents
- Changes in blood flow

These are known as Virchow's triad.

The thrombus is often cleared by the fibrinolytic system. In this process, plasminogen activator released from the endothelial cells converts plasminogen to plasmin, which dissolves the fibrin. The thrombosed vessel can undergo recanalisation – endothelial cells grow out from the vessel wall and create new channels through the thrombus. Alternatively, the thrombus occludes the vessel, resulting in infarction. Released fragments of thrombus sometimes travel via the bloodstream to occlude distal vessels.

Embolism

An embolus is material in the blood that has the ability to lodge in a vessel and block its lumen. An embolus arises either within or outside the circulatory system (**Table 9.3**). Embolism to the pulmonary arteries originates in the deep veins. Embolism to other organs and the limbs originates in the heart or large arteries.

Ischaemia and infarction

Ischaemia occurs when an organ or tissue has a perfusion lower than its metabolic needs. Arterial ischaemia occurs as a result of:

- Atheromatous narrowing
- Thrombosis
- Embolism
- Low-flow states (e.g cardiac failure)
- Vasculitis
- Hypertensive vascular disease
- Spasm

Its outcome is be influenced by various factors (**Figure 9.6**). Infarction occurs when tissue necrosis result from ischaemia. Both ischaemia and infarction can be the result of arterial, venous or capillary disease. Blocked or damaged capillaries can also cause tissue ischaemia, as in frostbite or diabetic microangiopathy in the absence of arterial disease.

After infarction, polymorphs and macrophages remove the dead tissue. Capillaries grow into the area, and granulation tissue forms. The growth of fibroblasts into the region creates a scar.

Sources of emboli	
Within the circulation	Outside the circulation
Thrombus	Fat
Atheromatous plaque	Gas
Infected thrombus	Amniotic fluid
Endocardial or cardiac valve vegetations	Tumour
	Foreign material

Table 9.3 Sources of emboli

Factors influencing the outcome of ischaemia	
Adequacy of cardiac function	Anatomy of the arterial supply
Speed of onset	Susceptibility of tissues

Figure 9.6 Factors influencing the outcome of ischaemia.

Causes of gangrene	
Cause	Examples
Arterial	Atheroma, thrombosis, embolism, diabetic microangiopathy, Buerger's disease
Venous	Acute venous occlusion
Infective	Gas gangrene, Fournier's disease
Traumatic	Vascular trauma, burns, chemicals, irradiation

Table 9.4 Causes of gangrene.

Gangrene

Gangrene is the term used to describe tissue death. Its the causes are shown in **Table 9.4**. Dry gangrene usually occurs following a gradual reduction in blood flow. Wet gangrene occurs when there is sudden tissue necrosis, often with superadded infection.

History, examination and investigation

Symptoms due to either arterial or venous disease depend on the vessels involved, the speed of onset of the underlying pathology and the state of the collateral circulation. Common symptoms and signs of vascular disease are shown in **Table 9.5**.

Common symptoms and signs of vascular disease	
Symptoms	Signs
Leg pain	Foot ulceration
Alteration in peripheral sensation	Peripheral oedema
	Absence of peripheral pulses
Foot ulceration	Muscle tenderness
Limb swelling	Varicose veins
	Lipodermatosclerosis

Table 9.5 Common symptoms and signs of vascular disease

History

Arterial disease usually presents with limb pain. Acute arterial occlusion causes a sudden onset of limb pain, often associated with loss of function and altered sensation. Gradual arterial occlusion presents with intermittent claudication – the development of pain in the muscles of the thigh or calf that is induced by exercise. The pain invariably starts after walking a particular distance and is relieved by rest. If the disease progresses, rest pain develops. This is often initially relieved by hanging the leg out of bed.

Venous disease often presents with swelling of the limb. Acute venous occlusion causes painful limb swelling. Chronic venous insufficiency causes painless swelling of the affected limb. The patient often notices brown discolouration or skin ulceration around the medial malleolus.

> When assessing a patient with vascular disease, enquire about risk factors (e.g. smoking, hypertension, diabetes and family history) and remember that vascular diseases can affect other parts of the circulation (e.g. cardiovascular and cerebrovascular).

Examination

Examination of the arterial system focuses on the presenting symptoms but also assesses the remainder the arterial tree. Examination of the venous system assesses both superficial and deep veins.

Arterial system

The following are assessed when examining the arterial system:

- The pulses
- Pulse rate and rhythm
- Pulse volume and character
- Arterial blood pressure
- Peripheral arterial sufficiency
- The aorta

The sites of the peripheral pulses are shown in **Figure 9.7**. An abdominal aortic aneurysm usually presents with an expansile epigastric lump. The expansile nature is best appreciated by placing a hand either side of the mass and

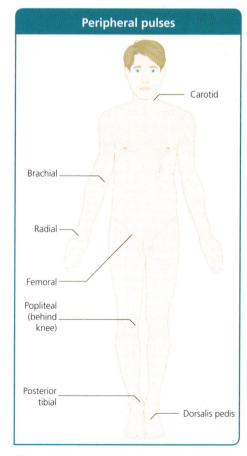

Peripheral pulses

- Carotid
- Brachial
- Radial
- Femoral
- Popliteal (behind knee)
- Posterior tibial
- Dorsalis pedis

Figure 9.7 Sites of the peripheral pulses.

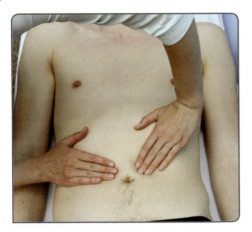

Figure 9.8 Examination for an abdominal aortic aneurysm.

> The vascular angle (Buerger's angle) is the angle to which the leg has to be raised before it develops pallor. With a healthy circulation, the toes stay pink even when the limb is raised by 90°. Raising an ischaemic leg for 30–60 seconds may cause pallor. A vascular angle of less than 20° indicates severe ischaemia.

feeling for increased diameter of the mass in time with the heart rate (**Figure 9.8**).

If there is acute obstruction of the arterial supply to the limb, it will look pale and feel cold. The skin becomes discoloured. If the obstruction is untreated, it leads to gangrene. Pressure on the skin will cause blanching with slow capillary return when the pressure is released. Peripheral pulses are usually absent, and muscle tenderness sometimes occurs.

In acute aterial occlusion, signs of chronic obstruction of the arterial supply, such as loss of hair and wasting of the muscles my be absent. If the occlusion progresses, discolouration of the skin (e.g. cyanosis) and skin ulceration over the heel or sole of the foot often occurs. Gentle pressure on the toes causes skin blanching, and the colour returns once the pressure is released. The normal capillary refill time is almost instantaneous and is abnormal if it is more than 2 seconds.

Venous system

Examination of the venous system should assess patency and check for the presence of varicose veins. Uncomplicated varicose veins are often asymptomatic. Examination begins by inspecting the veins with the patient standing. First look at the distribution of the veins – long or short saphenous on the medial and lateral aspects of the leg respectively (see page 213). Also note the possible presence of complications and the skin changes of varicose veins such as hyperpigmentation, peripheral oedema, and ulceration. The groin is inspected for a saphena varix, dilatation of the saphenofemoral junction, presenting as a groin lump. Next assess the competence of the valves (**Table 9.6**).

Acute venous occlusion causes a painful swollen limb. The overlying skin is often red, and palpation and sometimes the muscles are firm and indurated. There may be tenderness over the affected vein, and the superficial veins may be dilated. Pain can be induced on passive dorsiflexion of the ankle (Homan's sign).

Investigation

Peripheral vascular disease often remains clinically silent until late in life; it is more

Tests of valvular incompetence in varicose veins	
Test	Technique
Cough test	Place the fingers over the long saphenous vein just below the saphenous opening and ask the patient to cough. A palpable fluid thrill is felt if the saphenofemoral junction is incompetent
Percussion test	Place the fingers below the saphenous opening and tap the vein. Transmission of the tap indicates that the valves between the two fingers are incompetent
Trendelenburg test	Ask the patient to lie on the couch with the leg elevated. Place a tourniquet just below the saphenous opening. Lower the patient's leg and ask them to stand. If the veins do not refill, the saphenofemoral junction is incompetent

Table 9.6 Tests of valvular incompetence in varicose veins

common in men and usually presents beyond retirement. A significant degree of occlusion of the arterial tree is required before symptoms arise. The clinical condition progresses as the degree of stenosis increases. Arterial investigations are used to:

- Confirm the clinical impression of arterial disease
- Assess the severity of the disease
- Allow the preoperative planning of surgical or radiological interventions

Phlegmasia alba dolens describes a swollen pale limb due to thrombosis of the deep veins, with sparing of the superficial veins. **Phlegmasia cerulea dolens** describes a swollen cyanotic and congested limb caused by thrombosis of both the deep and the superficial veins.

Hand-held Doppler scanning

A hand-held Doppler probe is used to assess the arterial system. Measurements of arterial pressure are made both at rest and after exercise.

In a normal individual, arterial pressures are greater in the lower limb than the upper limb. A comparison of these measurements is used to assess the severity of peripheral vascular disease. The ankle–brachial pressure index (ABPI) is the ratio of the systolic pressure in the better foot to the brachial systolic pressure (**Figure 9.9**). It falls with increasing disease severity:

- In a healthy individual, the ankle–brachial pressure index is >1
- In patients with intermittent claudication, the ratio is usually 0.4–0.7
- In patients with critical limb ischaemia, it is usually 0.1–0.4

In healthy individuals, arterial pressures in the foot do not fall after exercise. In patients with intermittent claudication, the ankle–brachial pressure index decreases after exercise and recovery to normal values is delayed by several minutes. Lower limb pressures are sometimes falsely elevated in patients with

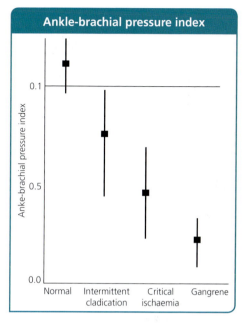

Figure 9.9 Relationship of clinical features to the ankle–brachial pressure index.

diabetes if there is calcification in the vessel walls.

Arterial pressures, also measured by Doppler scanning, in the toes provide an accurate assessment of the distal arterial circulation. Normal toe pressures are 90–100 mmHg. Pressures less than 30 mmHg suggest critical limb ischaemia. They are not influenced by calcification in the pedal vessels, which is particularly seen with diabetes.

Duplex ultrasonography

Duplex ultrasonography is a non-invasive combination of pulsed Doppler and real time B-mode ultrasound. It allows the vessels and any associated narrowing to be imaged.

The arterial blood flow and the waveform of the pressure wave can be simultaneously assessed. In healthy individuals, a 'triphasic' wave is obtained with a rapid antegrade flow during systole, a transient reverse flow in early diastole and a slow antegrade flow in late diastole. Arterial stenosis results in a 'biphasic' waveform. This shows a reduced rate of rise of the antegrade flow, a decreased amplitude of the forward velocity and a loss of reverse flow.

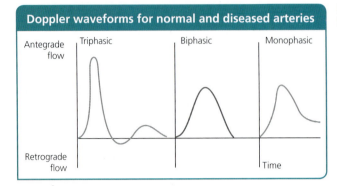

Doppler waveforms for normal and diseased arteries

Antegrade flow

Triphasic | Biphasic | Monophasic

Retrograde flow

Time

Figure 9.10 Doppler waveforms for normal and diseased arteries.

The velocity of the blood flow is increased at the site of the stenosis. Severe stenosis results in a 'monophasic' waveform (**Figure 9.10**).

Duplex ultrasound scanning has a sensitivity and specificity of 80% and 90%, respectively, for detecting stenotic lesions in the femoral and popliteal arteries.

Magnetic resonance angiography

Magnetic resonance angiography (MRA) is the use of MRI to image the blood vessels. A variety of techniques have been described based on flow effects and the use of intravenous contrast. The contrast medium is injected into a vein, and images are acquired during the first pass of the agent through the arteries. Unlike conventional or CT angiography, MRA does not display the lumen of the vessel; instead it indicates the blood flowing through the vessel.

Angiography

Angiography is usually performed under local anaesthesia using digital subtraction techniques. A catheter is inserted into an accessible artery, usually the femoral artery, using the Seldinger technique. Images are taken before and after the intra-arterial injection of contrast, with the patient in the same position, and the images subtracted from each other to visualise the arterial tree. Angiography is generally a safe procedure, and potential complications are related to either the technique or the contrast used (**Table 9.7**).

Complications of angiography

Local	Systemic
Haematoma	Embolisation
Arterial spasm	Anaphylactic reaction
Subintimal dissection	Toxic reactions
False aneurysm	Deterioration in renal function
Arteriovenous fistula	
Infection	

Table 9.7 Complications of angiography

> The Seldinger technique if used to place a cannula within a vessel. The vessel is punctured with a hollow needle, a guidewire is inserted through the needle, and the cannula is passed over it before the guidewire is removed.

CT angiography

CT angiography uses intravenous contrast and a significant dose of ionising radiation. The detailed images provided by spiral CT angiography and reconstruction are particularly useful for assessing aneurysmal disease.

> Peripheral vascular disease is often associated with impaired renal function. Caution is needed when radiological contrast is used in patients with arterial disease as it has the potential to further impair renal function.

Intermittent claudication and chronic limb ischaemia

Intermittent claudication is leg pain that is induced by exercise but relieved by rest and is caused by peripheral vascular disease. Critical limb ischaemia is defined as persistent ischaemic rest pain requiring regular analgesia. It is almost invariably associated with ulceration or gangrene of the foot or toes.

Epidemiology

About 5% of men over the age of 50 years have intermittent claudication. However, only 5% of patients with intermittent claudication progress to critical ischaemia each year. Peripheral vascular disease is an independent risk factor for other cardiovascular diseases.

Aetiology

Intermittent claudication and critical limb ischaemia occur when atheroma affects the lower limbs. Many patients have clinical features of other ischaemic conditions, including angina, myocardial infarction or cerebrovascular events.

Clinical features

The pain of intermittent claudication usually occurs after the patient has walked a predictable distance and is often described as 'cramp' or 'tightness'. The location depends on the vessels that are involved:

- Buttock and hip – aortoiliac disease
- Thigh – common femoral artery or aortoiliac disease
- Calf – superficial or popliteal femoral artery disease
- Foot claudication – tibial or peroneal artery disease

The rest pain that characterises critical limb ischaemia occurs or is worsened when the foot is elevated (e.g. in bed) and is improved with the foot dependent. It is almost invariably associated with foot ulceration or gangrene (**Figure 9.11**). Peripheral pulses are

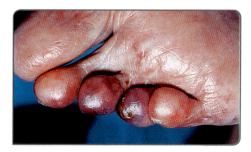

Figure 9.11 A critically ischaemic foot.

often present in patients with intermittent claudication but are invariably absent in patients with critical limb ischaemia.

Diagnostic approach

It is important to assess whether the symptoms are worsening, stable or improving. Clinical deterioration warrants further investigation and potential intervention. The impact on social function needs to be identified. By a careful history, vascular and neurological examination and the use of Doppler studies, intermittent claudication needs to be differentiated from spinal stenosis, which also causes exercise-induced leg pain. Spinal stenosis is, however, usually associated with neurological symptoms and the pain is relieved by spinal flexion. Critical limb ischaemia requires investigation to confirm the diagnosis and identify the site of the underlying vascular stenosis or occlusion.

Investigations

Intermittent claudication is essentially a clinical diagnosis. The severity of the underlying peripheral vascular disease is assessed by measuring the ankle–brachial pressure index. Investigation also aims to identify risk factors such as diabetes and hypercholesterolaemia.

The diagnosis of critical limb ischaemia is confirmed by measuring the ankle–brachial pressure index. Duplex ultrasonography can identify the site of the stenosis. MRA allows a more accurate non-invasive assessment of the arterial system and is especially useful when planning interventional radiological or surgical interventions.

Management

With appropriate management, more than 75% of patients with intermittent claudication remain stable or even show a clinical improvement over time.

Conservative management

The initial management is usually conservative. Reduction of risk factors includes advice to stop smoking, control of hypertension, the use of lipid-lowering drugs and antiplatelet medications, and good diabetic control as appropriate. Patients are advised to lose weight and undertake regular exercise as part of a supervised exercise programme. Indications for operative intervention in peripheral vascular disease are disabling claudication and critical limb ischaemia.

Revascularisation

There are two main approaches to the revascularisation of a critically ischaemic limb: balloon angioplasty with or without stenting, and bypass surgery. In recent years, however, expansion in the range of interventional radiological procedures have widened their indications and uses. Clinical outcomes are similar to those of balloon angioplasty and bypass surgery. As a result, the number of bypass operations performed for critical limb ischaemia has fallen.

Balloon angioplasty

In percutaneous transluminal angioplasty, a narrowed or obstructed blood vessel is mechanically widened. An empty, collapsed balloon on a guidewire is passed into the narrowed segment and inflated to a fixed size using water pressures around 75–500 times normal blood pressure. The balloon crushes the fatty deposits, opening up the blood vessel. The balloon is then deflated and withdrawn.

The best results are seen in those patients with short-segment stenoses (less than 2 cm long). Complications occur in fewer than 2% of patients and include:

- Wound haematoma
- Acute thrombosis
- Distal embolisation
- Rupture of the arterial wall

Bypass surgery

Long, multifocal or inaccessible lesions are better treated by surgery. In these complex situations, the arterial disease is not amenable to endovascular intervention. For superficial femoral disease, the surgical option is a femoropopliteal bypass. For popliteal or tibial vessel disease, the surgical option is usually a femorodistal bypass. The bypass is performed from the common femoral artery to either the anterior tibial, posterior tibial or peroneal arteries at the ankle or foot. Arterial bypass grafts can be either biological or synthetic, and various types are available (**Table 9.8**). Autologous vein is the best graft material but is not always available.

A late presentation of acute limb ischaemia or critical limb ischaemia that is not suitable for vascular reconstruction often necessitates amputation. The level of the amputation is influenced by the viability of the soft tissue and the ability to fit a prosthetic limb. The site of the amputation influences the patient's postoperative mobility. About 80% of below-knee amputees will walk, but this is reduced to 40% for patients undergoing above-knee amputation.

Options for the treatment of critical limb ischaemia are:

- Stent
- Angioplasty
- Graft
- Amputation

Types of vascular graft	
Biological grafts	Synthetic grafts
Long saphenous vein	Dacron
Internal mammary artery	Velour
Dacron-coated umbilical vein	Polyfluorotetraethylene (PTFE)

Table 9.8 Types of vascular graft

Prognosis

At 5 years of follow-up, 10% of patients with intermittent claudication and 50% of those with critical ischaemia will have undergone an amputation. In addition, 20% of patients with intermittent claudication and 50% of those with critical ischaemia will have died, usually from ischaemic heart disease.

Acute limb ischaemia

Acute limb ischaemia is defined as a sudden decrease in limb perfusion that causes a potential threat to limb viability. The effects of sudden arterial occlusion depend on the state of the collateral blood supply. The collateral supply in the leg is usually inadequate unless pre-existing occlusive disease has encouraged the collateral circulation to develop.

Epidemiology

Acute limb ischaemia affects about 1 per 1000 of the population per year and accounts for about 10% of the vascular surgery workload.

Aetiology

Acute limb ischaemia usually results from embolism. The source of the embolus is often from the left atrium in patients in atrial fibrillation, mural thrombus after a myocardial infarct, prosthetic or diseased heart valves, an aneurysm or atheromatous stenosis. Other common causes of acute limb ischaemia are thrombosis, trauma and arterial dissection, i.e. the passage if blood into the arterial wall, narrowing or occluding its lumen. Rare causes include tumour, foreign bodies or a paradoxical embolus arising in the venous system that enters the arterial system via an atrial or ventricular septal defect.

Clinical features

Acute limb ischaemia presents with a sudden onset of limb pain. It is most common in the lower limb but is occasionally seen in the upper limb. It may be associated with a lost or altered sensation and discolouration of the extremity. The severity of the symptoms depends on the adequacy of the collateral circulation.

> The clinical features of acute limb ischaemia can be remembered using the '6 Ps':
>
> - Pain
> - Pulselessness
> - Pallor
> - Paraesthesia
> - Paralysis
> - Perishingly cold

Attempting to differentiate an embolism from a thrombosis is vital to determine the best treatment. However, this is often difficult. Important clinical features include the rapidity of onset of the symptoms, features of pre-existing chronic arterial disease, a potential source of embolus and the state of pedal pulses in the contralateral limb. A sudden onset of symptoms in the absence of peripheral vascular disease favours the diagnosis of an embolus.

> Fixed staining of the skin and sensory loss are late signs of ischaemia and need urgent surgical intervention.

Diagnostic approach

Acute limb ischaemia is a surgical emergency and the diagnosis is usually clear from the history and examination. The patient should be anticoagulated with heparin and be given opiate opiate analgesia. Associated cardiac disease (e.g. arrythmias) should be investigated and a cardiology opinion obtained as required. The subsequent treatment options are different for embolic and thrombotic disease.

Investigations

There is usually no requirement for interventional radiological investigations before considering surgery. If there is diagnostic doubt, a Duplex ultrasound scan helps to confirm the presence and level of arterial occlusion. Arteriography with a view to balloon angioplasty should be considered in patients felt to have acute occlusion in the presence of chronic limb ischaemia.

Management

Patients shown to have embolic disease should be considered for embolectomy or intra-arterial thrombolysis. Those with thrombotic disease should undergo intra-arterial thrombolysis, and angioplasty and bypass surgery should be considered.

Emergency embolectomy

Emergency embolectomy is performed under general or local anaesthesia. The femoral vessels are exposed, and the inflow and outflow are both controlled. An arteriotomy (i.e. a surgical incision in the common femoral artery) is performed, and a Fogarty balloon embolectomy catheter is inserted with the balloon deflated. The balloon is then inflated and the catheter withdrawn to remove the embolus.

If the embolectomy fails, an on-table angiogram should be performed to decide whether a bypass graft or intraoperative thrombolysis will be carried out.

Intra-arterial thrombolysis

In this technique, an angiogram is first performed and a catheter is advanced into the thrombus. A thrombolytic agent (e.g. streptokinase) and heparin are then infused. The arteriogram is repeated 6–12 hours later. A chronic arterial stenosis can often be managed by balloon angioplasty. Success rates of 60–70% have been reported for balloon angioplasty after intra-arterial thrombolysis.

Prognosis

Despite technological advances, acute limb ischaemia is associated with limb loss in as many as 30% of patients, and has an in-hospital mortality of 20%. Cardiopulmonary complications (e.g. myocardial infarction) account for the majority of the deaths due to multiple cardiovascular co-morbidities of these patients.

Compartment syndromes

The muscles of the upper and lower limbs are enclosed by fascial planes that divide the limbs into compartments. There are two compartments in the forearm and three in the lower leg. These have a fixed volume so any muscle swelling within them results in an increase in compartmental pressure.

Compartment syndrome occurs when the circulation and function of the tissues within the closed space is compromised by an increase in pressure. Venous drainage is impeded before arterial inflow, further exacerbating the swelling (**Figure 9.12**). The most common causes of compartment syndrome are ischaemia–reperfusion injury and lower limb fractures.

Clinical features

Compartment syndromes usually present within 24 hours of the precipitating insult. The main clinical features are increasing pain and an altered sensation in the distribution of the nerves passing through the compartment. Muscle swelling, tenderness and pain on passive movement often occur.

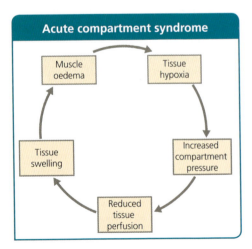

Figure 9.12 The vicious circle of acute compartment syndrome.

As the arterial inflow into a muscle compartment is rarely compromised in compartment syndrome, peripheral pulses may still be present.

Management

Compartment syndrome is a surgical emergency as failure to recognise a compartment syndrome will result in muscle necrosis and fibrosis. Constricting casts or splints must be removed. If there is no improvement, fasciotomies should be performed to decompress the compartment.

Diabetic foot

Foot problems are common in diabetes. About 30% of diabetics have a peripheral neuropathy. Many diabetics also have features of peripheral vascular disease. Approximately, 15% of diabetics develop foot ulceration, the incidence increasing with age.

Clinical features

A diabetic foot usually presents with either infection or ulceration. Infection is seen as cellulitis or osteomyelitis. Ulceration is due to a combination of vascular disease and neuropathy. The ulceration typically occurs over the tips of the toes and the heel (**Figure 9.13**).

Management

Diabetics should be monitored for foot problems. Education is given on washing the feet, care of corns and calluses, toenail cutting and suitable footwear. In those with ulceration, the presence of infection and vascular insufficiency is assessed.

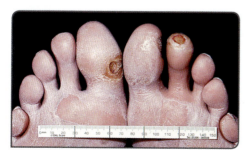

Figure 9.13 Ulceration of a diabetic foot

In patients with a diabetic foot, preventing complications is preferable to controlling infection and resorting to surgery.

Medication

Wound swabs often show Gram-negative, Gram-positive and anaerobic bacteria. Osteomyelitis is usually caused by *Staphylococcus aureus* infection. Plain radiography or MRI may demonstrate the extent of the infection. In order to reduce the risk of amputation, the threshold for antibiotic use should be low, and antibiotics should be selected based on culture sensitivities.

Surgery

Surgery, debridement or amputation, may be required if there is progression of the infection despite appropriate antibiotic treatment. Revascularisation should be considered if arterial insufficiency is present. Patients with diabetes have a predisposition for disease in the medium-sized vessels, especially at the popliteal trifurcation. However, the distal pedal vessels are often spared. Femorodistal bypass grafting may therefore be required.

All patients with diabetic ulceration should undergo non-invasive vascular assessment using Doppler ultrasound to assess the need for vascular intervention. The ankle–brachial pressure index is often falsely elevated due to arterial calcification, and normal values are often still be recorded even with diabetes with significant major vascular disease.

Carotid artery disease

Carotid artery disease is either asymptomatic or symptomatic. Symptomatic carotid artery disease results in either a transient ischaemic attack (TIA) or a stroke.

Epidemiology

A patient with an asymptomatic carotid stenosis with 50% narrowing of the artery, has a 1-2% annual risk of a stroke, which is higher than the risk in the general population. This risk increases with the degree of arterial stenosis. Once a stenosis has become symptomatic, the risk of a stroke is further increased. After a first ischaemic stroke, the risk of a further stroke is about 10% in the first year and 5% in subsequent years.

Aetiology

Atherosclerosis in the carotid arteries is most common at the bifurcation of the common carotid artery (**Figure 9.14**). Stenosis of the internal carotid artery is a potentially treatable cause of ischaemic stroke, TIAs and retinal infarction.

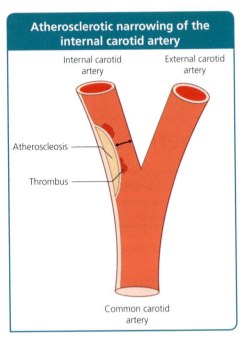

Atherosclerotic narrowing of the internal carotid artery

Internal carotid artery

External carotid artery

Atheroscleosis

Thrombus

Common carotid artery

Figure 9.14 Atherosclerotic narrowing of the internal carotid artery with adherent thrombus.

Clinical features

A TIA results from a sudden and temporary loss of blood flow to an area of the brain and usually lasts from only a few minutes to about 1 hour. The symptoms are dependent on the territory of the brain affected (**Table 9.9**). They usually resolve within 24 hours, with complete recovery. The heart and peripheral vascular system should be examined. In particular, the presence of atrial fibrillation, indicating a potential cardiac source of emboli, should be assessed. Examination sometimes shows a bruit at the bifurcation of the carotid artery.

Symptoms of carotid artery disease		
Territory	Vessels involved	Symptoms
Anterior	Anterior cerebral	Weakness or loss of sensation affecting the contralateral lower limb, loss of sense of smell
	Middle cerebral	Weakness or loss of sensation affecting the contralateral upper and lower limb, loss of sensation of the face, confusion and dizziness, loss of coordination and movement, changes in perception
Posterior	Posterior cerebral	Temporary loss of vision or blurred vision, homonymous hemianopia, cortical blindness
Vertebrobasilar	Vertebral	Inability to speak clearly or slurred speech, vertigo

Table 9.9 Symptoms of carotid artery disease

> **The presence of a carotid bruit is an unreliable guide to the severity of stenosis** as a bruit may be absent even in patients with severe stenosis.

Diagnostic approach

By the time the patient seeks medical help, the signs have often resolved. However, a concise history is nearly always able to diagnose a TIA. Subsequent investigation aims to identify any associated risk factors and the underlying cause.

Investigations

Most surgeons decide to operate on the basis of non-invasive assessments alone. These include the following:

- Duplex ultrasonography is the best method for the initial assessment of carotid artery disease
- Doppler recordings allow an assessment of the flow at the site of the stenosis
- Ultrasonography allows the arterial anatomy to be imaged (**Figure 9.15**)
- MRA is increasingly used as it provides detailed images of the carotid artery and an accurate assessment of the anatomy and extent of any stenosis

Carotid angiography was until recently the gold standard for assessing the degree of stenosis. Its use has rapidly decreased as it has

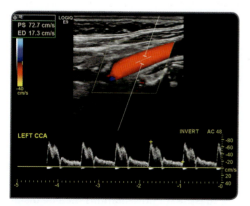

Figure 9.15 Duplex ultrasound scan of a left carotid artery stenosis

a 4% risk of inducing a further neurological event and a 1% risk of permanent paralysis from stroke.

Management

The initial management of carotid artery disease is medical, but surgery may be required in a carefully selected group of patients, where the benefit of surgery has been shown to outweigh the risk.

Medication

Patients are advised to smoking, and hypertension and diabetes are controlled. Prophylactic aspirin prevents 40 'vascular events' such as stroke or myocardial infarction, per 1000 patients treated over 3 years. It should be given to patients with asymptomatic stenoses and those in whom an ischaemic stroke has been confirmed by CT scanning.

Surgery

Symptomatic patients with a carotid stenosis should be assessed by a vascular surgeon within a week of onset of a stroke or symptoms of a TIA. Those with a symptomatic carotid stenosis of less than 50% should not undergo surgery as benefit has not been clearly demonstrated. Surgery is currently not indicated in asymptomatic patients as the risks of surgery outweigh the benefits.

Carotid endarterectomy

This procedure corrects a stenosis in the common carotid artery and is used to prevent a stroke. It is performed under local anaesthesia to allow direct monitoring of the neurological status in an awake patient. With general anaesthesia, indirect methods of assessing cerebral perfusion must be used, for example transcranial Doppler analysis.

In carotid endarterectomy, the internal, common and external carotid arteries are clamped. The lumen of the internal carotid artery is then opened, and the atheromatous plaque is removed. Some surgeons use a temporary shunt to maintain the blood supply to the brain during the procedure.

Carotid angioplasty and stenting

Carotid angioplasty is being increasingly used to dilate stenoses. It involves the selective catheterisation of the common carotid artery and often the deployment of a stent.

In this technique, a guidewire is advanced into external carotid artery, and a protective sheath is placed in the normal segment of the common carotid artery. The stenotic lesion is negotiated with a distal protection device. This is placed in the internal carotid artery and is either a balloon occlusion system or polyurethane sac used to prevent any embolisation of thrombus during the angioplasty procedure. Angioplasty is then performed, a stent is deployed and the distal protection device is retrieved.

Abdominal aortic aneurysm

An aneurysm is an abnormal dilatation of a blood vessel, classified as either a true or a false aneurysm. A true aneurysm involves one or more layers of the vessel wall. The wall of a false aneurysm is made up of connective tissue, and the condition is often the result of trauma or surgery (**Figure 9.16**). True aneurysms occur at several sites, for example the aorta and the iliac, femoral and popliteal arteries. The causes include:

- Congenital causes – Berry aneurysms on the circle of Willis
- Atheroma
- Trauma
- Infection – fungal infection or syphilis

An abdominal aortic aneurysm is an increase in aortic diameter of more than 50% greater than normal. In absolute terms, it is usually regarded as an aortic diameter of more than 3 cm.

Epidemiology

Abdominal aortic aneurysms are more prevalent in elderly men and account for 2% of deaths in men over the age of 55 years. The male-to-female ratio is 4:1. Approximately 3000 elective and 1500 emergency operations for abdominal aortic aneurysms are performed in the UK each year.

Aetiology

The risk factors include hypertension, peripheral vascular disease and a family history of an abdominal aortic aneurysm.

Clinical features

About 75% of abdominal aortic aneurysms are asymptomatic. Possible symptoms prior to rupture include epigastric and back pain. Malaise and weight loss are sometimes seen in patients with inflammatory aneurysms, which are a subtype of aneurysm characterised by a thickened and inflamed wall. Abdominal examination may show an expansile epigastric mass. A ruptured abdominal aortic aneurysms usually presents with sudden-onset abdominal pain, hypovolaemic shock and a pulsatile epigastric mass. Rare presentations include distal embolic features, an aortocaval fistula (with a continuous epigastric bruit) and a primary aortointestinal fistula (with an exsanguinat-

The difference between a true and a false aneurysm

True aneurysm   False aneurysm

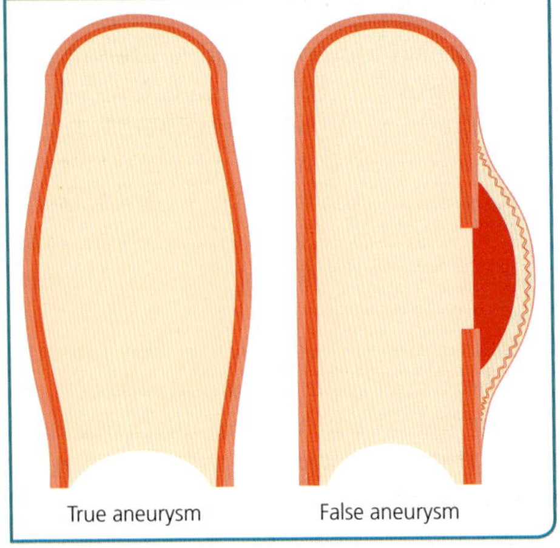

Figure 9.16 The difference between a true and a false aneurysm.

ing upper gastrointestinal bleed presenting with frank haematemesis, melaena or torrential fresh rectal blood loss).

> A ruptured abdominal aortic aneurysm occasionally presents with loin pain, similar to that of ureteric colic. Always be cautious about making a diagnosis of ureteric colic in an elderly man with risk factors for an abdominal aortic aneurysm.

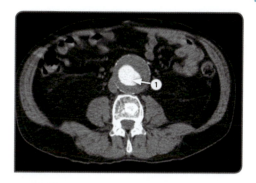

Figure 9.17 Abdominal CT scan showing ① an abdominal aortic aneurysm.

Diagnostic approach

The diagnosis can usually be confirmed by finding a pulsatile epigastric mass. An ultrasound scan will confirm the diagnosis if there is any diagnostic doubt.

Investigations

The preoperative investigation of patients being considered for elective surgery needs to determine the extent of the aneurysm and the patient's fitness for operation. Abdominal CT (**Figure 9.17**) with three-dimensional reconstruction (**Figure 9.18**) allows an assessment of the size of the aneurysm, its relation to the renal arteries and involvement of the iliac vessels, important in planning endovascular or surgical repair.

The most significant postoperative morbidity and mortality is related to cardiac disease. If the patient has preoperative symptoms of cardiac disease, a cardiological opinion will be required. Cardiac investigation with a view to coronary revascularisation is required in up to 10% patients before elective surgery for an abdominal aortic aneurysms.

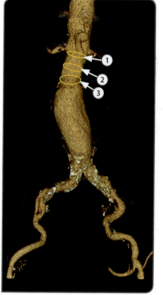

Figure 9.18 Three-dimensional reconstruction of a CT scan showing an abdominal aortic aneurysm. ① Patent renal arteries ② 15 mm infrarenal aorta ③ Proximal aneurysm.

Management

Conservative management

In patients with an abdominal aortic aneurysm, the aortic diameter expands at approximately 10% per year. The risk of rupture increases as the aneurysm expands. Overall, only 15% of aneurysms rupture, and about 85% of patients with an abdominal aortic aneurysm die from an unrelated cause.

Patients with small aneurysms (<6 cm in diameter) do not require surgery. They are observed and followed up with serial ultrasound scans. Surgery is considered if the aneurysm continues to increase in size.

Surgery

Indications for surgery include:

- Rupture
- A symptomatic aneurysm
- Rapid expansion
- An asymptomatic aneurysm that is more than 6 cm in diameter

Selection of patients for elective surgery, by either the open or endovasascular route, depends on an a comparison between the risk of rupture of the aneurysm and the risks of surgery.

Open aneurysm surgery

During open surgery, the aorta is clamped and the diseased section of aorta replaced with a prosthetic graft. Open aneurysm surgery presents a significant physiological challenge to the patient. The morbidity of open aneurysm surgery is related to the surgical exposure and cross-clamping of the infrarenal aorta in the abdomen, allowing continued perfusion of the kidneys during the surgical procedure. Late complications of an aortic graft include infection, an aortoenteric fistula and the formation of a false aneurysm.

Endovascular aneurysm repair

This technique is a recent development in the last decade in which a stent, inserted percutaneously through the femoral artery, is placed across the aneurysm. Proximal and distal cuffs deployed during expansion of the stent anchor the graft and exclude the aneurysm from the circulation. Endovascular repair is associated with reduced physiological stress compared with open surgery. However, due to the relationship of the anuerysm to the renal and iliac arteries, only about 40% of aneurysms are suitable for this type of repair.

Prognosis

The mortality after emergency surgery is more than 50%. The mortality following elective surgery should be less than 5%.

Vascular trauma

Vascular trauma occurs as a result of either blunt or penetrating injury. The pattern of injury differs according to the mechanism of injury. Blunt vascular trauma is often associated with fractures, tissue loss and an increased incidence of amputation. The signs of blunt vascular trauma are often subtle and the diagnosis is often delayed. Vascular injury is categorised as:

- Contusion
- Puncture
- Laceration
- Transection

Signs of vascular trauma	
Hard signs	Soft signs
Absent pulses	Haematoma
Bruit or palpable thrill	History of haemorrhage at scene of accident
Active haemorrhage	
Expanding haematoma	Unexplained hypotension
Distal ischaemia	Peripheral nerve deficit

Table 9.10 Signs of vascular trauma

Clinical features

The clinical features depend on the site, mechanism and extent of the injury. Signs of vascular injury are classically divided into 'hard' and 'soft' signs (**Table 9.10**).

Investigations

Hard signs of vascular injury often require urgent surgical exploration without prior investigation. If time permits, angiography is to confirm the extent of the injury in a patient who is stable but has equivocal signs. It is also used to exclude vascular injury when hard signs are absent but there is a strong suspicion of injury. The role of Doppler ultrasonography in vascular trauma has not yet been defined.

Management

The management of vascular trauma often requires a multidisciplinary approach including orthopaedic and plastic surgeons.

The aims of surgery are to control life-threatening haemorrhage and to prevent limb ischaemia. Revascularisation is unlikely to be successful if surgery is delayed for more than 6 hours.

Surgery

Vascular repair is usually performed once proximal control of the vessels has been gained and the wound has been debrided. The options include:

- Simple suture of a puncture hole or laceration
- Vein patch
- Resection and end-to-end anastomosis
- Interpositional graft (the use of vascular graft to bridge the defect)

The ideal interpositional graft is a section of the contralateral saphenous vein. Prosthetic graft material have to be used if the vein is poor or there is bilateral limb trauma. Primary amputation should be considered if there is severe damage with a significant risk of a reperfusion injury, or if the limb is likely to be painful and useless after surgery.

Reperfusion injury is systemic tissue damage caused when a blood supply is returned to ischaemic tissue. Tissue metabolites washed in to the circulation often result in significant systemic inflammation.

Complications of vascular trauma

The most common cause of a false aneurysm is catheterisation of the femoral artery. It often presents with pain, bruising and a pulsatile swelling. The diagnosis is confirmed by Doppler ultrasonography. It may be possible to obliterate the aneurysm using ultrasound-guided compression therapy, during which the aneurysm is compressed and occluded by pressure from the ultrasound probe. Alternatively, the puncture site occasionally needs to be sutured or a vein patch applied.

An arteriovenous fistula often presents several weeks after the injury. The patient complains of a swollen limb with dilated superficial veins. A 'machinery-type' bruit is often present throughout cardiac cycle. The diagnosis is confirmed by angiography. The fistula should be divided and both the vein and the artery sutured.

Varicose veins

Varicose veins are dilated superficial veins, usually of the lower limb, that arise due to incompetence of the venous valves. They usually occur in the distribution of the long and short saphenous veins.

Epidemiology

Varicose veins affects 20% and 10% of adult women and men, respectively. Until recently, 75,000 varicose vein operations were performed annually in UK. Surgery is now restricted to those with features of venous hypertension or ulceration.

Aetiology

Most cases are idiopathic but some are secondary to previous deep vein thrombosis. In addition, some individuals have congenital venous malformations that predispose to

varicose veins (e.g. Klippel–Trenaunay syndrome).

> **Klippel–Trenaunay syndrome is a rare condition characterised by cutaneous port wine stains, vascular malformations and excessive limb growth.** It is of autosomal dominant inheritance.

Clinical features

Varicose veins present as dilated superficial veins in the leg (**Figure 9.19**). Most are relatively asymptomatic. If symptoms occur, they are usually non-specific, for example leg pain and swelling. It is important to identify from the history features suggestive of a deep venous thrombosis (e.g. a previous lower limb fracture) as the dilated superficial veins may be the only venous drainage from the

Distribution of varicose veins

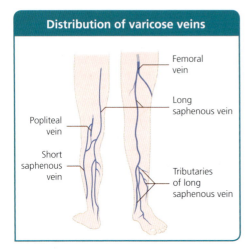

Femoral vein

Long saphenous vein

Popliteal vein

Short saphenous vein

Tributaries of long saphenous vein

Figure 9.19 Distribution of varicose veins

limb and surgery to the varicose veins is contraindicated.

Examination identifies the distribution of the varicose veins. The presence of complications such as varicose eczema (redness and flacking of the skin), lipodermatosclerosis (skin pigmentation around the medial malleolus) and venous ulceration must also be documented.

> **A saphena varix is a dilatation of the long saphenous vein at its junction with the femoral vein.** It presents as a groin lump and should be considered in the differential diagnosis of a femoral hernia.

Diagnostic approach

The diagnosis of varicose veins is clinical and can be confirmed by Doppler ultrasonography if surgery in particular is being considered.

Investigations

Duplex scanning should be considered if there is:

- Suspected incompetence of the short saphenous vein (to identify the site of the saphenofemoral junction which can have a variable position)

- Recurrent varicose veins
- Complications of the varicose veins (e.g. ulceration or lipodermatosclerosis)
- A history of deep venous thrombosis

Management

The management of varicose veins includes conservative measures, endovascular techniques and surgery. Absolute indications for intervention are:

- Lipodermatosclerosis leading to venous ulceration
- Recurrent superficial thrombophlebitis
- Bleeding from a ruptured saphena varix

Radiofrequency ablation

Radiofrequency ablation uses-high frequency alternating current delivered via a catheter that has been placed within the superficial vein under duplex ultrasound guidance. Local heating results in venous spasm and a collagen seal. It is associated with less pain than surgery. Complications include paraesthesia and skin burns. Recurrence rates are similar to those after open surgery.

Endovascular laser treatment

Endovascular laser treatment uses energy delivered via a narrow laser fibre, inserted in the superficial vein to cause heat injury of vessel wall and induce thrombosis. It is usually performed under local anaesthesia. Clinical and symptomatic improvement is seen in 95% of patients.

Sclerotherapy

Sclerotherapy is the intravenous injection of a chemical agent to induce thrombosis. It is suitable only for below-knee varicose veins. Before considering sclerotherapy, it is also necessary to exclude incompetence of the saphenofemoral junction and saphenopopliteal junction. Sclerotherapy alone in the presence of incompetence of the two junctions has a high incidence of recurrence.

In sclerotherapy, the needle is placed in the full vein with the patient standing. The vein is then emptied prior to injection. The principal sclerosants are 5% ethanolamine oleate and 0.5% sodium tetradecyl sulphate. Foam (a mixture of air and sclerosant) has recently been shown to be more effective than sclerosant alone. Compression is applied using grade compression stockings immediately after injection and is maintained for 6 weeks. The main complications of sclerotherapy are extravasation of the sclerosants, causing pigmentation or ulceration, and deep venous thrombosis.

Surgery

Surgery for varicose veins involves ligating the appropriate vein and removing ('stripping') the distal segment.

Stripping the long saphenous vein reduces the risk of recurrence of the varicose vein. The patient should be positioned supine with the head down at an angle of 20–30° (the Trendelenburg position), and the legs abducted 10–15°. The saphenofemoral junction is found 2 cm below and lateral to pubic tubercle and is the site for the surgical incision. Postoperative care should involve elevation of the foot of the bed for 12 hours. Class 2 varix stockings should be worn for at least 2 weeks.

For short saphenous vein surgery, the patient should be placed prone in a 20–30° head down position. The saphenopopliteal junction is ligated but has a very variable position so preoperative localisation with duplex ultrasonography is recommended.

> **Due to their close proximity, stripping of the short saphenous vein is associated with a risk of sural nerve damage.** This results in a loss of sensation on the lateral aspect of the foot.

Venous hypertension and leg ulceration

Leg ulceration is common, and its management imposes a considerable economic burden. Management of ulceration due to deep venous disease is difficult. However, healing is often promoted by surgical correction of superficial venous disease. Rare causes of leg ulceration include rheumatoid arthritis, malignancy and syphilis.

Epidemiology

Most cases of leg ulceration are caused by venous hypertension, which affects 1–2% of the population. About 40% of venous ulcers are due to hypertension in the superficial venous system.

Aetiology

Venous hypertension is the result of chronic venous insufficiency. Valves within both superficial and deep venous systems have an important role in maintaining normal venous pressure. Venous insufficiency usually occurs secondary to post-thrombotic syndrome causing damage to the deep venous valves. Occasionally, venous insufficiency is primary, with no obvious cause for the valvular dysfunction.

Venous insufficiency results in early refilling of the venous pool after muscle contraction. It causes a progressive and sustained increase in the pressure in the calf vein. This results in capillary dilatation and a leakage of plasma proteins and white cells into the tissues. The activation of the white cells damages the surrounding tissue.

Clinical features

Patients often have a history of leg swelling and skin changes consistent with chronic venous insufficiency. The history and examination should exclude other causes of leg ulceration. Signs of venous hypertension include:

- Perimalleolar oedema
- Pigmentation
- Lipodermatosclerosis
- Eczema
- Ulceration

Clinical assessment should identify previous deep vein thrombosis and assess the presence of arterial disease. It should also identify varicose veins and underlying valvular incompetencies.

Diagnostic approach

The diagnostic approach is to confirm the presence of venous hypertension and assess the presence of complications. The adequacy of the superficial and deep venous systems is then determined.

Investigations

Doppler scanning of the long and short saphenous veins and the perforators is used to assess the presence of venous reflux. The patency of the femoral and popliteal veins are also checked. Blood flow can be augmented by compressing the calf, deep inspiration or a Valsalva manoeuvre to assess flow and valvular function. Duplex ultrasonography allows both anatomical and functional assessments to be performed.

Management

Conservative management

The initial management is usually conservative. Elastic compression stockings provide graduated compression and produce a local alteration of venous flow and improve drainage of the superficial venous system. They have a minimal effect on deep vein dynamics. They do not cure hypertension but do protect the skin from its effects.

Surgery

Surgery is rarely required, and the outcome can be disappointing. The aims of surgery are to cure the venous hypertension and heal the ulceration. A combination of surgery of the superficial veins and compression is often required.

Marjolin ulceration

A Marjolin's ulcer is a squamous cell carcinoma arising at a site of chronic inflammation due to chronic venous ulceration, a burn or osteomyelitis. About 40% of Marjolin's ulcers occur on the lower limb. The malignant change is usually painless, and involvement of the lymph nodes is uncommon. The diagnosis is confirmed by a biopsy of the edge of the ulcer. Management involves adequate excision and skin grafting. Amputation is sometimes required for tumours that have invaded the deep tissues.

> In Marjolin's ulceration, there is usually a long period between the initiating injury and the malignant transformation. This is often as long as 10–25 years.

Lymphatic conditions

Lymphatic conditions present with either limb swelling (lymphoedema) or enlargement of the lymph nodes (lymphadenopathy).

Lymphoedema

Lymphoedema is due to progressive failure of the lymphatic system. It presents with gradual, often bilateral limb swelling (**Table 9.11**). Lymphoedema is primary, with no obvious or secondary cause to an underlying disease or medical intervention (**Table 9.12**).

Causes of lower limb swelling		
Bilateral pitting oedema	Painful unilateral oedema	Painless unilateral oedema
Heart failure	Deep venous thrombosis	Post-phlebitic limb
Renal disease	Superficial thrombophlebitis	Deep venous incompetence
Proteinuria	Cellulitis	Lymphoedema
Cirrhosis	Trauma	Immobility
Carcinomatosis	Ischaemia	
Nutritional		

Table 9.11 Causes of lower limb swelling

Causes of lymphoedema	
Primary lymphoedema	Secondary lymphoedema
Congenital (age <1 year) – familial or non-familial	Malignant disease
Praecox (age <35 years) – familial or non-familial	Surgery – axillary surgery or groin dissection
	Radiotherapy
Tarda (age >35 years)	Infection – parasitic (e.g. filariasis)

Table 9.12 Causes of lymphoedema

Epidemiology

Primary lymphoedema is rare and affects about 1 in 100,000 of the population. It is more common in women. The most common reason for secondary lymphoedema is surgery or radiotherapy for cancer.

> Lymphoedema of the arm occurs in about 10% of women undergoing an axillary node clearance for breast cancer.

Aetiology

Primary lymphoedema is usually bilateral. A proportion of patients have a family history of primary lymphoedema (Milroy's disease). It is due to aplasia, hypoplasia or hyperplasia of the lymphatics. In 80% of patients, there is obliteration of the distal lymphatics. In 10% of patients, proximal occlusion of the lymphatics in the abdomen and pelvis occurs. About 10% of patients develop incompetence of the lymphatic valves.

Chronic lymphoedema results in subcutaneous fibrosis, which can be worsened by secondary infection.

Clinical features

The presentation of either primary or secondary lymphoedema is usually with peripheral oedema that is worse on standing. This begins distally and progresses proximally. The affected limb usually feels heavy. With secondary lymphoedema, the underlying cause is often apparent. Examination shows non-pitting oedema. Skin examination often reveals hyperkeratosis, fissuring and secondary infection. Ulceration is rare.

Diagnostic approach

Lymphoedema is usually an obvious clinical diagnosis. The diagnostic approach aims to differentiate primary and secondary causes.

Investigations

Chronic venous insufficiency should be excluded using Doppler ultrasonography. Lymphoedema and its cause can be confirmed with lymphoscintigraphy and CT or MRI scanning. A normal result on lymphoscintigraphy essentially excludes a diagnosis of lymphoedema. Lymphangiography is painful and is no longer performed.

Management

The treatment is to reduce limb swelling, improve limb function and reduce the risk of infection. Swelling and limb function are treated by elevation, physiotherapy and manual lymphatic drainage, and external pneumatic compression. General skin care reduces the risk of infection.

Compression stockings should be applied once the swelling has reduced. Antibiotics should be given at the first sign of infection. Drugs (e.g. diuretics) are of no proven benefit. Surgery consists of two approaches: debulking (to excise the excess skin and subcutaneous tissue) and bypass procedures (to improve the lymphatic drainage).

Lymphadenopathy

Lymphadenopathy results from either neoplastic or inflammatory processes (**Table 9.13**).

Epidemiology

In adults in the developed world, 50% of cases of lymphadenopathy are neoplastic and 50% are inflammatory. In children, only 20% of cases are due to neoplasia. In the developing world, infective causes are more common, such as filariasis due to roundworm infection.

Causes of lymphadenopathy	
Cause	Examples
Neoplastic	Solid tumours – melanoma, breast, head and neck cancer
	Haematological – lymphoma, leukaemia, myeloproliferative disease
Inflammatory	Infection – bacterial, viral, fungal, tuberculous
	Autoimmune – rheumatoid arthritis, systemic lupus erythematosus
	Miscellaneous – e.g. dermatopathic lymphadenitis

Table 9.13 Causes of lymphadenopathy

Clinical features

The clinical assessment of patients presenting with lymphadenopathy includes:

- Duration of symptoms
- Distribution of lymphadenopathy
- Presence of pain
- Associated symptoms – fever, malaise and weight loss
- Examination – firm or rubbery, discrete or matted
- Presence of hepatosplenomegaly

Diagnostic approach

The diagnostic approach is to determine the cause and extent of the lymphadenopathy. Initially, a detailed history seeks out either an infective or a malignant cause. Clinical examination determines the extent of the lymphadenopathy. Abdominal examination for the presence of hepatosplenomegaly is important and may indicate a haematological disorder. Radiological and pathological investigations are then used to confirm the cause.

Investigations

Fine-needle aspiration cytology is used if there is a suspicion that the lymphadenopathy is due to metastatic solid tumours. Excision biopsy is usually required if there is suspicion of a haematological disorder.

> **When performing a lymph node biopsy, specimens should be sent 'dry' to laboratory.** This allows samples to be obtained for imprint cytology , where cells are pressed on to a microscope slide, or microbiological culture.

Raynaud's disease

Raynaud's phenomenon refers to the clinical picture that occurs as a result of episodic digital ischaemia.

Primary Raynaud's disease

Primary Raynaud's disease is due to excessive vasoconstriction of the digital arteries as a response to cooling of the hands and feet and sometimes the nose, ears and lips (**Figure 9.20**). Flow in the digital arteries ceases at a critical closing temperature. Reopening of the blood vessels requires a rise in perfusion pressure as vasodilatation occurs. A drop in skin temperature also occurs. The

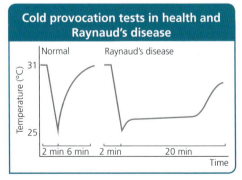

Figure 9.20 Results of a cold provocation test in a healthy individual and a patient with Raynaud's disease Skin temperature falls due to vasoconstriction following the cold insult.

vessels are normal between episodes. Pathophysiological mechanisms include:

- Increased sympathetic activity
- An increased number of alpha-receptors in the vessel wall

Secondary Raynaud's disease

Secondary Raynaud's disease results from conditions associated with abnormal vessel walls or increased blood viscosity. These include connective tissue (e.g. scleroderma, rheumatoid arthritis and Sjögren's syndrome), haematological and arterial diseases. It also results from neurovascular compression (e.g. cervical rib) and drugs (e.g. sumatriptan, ergotamine, beta-blockers).

Epidemiology

Raynaud's disease is more common in women and usually presents before the age of 35 years. The population prevalence is as high as 5%. Most patients have primary disease and have normal arteries.

Clinical features

The diagnosis is often made from the clinical history. A triphasic response occurs provoked by exposure to cold:

- Phase 1 – pallor due to intense vasoconstriction
- Phase 2 – cyanosis due to desaturation of haemoglobin and tissue ischaemia
- Phase 3 – erythema due to hyperaemia and restoration of the circulation

Primary disease is usually bilateral, symmetrical and involves all the fingers. Secondary disease is usually patchy and asymmetrical. The symptoms are often milder in primary disease. Examination often shows that the peripheral pulses are normal. Clinical features of connective tissue disorders are occasionally present.

Investigations

Investigations should be guided by the clinical features. Blood tests include a full blood count, erythrocyte sedimentation rate and anti-nuclear antibodies suggesting a connective tissue disorder. Electrophoresis, cold agglutinins and fibrinogen levels are used to identify hyperviscosity states, impairing blood flow and predispoing to Raynaud's phenomenon. A chest radiograph and thoracic outlet views are used to identify a cervical rib. Duplex ultrasonography and arteriography are indicated if there is a suspicion of arterial disease.

Management

Preventive measures include warm clothing, the use of hand warmers and smoking cessation. Occupational factors such as the temperature in which an individual is asked to work in, or the machinery they need to use may need to be taken into consideration. Sympathetic stimulants should be avoided. Vasodilating drugs such as alpha- or calcium-channel blockers have a limited role in this condition. Surgery to remove a cervical rib are required.

Answers to starter questions

1. Atheroma is the single most important cause of morbidity and mortality in Western countries. It affects medium-sized arteries resulting in vessel narrowing. Risk factors include smoking, hypertension, diabetes and hyperlipidaemia, all prevalent in the population. Depending on the circulation affected the results are ischaemic heart disease, cerebrovascular disease and peripheral vascular disease resulting in death from myocardial infarction and stroke.

2. Acute limb ischemia is defined as a sudden decrease in limb perfusion that causes a potential threat to limb viability. The effects of sudden arterial occlusion depend on the state of the collateral blood supply. In patients with embolic acute limb ischaemia the arterial tree is often normal and in order to maintain blood flow to the limb there has been no need for the collateral supply to compensate for a chronic reduction in blood flow. In patients with chronic limb ischaemia there is invariably narrowing of the main arteries with flow already maintained by dilation of the collateral blood supply. Therefore, if thrombotic occlusion occurs against this background a degree of blood flow distal to the occlusion is already maintained.

3. A compartment syndrome occurs when the circulation and function of the tissues within the closed space are compromised by an increase in pressure. The commonest causes are ischaemia-reperfusion injuries and lower limb fractures. The initiating insult causes muscle swelling within a compartment of fixed volume. As a result the pressure within the compartment increases, initially impairing the venous drainage. This induces a vicious circle of increasing tissue hypoxia, muscle oedema and impaired circulation.

4. Foot problems are common in diabetics. About 30% of diabetics have a peripheral neuropathy and many of these patients also have features of peripheral vascular disease. Approximately 15% of diabetics will develop foot ulceration with the incidence increasing with age. Superadded infection is also a problem. In diabetic feet, wound swabs often show both gram-negative, gram-positive and anaerobic bacteria. If osteomyelitis occurs, it is usually due to *Staphylococcus aureus* infection.

5. Abdominal aortic aneurysms have historically been treated by open surgery. The morbidity of open surgery is related to the surgical exposure and the cross clamping of the infra-renal aorta, massively increasing the afterload on the heart. Endovascular repair is performed using a minimally invasive technique with a stent placed across the aneurysm, having being inserted through the femoral artery. This avoids aortic clamping and is associated with reduced physiological stress. However, only about 40% of aneurysms are suitable for this type of repair.

6. Venous insufficiency results in early refilling of the venous pool after muscle contraction. It causes a progressive and sustained increase in calf vein pressure. This is known as ambulatory venous hypertension and results in capillary dilatation and leakage of plasma proteins. Incompetent perforating veins expose the superficial veins to high pressures during muscle contraction. Accumulation of leucocytes occurs in dependent limbs of those with venous hypertension. Trapping of white cells is associated with activation. Following activation they release O_2 radicals, collagenases and elastases which injure the surrounding tissue.

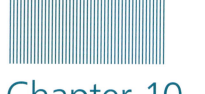

Chapter 10
Surgical emergencies

Introduction. 221
Acute appendicitis 222
Acute mesenteric ischaemia 224
Upper gastrointestinal
haemorrhage 225

Lower gastrointestinal
haemorrhage 227
Intestinal obstruction 229
Sigmoid volvulus 231
Gastrointestinal perforation 232
Acute pancreatitis 234

Introduction

Surgical emergencies account for about 20% of all general surgical operations. The most common presentation is with acute abdominal pain (**Figure 10.1**). A detailed history and thorough clinical examination often suggest the likely diagnosis. However, the underlying cause sometimes remains unclear in patients with multiple co-morbidities.

Unlike patients presenting electively, emergency patients are often unwell with significant physiological derangement. Prompt recognition of this allows early intervention to correct it. The measurement of vital signs, supplemented by simple investigations, enables a rapid assessment of the extent of the systemic response. Repeated observation then allows the adequacy of resuscitation to be measured. Surgical intervention sometimes needs to be delayed until the patient's condition has been optimised so that the risk of complications and death is reduced.

Figure 10.1 Causes of abdominal pain.

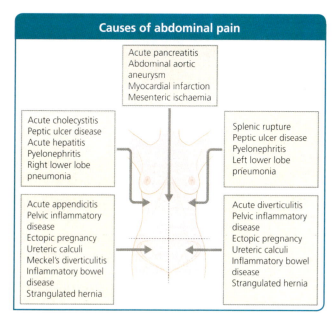

Causes of abdominal pain

Acute pancreatitis
Abdominal aortic aneurysm
Myocardial infarction
Mesenteric ischaemia

Acute cholecystitis
Peptic ulcer disease
Acute hepatitis
Pyelonephritis
Right lower lobe pneumonia

Splenic rupture
Peptic ulcer disease
Pyelonephritis
Left lower lobe pneumonia

Acute appendicitis
Pelvic inflammatory disease
Ectopic pregnancy
Ureteric calculi
Meckel's diverticulitis
Inflammatory bowel disease
Strangulated hernia

Acute diverticulitis
Pelvic inflammatory disease
Ectopic pregnancy
Ureteric calculi
Inflammatory bowel disease
Strangulated hernia

Acute appendicitis

Presentation

A 15-year-old previously healthy boy presents to the hospital having been generally unwell for 2 days. He first developed vague central colicky abdominal pain associated with nausea and anorexia. Over the next 24 hours, he vomited on a couple of occasions and the pain moved to the right iliac fossa. Examination shows him to be flushed with a temperature of 37.5°C and a pulse of 105 beats per minute. There is tenderness in the right iliac fossa.

Initial interpretation

This boy's history of initial central abdominal pain that migrates to the right iliac fossa is suggestive of acute appendicitis.

History and examination

The boy appears septic and unwell with a fever and tachycardia. The initial colicky central abdominal pain has migrated to the right iliac fossa and become localised and constant. He prefers to lie still and movement worsens his symptoms. He has lost his appetite and has vomited on two occasions. There is no diarrhoea or constipation, and no urinary symptoms.

Examination shows that the boy is lying quietly in bed. His face is flushed and he has a foetor oris (malodour of his breath). He is pyrexial and tachycardic. Abdominal examination shows localised tenderness in the right iliac fossa. There is tenderness on percussion. Rovsing's sign – pain in the right iliac fossa with pressure in the left – is positive. No abdominal mass is felt.

> **Acute appendicitis does not always present with the typical clinical features,** especially at the extremes of life. Consider the diagnosis in children with diarrhoea and vomiting, and in confused elderly patients with minimal abdominal pain.

Differential diagnosis of right iliac fossa pain and mass	
Right iliac fossa pain	Right iliac fossa mass
Appendicitis	Crohn's disease
Urinary tract infection	Caecal carcinoma
Non-specific abdominal pain	Mucocele of the gallbladder
Pelvic inflammatory disease	Psoas abscess
Renal colic	Pelvic kidney
Ectopic pregnancy	Ovarian cyst
Constipation	

Table 10.1 Differential diagnosis of right iliac fossa pain and mass

Differential diagnosis

The differential diagnosis of right iliac fossa pain and mass is shown in **Table 10.1**.

Immediate intervention

Acute appendicitis is essentially a clinical diagnosis and investigations are primarily used to exclude an alternative diagnosis. Urinalysis is performed to exclude a urinary tract infection. A blood sample is taken to measure the white cell count in support of the diagnosis.

> **Patients with acute appendicitis often have a raised white cell count.** However, it should be noted that inflammatory markers are sometimes normal in appendicitis.

Patients need intravenous fluids and analgesia. Opiates can safely be given as they do not mask the signs of peritonism (i.e. guarding and percussion tenderness). However, antibiotics should not be given until a decision to operate has been made as they can mask the clinical features.

An ultrasound scan may help in the assessment and confirmation of an appendix mass or abscess. An abdominal CT scan should be considered in adults particularly if the diagnosis is unclear. CT scanning has a greater utility as it may identify an alternative pathology (e.g caecal carcinoma or diverticulitis). Laparoscopy may be used as a diagnostic procedure and also offers the opportunity to proceed to a laparoscopic appendicectomy if an inflamed appendix is seen.

Acute appendicitis

If the diagnosis is in doubt, a period of 'active observation' is useful. This reduces the risk of negative appendicectomy (i.e. removal of a normal appendix) but without increasing the risk of perforation in those with subsequently proven appendicitis.

Open appendicectomy is usually performed via the right iliac fossa using a muscle-splitting approach. However, a midline incision is considered in elderly patients, especially if the diagnosis is uncertain. In both approaches, vessels in the mesoappendix should be ligated. The base of the appendix is then ligated and the appendix excised. Pus is sent for microbiological assessment.

Laparoscopic appendicectomy is associated with a shorter hospital stay and a more rapid return to normal activity. The potential complications of acute appendicitis are shown in **Figure 10.2**.

Appendix mass

An appendix mass usually presents with a history of several days of pain in the right iliac fossa. The inflammation is localised to the right iliac fossa by the omentum becoming adherent to the inflamed appendix. The patient is usually pyrexial with a palpable mass. Initial treatment is conservative with fluids, analgesia and antibiotics. The patient's general condition and the size of the mass are observed. Conservative management continues and appendicectomy can be avoided when there is evidence of clinical improvement.

Appendix abscess

An appendix abscess results from perforation of the appendix with the infection also localised to the right iliac fossa by the omentum. The abscess is drained surgically or percutaneously. It can be difficult to remove the appendix during the initial operation as the appendix is often destroyed when the abscess forms. Following recovery from either an appendix abscess or mass, and if the patient remains symptom free, there is no absolute indication to perform an interval appendicectomy after a few months as many patients remain symptom-free with no need for surgery.

A Meckel's diverticulum is a congenital anomaly found in the distal small bowel. Inflammation of the diverticulum mimics acute appendicitis. Therefore if the appendix appears normal during surgery, the distal small bowel is inspected to exclude a diagnosis of Meckel's diverticulitis.

If a normal appendix is identified during an open appendicectomy, the appendix should be removed to avoid future confusion. There is no need to remove a normal appendix seen during a diagnostic laparoscopy if an alternative cause for the abdominal pain is identified.

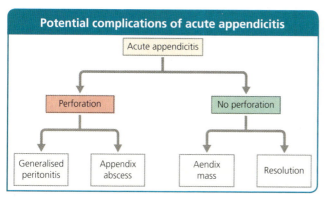

Figure 10.2 Potential complications of acute appendicitis.

Acute mesenteric ischaemia

Presentation

An 85-year-old man presents to hospital with a sudden onset of severe abdominal pain. The pain is poorly localised and involves the whole of his abdomen. On examination, he is distressed and is also in atrial fibrillation. Abdominal examination shows generalised tenderness but no signs of peritonitis.

Initial interpretation

The patient has had a sudden onset of severe abdominal pain. He is known to have cardiovascular disease and is in atrial fibrillation. The pain seems severe but the abdominal signs are few. This suggests a diagnosis of acute mesenteric ischaemia.

History and examination

The patient has presented with a 6-hour history of sudden-onset abdominal pain. This is poorly localised but seems to be in the centre of the abdomen. He has vomited three times. He has no diarrhoea or constipation. There is a past history of ischaemic heart disease and of a myocardial infarction 6 months previously. The patient is an ex-smoker. He is taking a beta-blocker and aspirin.

On examination, the patient appears distressed and in severe pain. He is apyrexial and in atrial fibrillation. An abdominal examination shows generalised tenderness but no signs of peritonitis. Bowel sounds are present.

Differential diagnosis

Acute mesenteric ischaemia should be considered as part of the differential diagnosis of any patient presenting with a sudden onset of abdominal pain. The differential diagnosis also includes acute pancreatitis, a perforated peptic ulcer and a leaking abdominal aortic aneurysm. Severe central abdominal pain is a common presentation. The pain is often out of proportion to the apparent clinical signs. Vomiting and rectal bleeding sometimes also occur.

Immediate intervention

An infusion of intravenous crystalloid is started, and the patient is given opiate analgesia.

No single investigation provides pathognomonic evidence of mesenteric ischaemia. Blood samples are taken to measure the white cell count, which is often raised with this condition. The serum amylase level is raised in 50% of patients. Arterial blood gases often show a metabolic acidosis. An ECG will confirm that the patient is in atrial fibrillation. An abdominal radiograph may be normal early in the disease process. Late radiological features include dilated small bowel and 'thumb[14]-printing' (i.e the impression of indentations by the thumb) of the bowel wall due to mucosal oedema. Mesenteric angiography is sometimes used to confirm the diagnosis.

> **No single clinical feature provides conclusive evidence of the diagnosis of acute mesenteric ischaemia.** As a result, the diagnosis is difficult and often delayed. Early diagnosis requires a high index of suspicion.

Acute mesenteric ischaemia

Acute mesenteric ischaemia occurs as result of superior mesenteric arterial or venous occlusion. It affects any part of the bowel either in continuity or in a patch nature in from the second part of the duodenum to the transverse colon. Whatever the underlying aetiology, reduced capillary flow causes intestinal necrosis. The overall mortality is approximately 90%.

After angiography, papaverine is sometimes infused into the superior mesenteric artery. Papaverine is a smooth muscle relaxant that induces arterial dilatation. If this fails rapidly to improve the symptoms, a laparotomy is considered. This confirms the diagnosis and allows the extent of the ischaemia to be assessed. It also provides an opportunity to revascularise the superior mesenteric artery if appropriate, and to resect necrotic bowel. Small bowel resection and primary anasto-mosis may be possible. If there is extensive necrosis of the small bowel in an elderly patient, palliative care is the preferred option.

Upper gastrointestinal haemorrhage

Presentation

A 70-year-old man with a history of indigestion has been brought to the hospital having collapsed at home. He has been vomiting 'coffee-ground' fluid and has passed black stools. On examination, he is pale and tachycardic. His pulse rate is 120 beats per minute. His blood pressure is 90/65 mmHg.

Initial interpretation

The patient appears to be having an upper gastrointestinal haemorrhage presenting with both haematemesis and melaena. The pallor and tachycardia suggest that he is shocked as a result of hypovolaemia.

History and examination

The patient admits to having had indigestion for the past few weeks, since he started on anti-inflammatory medication for arthritis. His general health is good with no abdominal pain or weight loss. He is not jaundiced, and there are no features of chronic liver disease. There are no abnormal findings on abdominal examination. Rectal examination reveals soft jet-black stools with an offensive smell.

> A patient's blood pressure may remain normal despite substantial bleeding and hypovolaemia.

Differential diagnosis

The differential diagnosis of an upper gastrointestinal haemorrhage includes bleeding from a peptic ulcer, oesophageal varices, a gastric malignancy and a Mallory–Weiss tear. Bleeding oesophageal varices are unlikely if there are no features of chronic liver disease.

Immediate intervention

The recent use of anti-inflammatories and the history of indigestion suggest that the bleeding is an upper gastrointestinal haemorrhage from a peptic ulcer. Peptic ulcer disease is the most common cause of upper gastrointestinal bleeding and is usually seen in elderly patients, particularly those taking non-steroidal inflammatory drugs.

Urgent investigation is required to both assess and correct the hypovolaemic shock resulting from blood loss. Blood samples are taken for full blood count, clotting studies, urea and electrolytes and cross-matching. The patient is given 1 L of crystalloid over 15 minutes via an intravenous cannula. The pulse and blood pressure are checked every 15 minutes. A urinary catheter is inserted and the urine output monitored hourly. The haemoglobin level is reported to be 70 g/L and 4 units of cross-matched blood are transfused.

Once the patient's clinical condition has stabilised, he requires an upper gastrointestinal endoscopy. Endoscopy allows direct visualisation of the oesophagus, stomach and proximal duodenum. It is both a diagnostic and a therapeutic investigation. If the source of the bleeding is identified, it is often possible to control it by endoscopic intervention (e.g. the injection of adrenaline into a bleeding peptic ulcer) without the need for surgery.

> Profuse bleeding from either a peptic ulcer or oesophageal varices often results in the passage of free blood per rectum. Fresh or altered rectal bleeding does not always indicate a lower gastrointestinal bleed.

Bleeding peptic ulcer

Peptic ulceration usually occurs in the gastric antrum or proximal duodenum. It presents as an emergency with either perforation or gastrointestinal bleeding. A bleeding peptic ulcer is a medical emergency requiring prompt resuscitation and investigation. Risk factors associated with a poor outcome included increasing age, co-morbidity, shock, the number of units of blood transfused and an increased blood urea level resulting from the breakdown of haemoglobin and the absorption of protein from the gastrointestinal tract.

Upper gastrointestinal endoscopy is both a diagnostic and a therapeutic procedure. It aims to identify the cause and the site of the bleeding. Endoscopic features of recent or active bleeding include the presence of fresh blood, adherent clot and a visible vessel in the ulcer base.

Endoscopy

Bleeding is often arrested by the endoscopic injection of adrenaline/epinephrine. If this is successful, patients should be monitored in a high-dependency environment for signs of cardiovascular instability suggesting a possible re-bleed. Treatment comprises a proton pump inhibitor and triple antibiotic therapy to eradicate *Helicobacter pylori* infection if it is detected on a urease test.

Surgery

If the bleeding cannot be stopped or there is rebleeding after endoscopic intervention, the patient is sent for surgery. Patients with a bleeding gastric ulcer usually require a local resection of the ulcer. A duodenal ulcer must be underrun with a non-absorbable suture, allowing the vessel in the base of the ulcer to be ligated but with care being taken to avoid damaging the underlying common bile duct.

Oesophagitis

Oesophagitis is a relatively rare cause of significant upper gastrointestinal haemorrhage. It usually presents with symptoms of gastro-oesophageal reflux. The principal symptom is heartburn – short-lived, intermittent, retrosternal chest pain often associated with an acid taste in the mouth. Upper gastrointestinal endoscopy confirms the presence of oesophagitis and allows a grading of the severity. Most patients gain symptomatic relief with conservative treatment with a proton pump inhibitor, and surgery (i.e. fundoplication) is rarely required.

Oesophageal varices

Approximately 90% of patients with portal hypertension have oesophageal varices, and 30% of patients with varices have an upper gastrointestinal bleed at some time. About 80% of upper gastrointestinal bleeds in patients with portal hypertension are from oesophageal varices, but other causes of upper gastrointestinal bleeding occur.

Patients with presumed bleeding from oesophageal varices are resuscitated with intravenous fluids and blood as for any other cause of upper gastrointestinal haemorrhage. Emergency endoscopic therapy employs endoscopic banding of the varices or paravariceal sclerotherapy. Upper gastrointestinal endoscopy is performed to confirm the site of haemorrhage. Temporary tamponade of the haemorrhage can be achieved with a Sengstaken–Blakemore tube (**Figure 10.3**). Tamponade successfully stops haemorrhage in 90% of cases. However, 50% of patients rebleed within 24 hours of the balloon being removed with little option to consider emergency surgical intervention. Vasopressin and octreotide can be used to decrease the splanchnic blood flow and reduce the portal venous pressure, reducing the risk of further variceal bleeding.

If tamponade or endoscopic methods fail, oesophageal transection, devascularisation and portocaval or mesenterico-caval shunting are considered.

Upper gastrointestinal malignancy

Oesophageal and gastric malignancy are rare causes of significant upper gastrointestinal haemorrhage. Oesophageal cancer usually

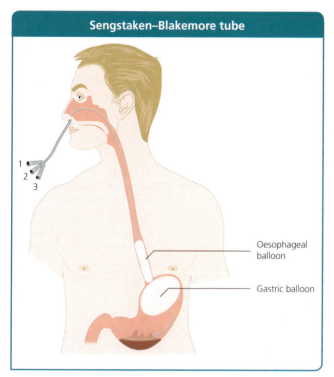

Sengstaken–Blakemore tube

1
2
3

Oesophageal balloon

Gastric balloon

Figure 10.3 A Sengstaken–Blakemore tube, with three channels to inflate the oesophageal and gastric balloons and aspirate the stomach.

presents with increasing dysphagia. Gastric cancer usually presents with persistent epigastric pain. The symptoms are chronic and progressive for both cancers. Vomiting with haematemesis is more likely in patients with gastric malignancy.

Patients are usually cardiovascularly stable, and aggressive resuscitation is rarely required. Gastrointestinal endoscopy confirms the diagnosis and allows biopsies to be taken if cancer is suspected.

Mallory–Weiss tear

A Mallory–Weiss tear is a longitudinal laceration of the gastrointestinal mucosa at the gastro-oesophageal junction. It usually occurs after persistent retching or vomiting. The main aetiological factor is a rapid increase in pressure across the gastro-oesophageal junction.

Patients usually present with haematemesis after an episode of severe vomiting. A significant degree of blood loss and systemic signs of hypovolaemia are both uncommon. The diagnosis is confirmed by endoscopy.

Lower gastrointestinal haemorrhage

Presentation

An 80-year-old woman is brought to the hospital after sudden per rectum bleeding. While performing her household chores, she suddenly had the urge to open her bowels. She describes passing dark blood containing clots into the toilet. On examination, she appears well, and both her pulse and blood pressure are normal.

Initial interpretation

This history suggests a lower gastrointestinal bleed. The patient has remained well, and there is no clinical evidence of hypovolaemia.

History and examination

The patient comments that this is the first time she has had rectal bleeding. Until this acute presentation, she had no other bowel symptoms of note. In particular, her bowels have been open regularly. She has been taking warfarin for atrial fibrillation for 5 years. She has not had previous abdominal surgery.

Examination shows her to be alert and comfortable. There are no abnormal findings on abdominal examination. Digital rectal examination indicates an empty rectum. Inspection of the gloved finger shows altered blood.

Differential diagnosis

Acute lower gastrointestinal haemorrhage is a common reason for acute surgical admission and accounts for 20% of cases of gastrointestinal bleeding. Most bleeding settles spontaneously and can is investigated electively. The usually site of the bleed is the distal colon, and the most common cause is diverticular disease. Other causes include neoplasms of the gastrointestinal tract, inflammatory bowel disease and angiodysplasia.

> Angiodysplasia refers to vascular malformations of the gastrointestinal tract. The lesions are often multiple and are most frequently found in the right colon. They are invariably asymptomatic until they present with an acute lower gastrointestinal bleed.

Immediate intervention

The patient appears to have had an acute lower gastrointestinal haemorrhage. The anticoagulatory medication she is taking for her atrial fibrillation may be a contributory factor. The priority is fluid resuscitation. Blood samples are sent for full blood count, urea and electrolytes and clotting studies. If the international normalised ratio is high, the warfarin should be omitted until the bleeding settles or can be rapidly reversed using an intravenous infusion of fresh frozen plasma if the patient is cardiovascularly unstable. A blood transfusion is set up if the patient is anaemic.

Further investigation aims to identify the source of the bleeding. Very few patients present with cardiovascular instability so investigations is performed once the bleeding has stopped and the blood has cleared from the bowel.

The investigation of choice is colonoscopy. This allows direct visualisation of the bowel lumen. Colonic neoplasms should be biopsied. In the small number of patients who present with hypovolaemic shock, selective mesenteric angiography is considered. This will only identify the source of the bleeding is there is a blood loss of over 1 mL per minute. However, it allows arterial embolisation to stop the bleeding if the source of bleeding is clearly identified. Surgical intervention can often be avoided.

> Before proceeding with surgery for what is clinically suggested to be an acute lower gastrointestinal bleed, an upper gastrointestinal endoscopy is considered to exclude a bleeding peptic ulcer.

In some patients, significant bleeding occurs and the source remains occult. In this case, appropriate resuscitation and a laparotomy are necessary. If the source of the bleeding is not identified by direct inspection of the bowel, a resection is required based on the most likely source of the bleeding.

Diverticular disease

One of the most common complications of diverticular disease is an acute lower gastrointestinal bleed, particularly in elderly patients. It results from rupture of a transmural vessel at the neck of a diverticulum. Patients usually present with rectal bleeding that is either bright or dark red in colour. They usually pass clots per rectum. Other gastrointestinal symptoms are rare. Abdominal examination is often normal, and rectal examination frequently shows altered blood on the glove.

Patients are usually cardiovascularly stable and only rarely require blood transfusion.

The bleeding usually stops spontaneously. A subsequent colonoscopy will confirm the presence of diverticular disease. Surgical intervention is rarely required.

Inflammatory bowel disease

Patients who have acute colitis with an inflammatory or infective cause also present with rectal bleeding. The bleeding is often neither acute nor torrential. It is often associated with other symptoms such as abdominal pain, diarrhoea and the passage of mucous per rectum. The stool frequency is often increased.

Abdominal examination often shows tenderness over the colon, and rectal examination sometimes shows both mucous and blood on the glove. The diagnosis is confirmed by cautious flexible sigmoidoscopy and colonic biopsies. Stool samples are taken to assess for an infective cause and the presence of *Clostridium difficile* toxin, indicating pseudomembranous colitis.

The initial treatment of acute colitis is steroids or antibiotics, depending on the cause. Surgery is considered if complications (e.g perforation, toxic megacolon) occur or medical management fails.

Colorectal malignancy

Colorectal malignancy rarely presents with an acute lower gastrointestinal haemorrhage. The blood loss from a tumour is usually minimal but, in the absence of other symptoms, is more likely to cause iron deficiency anaemia than acute blood loss. Right-sided colonic tumours often present with anaemia and a colonic mass. Left-sided colonic and rectal tumours cause a change in bowel habit. Rectal bleeding is usually minimal and is associated with the passage of mucous per rectum. The diagnosis is confirmed by colonoscopy and a colonic biopsy, which allows elective surgery to be planned.

Intestinal obstruction

Presentation

A 53-year-old man has been brought to hospital with a 24-hour history of colicky abdominal pain. During this time, he has vomited on several occasions. He feels that his abdomen has become distended. He has not had his bowels open for 48 hours.

Initial interpretation

The clinical picture suggests small bowel obstruction, based on the symptoms of colicky abdominal pain, vomiting, constipation and the feeling of abdominal distension.

History and examination

The patient comments that he has pain in the centre of his abdomen that comes and goes every few minutes. His vomit is bile stained. He has had absolute constipation and has not passed either stool or wind since the onset of the symptoms. He was previously relatively fit and healthy. He has not had previous abdominal surgery.

Examination shows that the patient is dehydrated (i.e. sunken eyes, reduced skin turgor). He is slightly tachycardic with a pulse rate of 105 beats per minute. The abdomen is distended with no surgical scars. Palpation showed the abdomen to be minimally tender. A mass is palpable in the right iliac fossa. No hernias are present in the groins. The bowel sounds are high pitched and tinkling. There are no abnormal findings on digital rectal examination.

> **The four cardinal features of intestinal obstruction are colicky abdominal pain, distension, vomiting and absolute constipation.** The symptoms and signs depend on the site of obstruction. Small bowel obstruction presents with colicky pain, vomiting and variable distension; constipation is a late feature. Large bowel obstruction presents with distension and constipation; pain is often minimal, and vomiting is a late feature.

Differential diagnosis

The suggested diagnosis is small bowel obstruction. The most common causes of mechanical obstruction are adhesions, a malignant tumour, an internal or external hernia and a stricture due to inflammatory bowel disease. Other causes of small and large bowel obstruction are shown in **Table 10.2**. Adhesional obstruction is unlikely is there has been no previous surgery. The presence of a right iliac fossa mass suggests either a malignant tumour or inflammatory bowel disease.

Immediate intervention

The suggested diagnosis is small bowel obstruction due to a mass in the right iliac fossa, which is likely to be either malignant or inflammatory. Fluids losses through either vomiting or sequestration in the dilated bowel can be significant and result in dehydration and hypovolaemia. The initial priority is fluid resuscitation. Blood samples are taken for a full blood count and urea and electrolytes. A urinary catheter and nasogastric tube are inserted to monitor the urine output and make the patient more comfortable, respectively. Crystalloid should be given to replace the maintenance requirements and ongoing losses.

Further investigation aims to confirm the clinical impression of small bowel obstruction and determine the underlying cause. A plain abdominal radiograph helps to confirm the dilated small intestine (**Figure 10.4**).

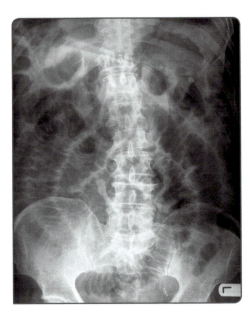

Figure 10.4 Plain abdominal radiograph showing numerous loops of dilated small bowel as a result of small bowel obstruction.

A contrast-enhanced abdominal CT scan usually identifies the underlying cause.

> **Dilated large bowel and the absence of small bowel dilatation on a plain abdominal radiograph are worrying radiological features** as they indicate a competent ileocaecal valve and closed loop large bowel obstruction. The patent ileocaecal valve prevents the pressure in the large bowel being released into the small bowel and if the obstruction is not relieved, perforation of the caecum and generalised peritonitis eventually occur.

Adhesional small bowel obstruction

Adhesional small bowel obstruction often resolves with conservative management, limitation of oral intake, intravenous fluids and regularly aspiration of the nasogastric tube. Resolution is often heralded by the passage of flatus, a reduced volume of nasogastric aspirate and resolution of the distension.

Causes of intestinal obstruction	
Small bowel obstruction	Large bowel obstruction
Adhesions from previous surgery	Malignant neoplasms
Hernias – internal or external	Diverticular strictures
Malignant neoplasms	Sigmoid volvulus
Crohn's disease	Hernias – internal or external
Intussusception	Pseudo-obstruction
Small bowel volvulus	
Foreign bodies (e.g. gallstones)	

Table 10.2 Causes of intestinal obstruction

> **Surgery should be the last resort in patients with adhesional small bowel obstruction** as it often results in the formation of further adhesions with the risk of further episodes of intestinal obstruction.

Non-adhesional small bowel obstruction

Non-adhesional small bowel obstruction often requires surgery involving a laparotomy and resection of the affected segment of bowel. A primary anastomosis may be possible, but in some patients the safest option will be well be fashioning a stoma. Patients who have a carcinoma obstructing the caecum will require a right hemicolectomy with an ileocolic anastomosis (**Figure 10.5**).

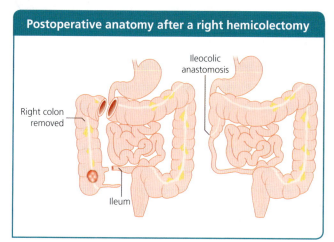

Postoperative anatomy after a right hemicolectomy

Ileocolic anastomosis

Right colon removed

Ileum

Figure 10.5 Postoperative anatomy after a right hemicolectomy.

Sigmoid volvulus

Presentation

A frail 90-year-old man is brought to the hospital with a 3-day history of painless abdominal distension. He is has not had his bowels open over this time. Examination shows his abdomen to be grossly distended but not tender.

Initial interpretation

The clinical picture suggests large bowel obstruction, based on the findings of constipation, distension and the absence of abdominal pain.

History and examination

The patient lives in a nursing home. He has dementia and numerous other medical problems including ischaemic heart disease, diabetes and chronic kidney disease. He has had several previous episodes of abdominal distension and constipation, but these have usually settled spontaneously. He has not had previous abdominal surgery.

Examination shows him to be confused with normal vital signs. The abdomen is grossly distended and non-tender. Digital rectal examination shows no rectal masses. The rectum contains soft stool.

Differential diagnosis

The differential diagnosis of large bowel obstruction is between mechanical and functional obstruction (pseudo-obstruction). The most common causes of mechanical large bowel obstruction in an elderly patient are colonic neoplasm and sigmoid volvulus.

> **Colonic pseudo-obstruction is characterised by reduced colonic mobility and dilatation.** It presents with the symptoms and signs of large bowel obstruction. The diagnosis is confirmed by excluding an obstructing lesion on CT scanning.

Immediate intervention

The patient's oral intake is restricted and he is maintained on intravenous fluids while investigation proceeds. Blood samples are taken for a full blood count and urea and electrolytes. A plain abdominal radiograph shows the characteristic appearance of a sigmoid volvulus with a large 'bean'-shaped loop of large bowel arising from the pelvis (**Figure 10.6**). If the diagnosis is in doubt, an abdominal CT scan helps to confirm it. Extensive further investigation is usually not required.

Sigmoid volvulus

A volvulus is defined as rotation of the gut on its own mesenteric access, producing partial or complete intestinal obstruction. Intestinal ischaemia occurs if the blood supply to that segment of bowel is compromised. Venous congestion eventually leads to infarction. The arterial supply is rarely compromised.

The sigmoid colon is the most common site of a colonic volvulus and accounts for 5% of cases of large bowel obstruction. It is usually seen in very elderly individuals and in those with multiple co-morbidities. About 50% of patients have had a previous episode. Severe pain and tenderness suggest intestinal ischaemia.

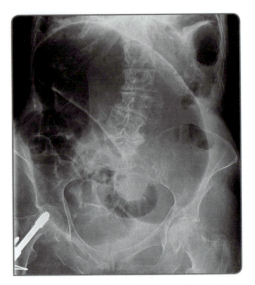

Figure 10.6 Plain abdominal radiograph showing typical 'kidney bean' appearance of a sigmoid volvulus.

Management of volvulus

Conservative management is usually appropriate if there are no features of perforation or infarction. Flexible sigmoidoscopy can be both diagnostic and therapeutic – passage of the scope beyond the obstruction often results in a dramatic release of flatus and liquid stool.

Overall, 80% of patients with a sigmoid volvulus settle with conservative management. If decompression fails or there are clinical features of peritonitis, surgical intervention needs to be considered. Surgery for a sigmoid volvulus is often high-risk due to the age and frailty of patients and a sigmoid resection with end colostomy (Hartmann's procedure) is usually the operation of choice. This procedure removes the diseased bowel and spares the risk of leak associated with fashioning a colonic anastomosis.

Gastrointestinal perforation

Presentation

A 75-year-old man is brought to the hospital after a sudden onset of epigastric pain. He was sitting in his chair watching television and remembers the exact moment the pain started. It was very severe and spread rapidly across the whole of his abdomen. Any movement was excruciatingly painful.

Initial interpretation

A sudden onset of severe epigastric pain that rapidly generalises to the whole of the abdomen is highly suggestive of a perforation of the gastrointestinal tract. The gastrointestinal contents then leak from the lumen of the bowel and irritate the perineum. Pain beginning in the epigastrium and rapidly generalising to the whole abdomen is most likely caused by a perforated peptic ulcer.

History and examination

The patient was remarkably well before the onset of the abdominal pain. He has no significant past medical history and does not drink alcohol. He has been taking non-steroidal anti-inflammatory drugs for mild osteoarthritis and has suffered no side effects from these.

Despite having been given analgesia by the ambulance crew, the patient is still clearly in pain when he reaches hospital. He is tachycardic with a pulse rate of 110 beats per minute. His blood pressure is normal. Examination shows his abdomen to be distended and generally tender. There is tenderness on percussion in all four quadrants of the abdomen. Bowel sounds are absent. These are all features of generalised peritonitis.

> **Non-steroidal anti-inflammatory drugs impair the mucosal defence of the gastrointestinal tract and are associated with peptic ulcer disease.** They are good analgesics due to their inhibitory effects on cyclooygenase-2. However, they also inhibit cyclooxygenase-1, which has a role in maintaining mucosal integrity.

Differential diagnosis

The differential diagnosis of a sudden onset of severe generalised abdominal pain is usually between a gastrointestinal perforation and acute pancreatitis. When the onset of pain is in the epigastrium, the most common cause of perforation is a peptic ulcer in either the duodenum or distal stomach. Other possible causes of perforation are a malignancy and a sigmoid diverticulum.

Immediate intervention

The immediate priority is to administer analgesia and fluid resuscitation. The patient is given intravenous morphine, and the pain settles rapidly. Blood samples are taken for full blood count, clotting studies, urea and electrolytes, amylase levels and cross-matching. Measurement of the serum amylase is important to exclude a diagnosis of acute pancreatitis. An intravenous cannula is inserted and 1 L of crystalloid is given over 15 minutes. A urinary catheter is inserted and the urine output is monitored hourly. High-flow oxygen is administered via a rebreathing bag.

The full blood count shows a raised white cell count, confirming the presence of inflammatiion. Renal function and amylase levels are normal. Once the patient has been stabilised, an erect chest radiograph is taken. This shows free gas under the diaphragm (**Figure 10.7**). An abdominal CT scan indicates free fluid and air free within the abdomen (**Figure 10.8**). The site of the perforation has not been identified but a perforated peptic ulcer is

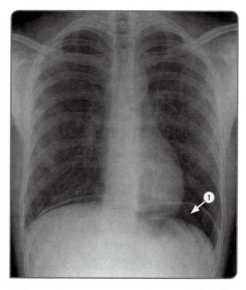

Figure 10.7 Erect chest X-ray showing free gas ① under the diaphragm.

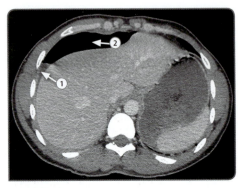

Figure 10.8 Abdominal CT scan showing free fluid ① and air ② after a perforated duodenal ulcer.

suspected as most of the fluid is in the right upper quadrant. The serum amylase level is normal.

> An erect chest radiograph may be normal in patients with a pneumoperitoneum (free gas within the peritoneal cavity). A CT scan is considered if there is diagnostic doubt.

Perforated peptic ulcer

Surgery is required if generalised peritonitis is present. After fluid resuscitation, laparotomy is performed through a midline incision. This allows lavage of the gastrointestinal

contents from the peritoneal cavity. The site of the perforation is then confirmed.

In patients presenting with a perforated peptic ulcer, the most common sites of perforation are the anterior wall of the first or second part of the duodenum, and the pre-pyloric region of the stomach. The perforation is usually a small hole that is surgically sealed using an 'omental patch' – the hole is oversewn using a portion of greater omentum.

The patient's oral intake should be restricted for a few days after surgery. Most perforated peptic ulcers occur in gastric or duodenal mucosa that is positive for *H. pylori*, and patients should be given *H. pylori* eradication therapy once oral intake has been re-established. This usually involves 'triple therapy' for 1 week (**Table 10.3**).

First-line triple therapy regimens to eradicate *H. pylori*		
Proton pump inhibitor	Antibiotic 1	Antibiotic 2
Omeprazole Or lansoprazole	Amoxicillin	Clarithromycin
Omeprazole Or lansoprazole	Clarithromycin	Metronidazole

Table 10.3 First-line triple therapy regimens to eradicate *H. pylori*

Acute pancreatitis

Presentation

A 40-year-old man is brought to hospital with a sudden onset of epigastric pain. The pain is severe and is radiating directly through to his back. He has vomited several times.

Initial interpretation

A sudden onset of epigastric pain radiating through to the back is highly suggestive of acute pancreatitis.

History and examination

The patient reports that the pain started at about 3 a.m. and woke him from sleep. He

had been out drinking with friends the previous evening and had consumed about 10 units of alcohol. His normal alcohol intake is about 50 units per week. He has not previously experienced similar symptoms. He is taking medication for hypertension but has no significant past medical history.

On examination, the patient is clearly distressed and in pain. He is flushed and tachycardic, with a pulse rate of 120 beats per minute. The abdomen is distended and is generally tender. Bowel sounds are absent.

Two late eponymous signs of retroperitoneal haemorrhage are sometimes seen in patients with acute pancreatitis. Grey Turner's sign is bruising in the flanks. Cullen's sign is oedema and bruising around the umbilicus.

High-flow oxygen via a rebreathing bag is commenced.

With acutely ill patients, the administration of high-flow oxygen does not run the risk of respiratory failure, even in patients with pre-existing respiratory disease.

Differential diagnosis

The differential diagnosis of a sudden onset of severe generalised abdominal pain is usually between a gastrointestinal perforation and acute pancreatitis. A history of previous episodes of pain, gallstones or high alcohol intake favours a diagnosis of acute pancreatitis. The causes of acute pancreatitis are shown in **Figure 10.9**.

Immediate intervention

The immediate priority is to administer analgesia and commence fluid resuscitation. The patient is given intravenous morphine but with little effect. This is repeated after 30 minutes. Blood samples are taken for full blood count, clotting studies, urea and electrolytes, liver function tests and amylase level. An intravenous cannula is inserted and 1 L of crystalloid administered over 15 minutes. A urinary catheter is inserted and the urine output monitored hourly.

The full blood count shows that the white cell count is raised, which is a sign of inflammation. Liver function tests are normal but the amylase level is raised to 5500 U/L. Serum amylase has a low sensitivity and low specificity for the diagnosis of acute pancreatitis. However, a serum amylase level four times the upper limit of normal suggests this diagnosis. Other causes of hyperamylasaemia are shown in **Table 10.4**.

About 20% of patients with acute pancreatitis have normal serum amylase values, particularly if alcohol is the aetiological factor.

Abdominal CT scanning is the standard imaging modality for evaluating acute pancreatitis and its complications (**Figure 10.10**). Typical CT findings in acute pancreatitis include focal or diffuse enlargement of the pancreas, heterogeneous enhancement of the gland, blurring of the peripancreatic fat planes and the presence of intraperitoneal or retroperitoneal fluid collections.

It is important to identify those patients with gallstone pancreatitis, in order to offer them a laparoscopic cholecystectomy

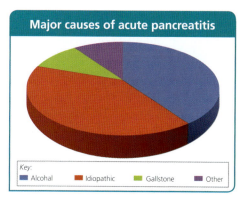

Major causes of acute pancreatitis

Key:
- Alcohal
- Idiopathic
- Gallstone
- Other

Figure 10.9 Major causes of acute pancreatitis. Other causes include hereditary pancreatitis, hyperparathyroidism, hyperlipidaemia, trauma, autoimmune disease and structural abnormalities of the pancreas or biliary tree.

Causes of hyperamylasaemia	
Hepatobiliary causes	Non-hepatobiliary causes
Acute pancreatitis	Perforated peptic ulcer
Acute cholecystitis	Intestinal obstruction
Acute cholangitis	Mesenteric infarction
	Ruptured abdominal aortic aneurysm
	Ectopic pregnancy

Table 10.4 Causes of hyperamylasaemia

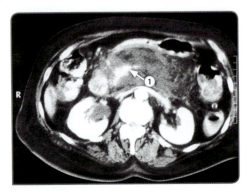

Figure 10.10 Abdominal CT scan showing acute pancreatitis. ① Oedematous pancreas.

preferably during their index admission. Abdominal ultrasound is the investigation of choice for the demonstrating or excluding the presence of gallstones.

Management

The treatment of acute pancreatitis aims to halt the progression of local disease and prevent remote organ failure. In severe disease, this requires full supportive therapy, often in an intensive care or high-dependency environment.

The key steps in the management of acute pancreatitis are summarised by the mnemonic MACHINES:

- Monitor vital signs
- Analgesia and antibiotics
- Calcium gluconate if necessary to treat hypocalcaemia
- H₂ receptor antagonist or proton pump inhibitor to reduce the risk of peptic ulceration
- Intravenous fluids
- Nil by mouth
- Empty stomach
- Surgery, if required

A urinary catheter is inserted to measure urine output and assess fluid balance. Serum electrolytes, calcium and blood sugar levels, and liver function tests are regularly assessed. Hypocalcaemia occurs in some patients with acute pancreatitis due to calcium binding to

released fatty acids. Patients require fluid resuscitation, correction of hypoxia using an increased fraction of inspired oxygen, and adequate analgesia. Antibiotic prophylaxis to prevent infected pancreatic necrosis is useful in those with severe pancreatitis. Endoscopic retrograde cholangiopancreatography has been shown to be of benefit within the first 48 hours in patients with predicted severe pancreatitis due to gallstones. Removal of stones from the common bile duct speeds up resolution of the pancreatic inflammation.

Prognostic factors

The aim of prognostic scores is to identify patients with severe disease, allowing them to be more closely monitored. Any scoring system must have a high sensitivity and specificity and can ideally be carried out on admission.

Ranson's criteria can be measured both on admission and at 48 hours (**Table 10.5**). They are, however, not ideal as they cannot be fully applied for 48 hours and are also a poor predictor later in the disease. They have been described as a 'single snapshot in a whole feature length of the film'.

APACHE (Acute Physiology and Chronic Health Evaluation) II is a multivariate scoring system that measures objective parameters – vital signs and biochemical variables (**Table 10.6**). It has the advantage that it takes account of the patient's age and premorbid state, and can be used throughout the course of the illness.

Ranson's prognostic criteria for acute pancreatitis	
On admission	Within 48 hours
Age >55 years	Fall in haematocrit of more than 10%
White cell count >16,000 U/mL	Rise in blood urea of more than 0.9 mmol/L
Lactate dehydrogenase >600 U/L	Calcium <2 mmol/L
Aspartate aminotransferase >120 U/L	pO₂ <8 kPa
	Base deficit >>4
Glucose >10 mmol/L	Fluid sequestration >6 L

Table 10.5 Ranson's prognostic criteria for acute pancreatitis

Variables measured in the APACHE II score	
Vital signs	Physiological measurements
Temperature	Arterial partial pressure of oxygen
Heart rate	
Mean arterial pressure	Arterial pH
Respiratory rate	Serum sodium
	Serum potassium
	Serum creatinine
	Haematocrit
	White cell count

Table 10.6 Variables measured in the APACHE II score

Local and systemic complications of acute pancreatitis	
Local complications	Systemic complications
Necrosis, possibly with infection	Hypovolaemic and shock
	Coagulopathy
Pancreatic fluid collections	Respiratory failure
Colonic necrosis	Acute renal failure
Gastrointestinal haemorrhage	Hyperglycaemia
	Hypocalcaemia
Splenic artery aneurysm	

Table 10.7 Local and systemic complications of acute pancreatitis

Complications

About 80% of patients have mild disease with a low risk of complications However, a small proportion have severe disease, and about 40% of these develop life-threatening complications. Half of all deaths from acute pancreatitis occur within the first week due to multiorgan failure. This usually occurs in the absence of local complications. Late deaths are often due to local complications. The local and systemic complications of acute pancreatitis are shown in **Table 10.7**.

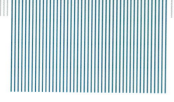

Chapter 11
Self-assessment

SBA questions

First principles

1. A 14 year-old boy has central abdominal pain that migrates to the right iliac fossa. On examination he appears unwell. He is pyrexial and locally tender in the right iliac fossa. Clinically he appears to have acute appendicitis and requires an operation. His parents are away on holiday and cannot be contacted. He has been brought to the hospital by aunt who has been looking after him. Which single statement best describes the situation in relation to informed consent?

A It is necessary to obtain consent from a social worker

B The aunt can give consent and sign the consent form

C The patient can consent to surgery if he understands the nature of the procedure

D The patient is a child and no consent is required

E The surgery cannot proceed until his parents return from holiday

2. A 60 year-old man has a sudden onset of abdominal pain. He appears dehydrated, is tachycardic and has generalised peritonitis. Following initial assessment, an intravenous cannula is inserted and he is given 1L of normal saline.
Which single statement regarding the normal saline is true?

A He has been given a colloid solution

B He will have received 30 mmol of sodium

C He will have received 29 mmol of bicarbonate

D No calcium will have been given

E He will have received 5 mmol of potassium

3. A 73 year-old woman has a caecal carcinoma and is admitted for an elective right hemicolectomy. She has no significant past medical history and is on no regular medications. As part of her preoperative preparation investigations are performed.

Which single statement regarding her tests is true?

A A chest X-ray is essential

B A colonoscopy should be performed the day prior to surgery

C All blood tests should be avoided

D An ECG should be performed

E At least 6 units of blood should be cross-matched

4. An 84 year-old woman has an open cholecystectomy. Her initial postoperative recovery has been uncomplicated, but approximately 10 days after her surgery she develops right calf pain. Walking is painful. Examination shows her to be pyrexial. Her calf is swollen and tender.
What single statement is true?

A Clinically she has developed acute limb ischaemia

B Diagnosis can be confirmed with femoral angiography

C Her symptoms are minor and can safely be ignored

D Homan's sign may be positive

E She should not be treated until a diagnosis has been confirmed

5. A 45 year-old woman is scheduled to undergo a laparoscopic cholecystectomy. She weighs 120 kg and has a BMI over 40.
Which single statement regarding her surgery is true?

A Intubation and ventilation should not prove technically difficult

B Pain control will be as effective as with someone of normal weight

C Surgery can safely be performed as a day case

D There is a high risk of postoperative hypoxaemia

E With adequate thromboprophylaxis she is at no higher risk of a DVT

Clinical essentials

6. A 70 year-old man collapses at home. His daughter reports that over the preceding 2 days he has had increasing abdominal pain. His vital signs are measured.
Which single statement is true?

A A pulse rate of 100 indicates a bradycardia
B A respiratory rate of 30 breaths per minute is normal
C A systolic blood pressure of less than 120 mmHg indicates hypotension
D A temperature of 38.0 °C is normal
E Vital signs can be scored and summated to provide an Early Warning Score

7. A 67 year-old notices a painful lump in his right groin. Examination shows a lump that extends in to the scrotum but is separate from the testis. It is impossible to get above the lump. It can be reduced with gentle pressure.
Which single statement is true?

A A cough impulse is likely to be absent
B The lump is a strangulated femoral hernia
C The lump is a reducible inguinal hernia
D The lump is likely to be very tender
E The lump will transilluminate brightly

8. A 45 year-old man has a sudden onset of severe epigastric pain. It rapidly spreads to all of his abdomen. Examination shows him to pyrexial and tachycardic. Abdominal examination shows generalised tenderness and absent bowel sounds. As part of his investigation, an arterial blood gas is taken.
What is the single most likely finding?

A Respiratory acidosis
B Respiratory alkalosis
C Metabolic acidosis with a normal lactate
D Metabolic acidosis with a raised lactate
E Metabolic alkalosis with a raised lactate

9. An 80 year-old man has a sudden inability to pass urine. He develops increasing lower abdominal pain. Examination shows his bladder to palpable up to the umbilicus and tender. He requires a urinary catheter.
Which single statement is true?

A All catheters are the same length and suitable for all patients
B The catheter balloon should not be inflated until urine is seen draining from the catheter
C The catheter should always be inserted via the suprapubic route
D The catheter should be removed as soon as it is no longer required
E The use of local anaesthesia with lignocaine gel is appropriate

10. A 28 year-old man has a 3-day history of a painful red lump on his back. Prior to this he had a small sebaceous cyst at the same site. Examination shows a tender, red and fluctuant lump.
Which single statement is true?

A Fluctuation shows the lump is solid and surgery is not required
B He has a cold abscess due to tuberculosis
C If untreated the lump will 'point' and discharge pus
D Microbiological culture of the pus is unlikely to grow any organisms
E Redness and pain suggest chronic inflammation

11. A 64 year-old woman has a 1 week history of right iliac fossa pain. Over the last 24 hours the pain has increased in severity and spread to the whole of her abdomen. Examination shows her to be pyrexial, tachycardic and hypotensive. She is septic with generalised peritonitis.
Which single statement is true?

A A cannula can be avoided and fluids given orally
B Blood cultures should be taken after the administration of antibiotics
C Broad spectrum antibiotics can be given orally
D High-flow oxygen should be given
E No need to perform any blood tests

Breast disease

12. A 20 year-old woman has a 2-week history of a painless right breast lump. Examination shows a 2 cm well-defined and mobile lump in the upper outer quadrant of the right breast.
What is the single most likely diagnosis?

A Breast carcinoma
B Breast cyst
C Fat necrosis
D Fibroadenoma
E Galactocele

13. A 50 year-old woman has a left breast lump. She receives a letter informing her that when she attends the clinic she will undergo a 'Triple assessment'. She does not understand the information in the letter and consults her general practitioner.
What is the single most appropriate advice the general practitioner should give?

A All women have a biopsy
B All women have a mammogram
C If a biopsy is performed she definitely has cancer
D The investigations performed are the same in all women
E Triple assessment involves a clinical, radiological and pathological assessment

14. A 33 year-old woman has a 48 hour history of painful left breast lump. She is 2 weeks postpartum and is breast feeding. Examinations shows her breast to be red and inflamed with a 4 cm diameter tender lump towards the periphery of the breast. Clinically she appears to have a breast abscess.
Which single organisms is likely to be the underlying cause?

A Escherichia coli
B Haemophilus influenza
C Mycobacterium tuberculosis
D Staphylococcus aureus
E Streptococcus pyogenes

15. A 46 year-old woman has a left breast cancer. She has enlarged axillary lymph nodes with nodal metastases confirmed by a core biopsy. She has been advised that she needs an axillary node clearance.
What single anatomical structure should be identified and preserved during surgery?

A Long thoracic nerve
B Median nerve
C Subclavian artery
D Thoracic duct
E Ulna nerve

16. A 75 year-old woman has undergone a left wide local excision and sentinel node biopsy for a small palpable breast cancer. She has made an uncomplicated recovery and her postoperative results show the tumour is 2 cm in diameter, the resection margins are clear, the lymph nodes are clear and the tumour is oestrogen-receptor positive and HER2 negative.
Which single statement is true regarding her treatment?

A A mastectomy is needed
B Chemotherapy is always required
C Hormonal treatment (e.g. tamoxifen) will improve survival
D Radiotherapy can be avoided
E There will be benefit from treatment with trastuzumab (Herceptin)

17 A 14 year-old boy has noticed a small painless lump behind his right nipple. It has been present for about 1 month. He has no other concerns. Examination shows a 2 cm non-tender retroareolar lump.
Which single statements regarding the lump is most likely to be true?

A A core biopsy is always required to confirm the diagnosis
B It is a breast cancer that requires further investigation
C It is harmless physiological gynaecomastia
D The lump will gradually increase in size and surgery is inevitable

E There is always an associated endocrine abnormality

Endocrine disease

18. A 14 year-old girl has a lump in the midline of her next. It moves up when she protrudes her tongue.
Which single statement about the lump is true?

A It arose from the tip of the tongue
B It is in the line of descent of the thyroid gland
C It is most likely to be lymph node
D It moves on protruding the tongue as it is connected to the mandible
E Surgery involves removing part of the cricoid cartilage

19. A 24 year-old woman is feeling generally unwell. Investigations show her to have raised serum T4. Her TSH level is unrecordable. She has thyrotoxicosis.
What single combination of symptoms and signs is she most likely to have?

A Dyspnoea, insomnia and weight gain
B Hair loss, slow speech and slow thought
C Slow speech, insomnia and preference for warm weather
D Sweating, bradycardia and tremor
E Tachycardia, weight loss and irritability

20. A 43 year-old woman has swelling affecting both side of her neck. Examination shows swelling either side of the trachea. She appears to have a goitre.
Which single statement regarding her subsequent investigation is true?

A Anti-TSH antibodies will be increased in Hashimoto's thyroiditis
B Thyroid–stimulating hormone (TSH) will be normal in hypothyroidism
C Thyroid–stimulating hormone (TSH) will be unmeasurable in thyrotoxicosis
D Thyroxine (T4) may be normal in thyrotoxicosis
E Triiodothyronine (T3) is increased in all cases of thyrotoxicosis

21. A 60 year-old man has undergone a total thyroidectomy for papillary carcinoma of this thyroid gland. When he awakes from his surgery is noted to both have a hoarse voice and stridor.
What single structure in the neck is most likely to have been damaged during his surgery?

A Larynx
B Left recurrent laryngeal nerve
C Parathyroid glands
D Right vagus nerve
E Trachea

22. A 30 year-old woman has a 2 week history of a lump in the right side of her neck. She has a strong family history of the thyroid cancer. Examination shows that she has a large lump in the right lobe of her thyroid gland and she has enlarged cervical lymph nodes. Her serum calcitonin level is elevated.
Which single statement is most likely to be true?

   A Her condition is inherited in an autosomal recessive fashion
   B Her condition may be part of the MEN I syndrome
   C Her tumour has arisen from the parafollicular C cells of the thyroid gland
   D She has a thyroid lymphoma
   E Treatment should be by a thyroid lobectomy

23. A 45 year-old woman is investigated for abdominal pain. Her serum calcium is elevated. She has no significant past medical history.
Which single statement is most likely to be true?

   A Her serum parathyroid hormone level will be reduced
   B Her serum phosphate will always be normal
   C She has primary hyperparathyroidism
   D She will require surgery
   E The underlying cause is a parathyroid carcinoma

24. A 58 year-old woman has a 1 year history of weight gain. Her relatives have noticed changes to her facial appearance; it has become more rounded. She has also noticed an increased difficulty climbing stairs. She is hypertensive. She has abdominal adiposity and striae. A cranial nerve assessment is undertaken.
Which single clinical feature is most likely to be identified?

   A Drooping of one side of the face
   B Inability to shrug her shoulders
   C Homonymous hemianopia
   D Loss of sensation to the posterior third of the tongue
   E Ptosis

25. A 42 year-old woman has a 6 month history of intermittent palpitations, chest pain and sweating. The episodes occur at variable intervals and last about 1 hour. During one episode she was shown to be hypertensive and to be tachycardic.
Which single statement about her condition is true?

   A Her 24-hour urinary vanniyl mandelic acid levels will be elevated
   B It can be managed by drugs and surgery avoided
   C It is due to a problem with adrenal cortex
   D It results from a malignant tumour
   E Surgery involves removal of both adrenal glands

26. A 52 year-old man has a 3 year history of vague right-sided abdominal discomfort. More recently he has intermittent diarrhoea and episodes of facial flushing often induced by chocolate eating. Examination shows a right iliac fossa mass and hepatomegaly. Clinically he appears to have carcinoid syndrome.
Which single statement is true?

   A Carcinoid tumours most commonly occur in the large bowel
   B Carcinoid syndrome occurs when the tumour metastasises to the lungs
   C 111^{In} - octreotide scintigraphy may identify a primary or secondary tumour
   D The diagnosis can be confirmed by measuring the urinary vanniyl mandelic acid
   E Plasma chromogranin B levels may be increased

Upper gastrointestinal surgery

27. A 33 year-old woman has a 2 month history of intermittent epigastric pain. Her general practitioner is concerned that she has a peptic ulcer and refers her for an upper gastrointestinal endoscopy.
Which single statement regarding the investigation is true?

   A Interventional procedures such as biopsies can be performed
   B It aids visualisation of the stomach, duodenum, jejunum and proximal ileum
   C It will performed under a general anaesthetic
   D She can eat and drink until the investigation is performed
   E There is no risk of complications

28. A 48 year-old man has a 3 month history of heartburn. The pain he describes is retrosternal, short-lived and intermittent and is worse at night or when he lies flat. It is associated with an acid-like taste in the back of his throat.
What is the single most appropriate next step?

   A Abdominal CT scan and tumour markers
   B Abdominal ultrasound and full blood count
   C Barium swallow and abdominal CT scan
   D Upper GI endoscopy and colonoscopy
   E Upper GI endoscopy and oesophageal pH studies

29. A 78 year-old man has a 4 month history of increasing difficulty with swallowing. He initially had difficulty swallowing solids but is now struggling to swallow fluids. He has lost 10 Kg in weight. Examination shows him to be thin and cachectic. Abdominal examination is normal.

What is the single most likely diagnosis?

A Achalasia
B Barrett's oesophagus
C Benign oesophageal stricture
D Carcinoma of the bronchus
E Oesophageal carcinoma

Colorectal surgery

30. A 75 year-old man has a 1 week history of left iliac fossa pain. He is feverish and generally unwell, and has vomited on several occasions. He has a history of diverticular disease. On examination he is pyrexial and tachycardic. Abdominal examination shows a tender mass in the left iliac fossa. The remainder of his abdomen is non-tender.
What is the single most likely complication of diverticular disease to have occurred?

A Colonic stricture
B Diverticular haemorrhage
C Pericolic abscess
D Sigmoid perforation with generalised peritonitis
E Vesico-colic fistula

31. A 25 year-old woman has undergone emergency surgery for acute colitis. She now has a stoma in right iliac fossa.
Which single statement is true?

A Complications of stomas rarely occur
B The output from the stoma is likely to be formed stool
C The stoma is a loop colostomy
D The stoma is always permanent
E The stoma is an end ileostomy

32. A 73 year-old woman has a 2 month history of right iliac fossa pain. Examination shows her to be pale and abdominal examination shows a right iliac fossa mass. A full blood count shows her to have hypochromic microcytic anaemia.
What is the single most likely diagnosis?

A Appendix mass
B Caecal carcinoma
C Crohn's disease
D Mucocele of the gallbladder
E Ovarian carcinoma

33. A 65 year-old man has a 6 month history of a perianal lump. It has gradually increased in size and is becoming uncomfortable. He has a past history of perianal warts. Examination shows an ulcerating lesion at the anal margin and the inguinal lymph nodes are enlarged.
Which single statement is true?

A All patients with palpable lymph nodes have metastatic disease

B Human papilloma virus is important in the aetiology of this condition
C The lesion is almost certainly benign
D The tumour is most commonly a melanoma
E The tumour most commonly arises from the anal canal above the dentate line.

34. A 30 year-old man has a 3 day history of severe perianal pain. It occurs on defaecation and occurs for a few minutes after. He has had several similar episodes in the past but not sought medical advice. Inspection of his anus shows a sentinel pile. Digital rectal examination proves impossible due to the pain.
Which of the following single statements is true?

A Botulinum toxin can be used to relax the anal sphincter
B Few fissures heal with medical management
C GTN ointment can be used with no risk of side effects
D He has an anal fissure, most likely to be found in the anterior midline
E Surgical sphincterotomy allows healing with no risk of complications

Hepatobiliary surgery

35. A 41 year-old woman has a 6 month history of intermittent right upper quadrant abdominal pain. The pain occurs every few days and radiates around to her scapula. It lasts about 1 hour and in between she is symptom free. On examination, when pain free, she is not jaundiced and she has no abdominal tenderness.
What is the single most likely diagnosis?

A Acute cholangitis
B Acute cholecystitis
C Biliary colic
D Gallstone ileus
E Mirrizi's syndrome

36. An 83 year-old woman has a 1 week history of increasing painless jaundice. She also has dark urine and pale stools. She appears relatively well but is obviously jaundiced. Abdominal examination shows her gallbladder to be palpable in the right upper quadrant. She appears to have obstructive jaundice.
Which single statement is true?

A An abdominal CT scan will always show a mass in the head of the pancreas
B An abdominal ultrasound will show her common bile duct to be of normal diameter
C Her serum alkaline phosphatase will be normal
D Her serum conjugated bilirubin will be raised
E Her urine conjugated bilirubin will be low

37. A 68 year-old Caucasian woman has a 6 month history of increasing abdominal distension. She has noticed that her clothes have become increasingly tight. Despite this, she appears to be losing weight. She has no significant past medical and no history of alcohol excess. Examination shows her to cachectic but abdominal examination shows it to be grossly distended. She has shifting dullness and a fluid thrill.
What is the single most likely diagnosis?

   A Cardiac failure
   B Cirrhosis
   C Nephrotic syndrome
   D Ovarian carcinoma
   E Tuberculosis

38. A 50 year-old Chinese man has a 3 month history of right hypochondrial pain and weight loss. He has a past history of hepatitis B that has led to liver cirrhosis. Examination shows a low grade pyrexia and right upper quadrant abdominal mass.
What is the single most likely diagnosis?

   A Acute liver failure
   B Hepatocellular carcinoma
   C Multiple liver metastases
   D Pancreatic carcinoma
   E Pyogenic liver abscess

Urology

39. A 20 year-old woman has a 2 day history of urinary frequency, urgency and dysuria. She is sexually active. She is apyrexial and abdominal examination shows her to have suprapubic tenderness. Urinalysis shows red blood cells, white blood cells and leucocytes in her urine. She has acute cystitis.
What is the single most likely causative organism?

   A *Escherichia coli*
   B *Haemophilus influenzae*
   C *Proteus mirabilis*
   D *Staphylococcus aureus*
   E *Staphylococcus saprophyticus*

40. A 32 year-old man has a sudden onset of severe right loin pain. It is colicky in nature and is the most severe pain he has experienced. The pain moves down to his groin and is then associated with urinary frequency. On examination he is writhing around and is in obvious discomfort. Examinations shows right loin tenderness and urinalysis shows microscopic haematuria.
What is the single most likely diagnosis?

   A Acute appendicitis

   B Acute prostatitis
   C Testicular torsion
   D Ureteric colic
   E Urinary tract infection

41. A 25 year-old man has noticed a lump in his right testis. It is painless and his general health is good. He had a right orchidopexy for an undescended testis at the age of 5. Examination shows a 3cm firm and irregular lump arising from the right testis.
What is the single most likely diagnosis?

   A Acute epididymitis
   B Epididymal cyst
   C Hydrocele
   D Testicular tumour
   E Varicocele

42. A 73 year-old man has a 3 month history of right loin discomfort and on several occasions has noticed blood in his urine. Examination shows him to be pyrexial and hypertensive. Abdominal examination shows a right loin mass.
What is the single most likely diagnosis?

   A Acute pyonephrosis
   B Bladder carcinoma
   C Bladder calculi
   D Prostatic carcinoma
   E Renal cell carcinoma

43. An 85 year-old man has noticed a deterioration in his urinary stream over a number of years. He has observed that the stream is not as strong as previous and he has developed hesitancy and terminal dribbling. He now has to go more often and to get up several time per night to pass urine.
Which single statement regarding his investigations is true?

   A A renal ultrasound should be performed to exclude hydronephrosis
   B A serum PSA will always be normal
   C Serum electrolytes will always be normal
   D Urine cytology should always be performed to exclude malignancy
   E Uroflowmetry will show the same profile as in younger men

44. A 17 year-old boy has sudden onset of severe right testicular pain. He has no urinary symptoms. Examination shows an exquisitely tender high-riding testis with a small hydrocele.
What is the single most likely diagnosis?

   A Acute epididymitis
   B Strangulated inguinal hernia
   C Testicular torsion
   D Torted hydatid of Morgagni
   E Varicocele

Vascular surgery

45. A 75 year-old man has developed pain in his left calf when he walks. The pain occurs after about 100m and is relieved by rest. He is hypertensive and a heavy smoker. His pulse and blood pressures are normal. Examination shows normal femoral and popliteal pulses but his foot pulses are absent.
What is the single most appropriate next step?

A Blood tests should be requested to check his serum cholesterol
B He should be advised to rest in order to avoid pain
C He should be referred as an emergency to a vascular surgeon for surgery
D Stopping smoking will not improve the situation
E The situation is irreversible and no treatment is possible

46. A 93 year-old women has a sudden onset of a painful cold right foot. She has had no previous symptoms. She is non-smoker and is not hypertensive. Examination shows her to be in atrial fibrillation. She has no palpable pulses below the femoral artery on that side. All peripheral pulses are palpable in her left leg.
What is the single most likely cause of her symptoms?

A Deep venous thrombosis
B Dissection of the thoracic aorta
C Embolism from a mural thrombus in the left atrium
D Ruptured abdominal aortic aneurysm
E Thrombosis of the superficial femoral artery

47. A 75 year-old man collapses with a sudden onset of severe epigastric pain, radiating through to his back. He is tachycardic and hypotensive. Abdominal examination shows him to be tender with an 8cm pulsatile epigastric mass.
What is the single most likely diagnosis?

A Acute mesenteric ischaemia
B Acute pancreatitis
C Leaking abdominal aortic aneurysm
D Obstructing colonic carcinoma
E Perforated duodenal ulcer

48. A 40 year-old woman has dilated veins on the medial aspect of her left calf. They cause her mild discomfort but her main concern is their cosmetic appearance. Examination confirms the presence of varicose veins and the overlying skin appears healthy.
What single statement best describes the pathophysiology of her condition?

A A good correlation exists been symptoms and signs of the disease

B At some time in the past she had a deep vein thrombosis
C If she develops skin discolouration in the ankle region she is protected form the risk of skin ulceration
D She must have had a lower limb fracture in the past
E The veins are in the distribution of the long saphenous vein

49. A 25 year-old man has undergone emergency surgery for a fracture of his right tibia. An intramedullary nail was inserted. Following the surgery, he is initially comfortable but develops increasing calf pain and altered sensation on his toes over the next 6 hours.
What is the single most likely diagnosis?

A Acute osteomyelitis
B Compartment syndrome
C Deep venous thrombosis
D Necrotising fasciitis
E Wound haematoma

50. A 43 year-old diabetic woman has developed an ulcer over the heel of her right foot. It is relatively painless and has a purulent discharge.
Which single statement is true regarding the Most heal rapidly and spontaneously ulcer?

A A plain X-ray has no role in the management of this patient
B Antibiotics are not required
C The arterial supply to the foot should be assessed and the ankle-brachial pressure index measured
D The ulcer is due to venous insufficiency
E They are always due to infection with *Staphylococcus aureus*

51. A 55 year-old man undergoes an angioplasty of a coronary artery stenosis. The angiography catheter and angioplasty balloon are inserted through his right femoral artery. 1 week after the procedure he has notices a painful lump in his right groin. Examination shows a pulsatile swelling.
What is the single most likely diagnosis?

A Enlarged inguinal lymph node
B False aneurysm of the common femoral artery
C Saphena varix
D True aneurysm of the right external iliac artery
E Wound haematoma

Surgical emergencies

52. A 40 year-old man has a sudden onset of vomiting of fresh blood. He has previously drunk heavily and is known to have cirrhosis. Examination shows him to pale and clammy. He is tachycardic and hypotensive.

What is the single most likely cause of the bleeding?

A Acute oesophagitis
B Duodenal ulcer
C Mallory Weiss tear
D Meckel's diverticulum
E Oesophageal varices

53. A 20 year-old woman has central abdominal pain that migrates over the following 2 days to her right iliac fossa. She feels generally unwell, has a low-grade pyrexia and tachycardia. She has lost her appetite. Examination shows her to have lower abdominal tenderness, more so in the right iliac fossa. Her white cell count is raised and urinalysis shows her urine to be clear.
What is the single most likely diagnosis?

A Acute appendicitis
B Acute salpingitis
C Appendix abscess
D Ureteric colic
E Urinary tract infection

54. A 70 year-old woman has had colicky abdominal pain and vomiting for 3 days. She feels bloated and has not had her bowels open for 48 hours. She has had no previous abdominal surgery. Examination shows her abdomen to be distended, generally tender but with no evidence of peritonitis. She has a fullness in her right iliac fossa. She has high-pitched bowel sounds.
What is the single most likely cause of her presentation?

A Abdominal adhesions
B Obstructing caecal carcinoma
C Obstructing rectal carcinoma
D Pyloric stenosis due to a gastric carcinoma
E Strangulated femoral hernia

55. A 50 year-old man has sudden onset of severe epigastric pain and vomiting. He went to a wedding a 2 days previously where he drank alcohol to excess. He appears unwell, tachycardic and dehydrated. He has epigastric tenderness. His white cell count and serum amylase are raised. His liver function tests are normal.
What is the most like single cause of his raised serum amylase?

A Acute cholecystitis
B Acute mesenteric ischaemia
C Acute pancreatitis
D Perforated peptic ulcer
E Rupture abdominal aortic aneurysm

56. A 70 year-old man has a sudden onset of severe abdominal pain. He has vomited on several occasions. He is known to have angina and intermittent claudication. He is a heavy smoker. Examinations shows generalised abdominal tenderness. The admitting medical team are concerned he has acute mesenteric ischaemia. Which single statement regarding his investigations results is most likely to be true?

A An early radiological sign is 'thumb printing' of the bowel wall
B ECG will show sinus rhythm
C Serum amylase will be normal
D Serum lactate level will be raised
E White cell count will normal

57. An 89 year-old man has a sudden onset of rectal bleeding. It occurred spontaneously and caused him alarm due the apparent volume. He describes it as dark red and containing clots. He is on aspirin but no other regular medications. He remains cardiovascularly stable and the bleeding settles spontaneously.
What is the single most likely cause of the bleeding?

A Acute colitis
B Diverticular disease
C Haemorrhoids
D Rectal carcinoma E Upper gastrointestinal bleed

58. A 30 year-old man has a sudden onset of severe epigastric pain. It rapidly spreads throughout his abdomen. He vomits on several occasions. Examinations shows him to be pyrexial and tachycardic. He has generalised peritonitis. His bowel sounds are absent.
What single statement is true regarding his initial management?

A A urinary catheter should be inserted
B He should be given fluid resuscitation with oral fluids
C Opiate analgesia should be avoided
D Oxygen should not be given until a decision to operate has been made
E Surgery should be delayed until the following day

59. A 35 year-old man falls off the roof of his house. He has a large scalp laceration and displaced fracture of his right tibia and fibula.
What single statement is true regarding his management?

A A primary survey should be performed after tending to non-life threatening injuries
B A secondary survey is unnecessary if all injuries are obvious
C His Glasgow Coma Score should be measured before securing venous access
D Realignment of the fracture of his right leg is the highest priority
E Securing his airway is the first part of the primary survey

SBA answers

First principles

1. C

At the age of 16 years a child can be presumed to have the capacity to decide on treatment. Below this age, the child may have the capacity to decide depending on their ability to understand what the treatment involves. This is known as Gillick competence. Below the age of 16 years, if the child does not understand the advantages and risk of the proposed treatment only his parents have 'parental responsibility' and give consent. Family friends and relatives are unable. In an emergency, a doctor can act in the best interest of the child without consent.

2. D

Normal saline is a crystalloid solution. It is an isotonic solution. One litre contains 150 mmol of sodium and 150 mmol of chloride. It does not contain potassium, bicarbonate or calcium. Hartmann's solution is also a crystalloid. It contains less sodium and chloride but it does contain potassium, bicarbonate or calcium. Dextrose saline is also isotonic but contains both sodium, chloride and dextrose.

3. D

The aim of preoperative assessment is ensure the patient understands the surgery that is scheduled and to ensure that they are fit enough to undergo the procedure. The extent of preoperative investigation is determined by the age and medical history of the patient and the nature of the procedure to be undertaken. Young fit patients undergoing minor surgery usually required no investigation. In a more elderly patient undergoing major surgery the minimum of a full blood count, urea and electrolytes, clotting and an ECG is required. Cross matching of 6 units of blood for a right hemicolectomy is excessive.

4. B

The development of a painful red swollen calf following surgery is very suggestive of the development of a deep vein thrombosis. Homan's sign (calf pain on passive dorsiflexion of the foot) may be positive. As well as local symptoms, there is risk of the development of a pulmonary embolism and patients should be treated with a therapeutic dose of subcutaneous heparin as soon as the diagnosis is suspected. The diagnosis can be confirmed with the use of Doppler ultrasound showing clot within the vein. D-dimers are of limited use in postoperative surgical patients as the levels will be raised by clots/haematoma at the surgical site.

5. D

Morbidity and mortality after all surgery are increased in the obese. The risk is increased even in the absence of other disease. Obese patients are at risk of numerous complications often related to either the cardiovascular or respiratory system. Patients should be advised to lose weight before elective surgery. In those patients in whom surgery cannot be delayed it should performed as an inpatient with an appropriately experienced anaesthetist.

Clinical essentials

6. E

Vital signs should be recorded in all patients – temperature, pulse, blood pressure and respiratory rate. They provide objective evidence of physiological normality or derangement. Patients presenting with acute surgical emergencies are often septic and unwell. They are often pyrexial, tachycardic and hypotensive. Vital signs can be scored and summated to provide an Early Warning Score. Changes in the score can provide an objective assessment of the physiological response to resuscitation.

7. C

A groin lump that extends in to scrotum and is separate from the testis is mostly likely to be due to an inguinal hernia. Most uncomplicated inguinal hernias have a cough impulse and are reducible. The presence of a tender and irreducible lump suggests strangulation and is a surgical emergency. A scrotal swelling that is not separate from the testis and transilluminates brightly is most likely to be a hydrocele.

8. D

Derangement of the acid-base status is common in patients presenting with acute abdominal pathology. A lactic acidosis is a common finding. This presents with a metabolic acidosis with a raised serum lactate. This occurs as a result of reduced tissue perfusion, as consequence of hypovolaemia.

9. E

Urinary catheters vary in their length (22 or 38 cm), diameter (10 Fr to 24), volume of the balloon (5 mL to 30 mL) and the material from which they are made. A catheter should be selected appropriate for the use being considered. In male patients it is important to use a 'male' length catheter. A catheter is normally inserted via the urethra following installation of a local anaesthetic gel into the urethra. A catheter should be inserted suprapubically if the transurethral result fails or there is suspicion of a urethral injury. To avoid injury to the urethra, the balloon should not be inflated until urine is seen coming from the catheter. To reduce the risk of infection, a catheter should be removed as soon as it is no longer required.

10.C

Calor, rubor, dolor and tumour (heat, redness, pain and swelling) are signs of acute inflammation. An abscess is a localised collection of pus, usually in the subcutaneous tissues that arises a result of an acute inflammatory response to infection. An abscess contains pus – a yellow / green liquid containing dead tissue, white cells and bacteria. If untreated, an abscess will 'point' and discharge spontaneously. Resolution can be hastened by surgical drainage. Pus should be sent for microbiological culture and in subcutaneous infections, Staphylococcus aureus is most likely to be identified as the causative organism.

11.A

Sepsis is common in emergency surgical patients and delayed recognition, intervention and inadequate treatment results in increased mortality and preventable deaths. If sepsis is clinically suspected then the 'Sepsis six' should be initiated. Patients should be given high-flow oxygen and blood cultures taken. Intravenous fluids and broad spectrum antibiotics should be administered. The serum lactate should be measured and the patients response to treatment assessed by measuring the urine output.

Breast disease

12.D

Breast lumps are the commonest reason that women are referred for assessment in a breast clinic. The three most frequent causes of breast lumps are fibroadenomas, breast cysts and breast carcinoma. Each are more common in various age groups. Fibroadenomas are problem of breast development and occur in young women. Breast cysts occur during breast involution around the time of the menopause. Breast cancer is very uncommon below the age of 30 years.

13.D

Triple assessment is a standard approach to the assessment of patients with possible breast disease and, as its name implies, involves three aspects: a clinical, radiological and pathological assessment. All women will need a clinical assessment. The need for radiological (mammograms/ultrasound) and pathological (FNA/core biopsy) investigations will depend on the age of the patient, the presenting symptoms and physical signs. Mammography has a limited utility in premenopausal women. Many breast lesions are benign and the use of a biopsy does not necessarily imply clinical or radiological signs of breast cancer.

14.D

Lactational breast sepsis is a common complication of breast feeding. Generalised infection within the breast results in mastitis. If the infection becomes localised then an abscess can occur. The most common organism involved is Staphylococcus aureus. Non-lactational breast abscess usually occur in slightly older women usually as a result of duct ectasia or periductal mastitis. The organisms involved are usually Bacteroides species, anaerobic streptococci or enterococci.

15.A

An axillary node clearance should be performed in patients with known axillary lymph node metastases. The extent of the surgery performed (Level 1,2 or 3) can be defined in relation to the pectoralis minor muscle. It is important that various anatomical structures are clearly define and preserved at surgery. These include the long thoracic nerve (to serratus anterior), the thoracodorsal bundle (to latissimus dorsi) and the axillary vein.

16.C

All patients undergoing breast-conserving surgery for invasive breast cancer should be considered for breast radiotherapy to reduce the risk of local recurrence. Chemotherapy is of limited benefit in good prognosis tumours – low grade, node negative. There is however benefit of hormonal treatment in patients with oestrogen receptor positive tumours. Trastuzumab (Herceptin) is a monoclonal antibody against the HER2 receptor and is of benefit in addition to chemotherapy in HER2 positive patients.

17.C

A retroareolar lump in teenager is almost always due to gynaecomastia and is rarely the sign of any underlying endocrine disorder. The diagnosis is made on clinical grounds and extensive investigation is not required. The lump will often reduce in size during the teenage years and surgery is rarely required. Male breast cancer is rare and is very uncommon below the age of 50 years.

Endocrine surgery

18.B

A midline next lump that is elevated on protrusion of the tongue is most likely to be a thyroglossal cyst. They arise from remnants of thyroid tissue left in the line of descent of the thyroid gland from the base of the tongue. About of half of all thyroglossal cysts present in childhood. Surgery is by surgical excision. As the cyst is often still attached the hyoid bone, the mid portion this bone should be excised. This reduces the risk of recurrence.

19.E

Thyrotoxicosis presents with features of increased metabolic rate and increased sympathetic nervous system activity. The symptoms and signs of thyrotoxicosis are weight loss, nervousness, hyperactivity and irritability, insomnia, tremor, tachycardia and palpitations, dyspnoea, increased appetite, sweating, diarrhoea and a preference for cold weather. Hypothyroidism is often asymptomatic but clinical features include weight gain, slow thoughts, slow speech, hair loss, muscle fatigue and a preference for warm weather

20.C

Goitre is a non-specific term describing enlargement of the thyroid gland. It does not imply the presence of any specific pathology. Thyroid function tests are useful in the investigation of potential thyroid disease. Changes in levels of thyroxine (T4), triiodothyronine (T3) and thyroid-stimulating hormone can be understood in relation to the feedback mechanism. T4 may be normal in patients with T3-toxicosis, TSH will be unmeasurable in patients with thyrotoxicosis and elevated in those with hypothyroidism. Anti-TSH antibodies are increased in patients with Grave's disease.

21.B

There are two recurrent laryngeal nerves – left and right. They are branches of the vagus nerves and supply all the intrinsic muscles of the larynx, except the cricothyroid muscles. The nerves emerge from the vagus nerve at the level of the arch of aorta, and then travel up the side of the trachea to the larynx. The right and left nerves are not symmetrical, with the left nerve looping under the arch, and the right nerve travelling directly upwards. Close to the thyroid gland they pass in the groove between the trachea and oesophagus. Intraoperative damage to one or other of the recurrent laryngeal nerves results in hoarseness and stridor.

22.C

This patient has a medullary carcinoma of the thyroid gland. They arise from the para-follicular C-cells and about 20% of cases are familial with autosomal dominant inheritance. It can also occur as part of MEN IIa and MEN IIb syndromes. Medullary carcinoma metastasise to the regional nodes and also via blood to bone, liver and lung. About 50% of patients have lymph node metastases at presentation. Tumours produce calcitonin and serum calcitonin levels can be used in follow up to look for the presence of metastatic disease. Total thyroidectomy is the treatment of choice.

23.C

Hyperparathyroidism is increased parathyroid hormone production by the parathyroid. Primary hyperparathyroidism is due to autonomous overproduction of parathyroid hormone by the parathyroid glands, usually as a result of a parathyroid adenoma. Secondary hyperparathyroidism is a reactive increase in parathyroid hormone production to compensate for a hypocalcaemia, usually as a result of chronic renal failure. In most patients with primary hyperparathyroidism the serum phosphate level is increased. In many patients with minimally elevated calcium levels, surgery can be avoided.

24.E

This patient has Cushing's syndrome due to cortisol excess. Cushing's disease is the syndrome arising as a result of a pituitary microadenoma and can present with clinical features due to either the features of cortisol excess or pressure on adjacent structures. Pituitary tumours may press on the optic chiasma resulting in visual changes. The commonest visual field change is a bitemporal hemianopia. It can also cause a third nerve palsy which results in drooping of eye lid and the eye to move down and out.

25.A

This patient has a phaeochromocytoma, a neuroendocrine tumour usually arising from the adrenal medulla. Most secrete adrenaline and some noradrenaline and the clinical features are due intermittent catecholamine excess. Of all phaeochromocytomas 10% are malignant, 10% are bilateral and 10% are extra-adrenal. To confirm the diagnosis, it is necessary to demonstrate catecholamine excess by measuring 24-hour urinary vanniyl mandelic acid, 24-hour urinary total catecholamines and serum adrenaline or noradrenaline. Unilateral adrenalectomy of the affected adrenal gland is usually necessary.

26.C

Carcinoid tumours are neuroendocrine lesions of the gastrointestinal tract that arise from amine precursor uptake and decarboxylation (APUD) cells. They are most commonly found in the appendix and small bowel. Carcinoid syndrome occurs when they metastasise to the liver. The diagnosis can confirmed by finding increased 5-Hydroxy indol acetic acid (5HIAA) in a 24 hour urine specimen. Plasma chromogranin A levels may be increased. 111In - octreotide scintigraphy may identify the primary or secondary tumour.

Upper gastrointestinal surgery

27.A

Upper gastrointestinal endoscopy is a commonly performed investigation for the assessment of gastrointestinal symptoms. It usually performed as day case under sedation or topical local anaesthesia to the pharynx. The stomach needs to be empty and views are usually obtained as far as the second part of the duodenum. Interventional procedures can be performed such as biopsies, removal of foreign bodies or dilatation of strictures.

28.E

The patient has the typical symptoms of gastro-oesophageal reflux disease. It results from the reflux of either acid or bile from the stomach in to the oesophagus. It affects about 40% of the adult population. There is a poor correlation between the severity of symptoms and the extent of the reflux. An upper GI endoscopy may show the presence of oesophagitis. However, an upper GI endoscopy may be normal even in the presence of typical symptoms. The presence of reflux is best demonstrated by oesophageal pH studies. These can be used to correlate symptoms with an objective measure of reflux and is an essential investigation ahead of any surgical intervention.

29.E

This patient has dysphagia; difficulty in swallowing. It is often described as food 'sticking' after swallowing and is usually the result of obstruction at the lower end of the oesophagus. The symptoms may be progressive; initially with solids and then with liquids. Dysphagia results from either extrinsic or intrinsic mechanical oesophageal compression or neuromuscular problems. The commonest cause of progressive dysphagia associated with weight loss is oesophageal carcinoma. The disease often presents late and is often inoperable at presentation.

Colorectal surgery

30.C

Complications of diverticular disease are common reason for surgical admission and emergency surgery. Acute diverticulitis usually presents with left iliac fossa pain, fever, tachy-cardia and localised tenderness. If perforation of the diverticulum occurs then an abscess can develop with formation of a tender mass. If the infection fails to localise then generalised peritonitis can occur. A diverticular stricture causes large bowel obstruction. A vesico-colic fistula presents with recurrent urinary tract infections and the passage of air per urethra (pneumaturia).

31.E

A stoma is a surgically created communication between a hollow viscus and the skin. The commonest types encountered are colostomies and ileostomies. An ileostomy is usually situated in the right iliac fossa, has a spout and the bag will contain liquid small bowel contents. A colostomy is usually situated in the left iliac fossa, is flush with the skin and the bag contains firm stool. Complications such a prolapse, retraction and parastomal hernias do occur. Some stomas are potentially reversible but surgery is often complex and risky.

32.B

In an elderly patient presenting with right iliac fossa pain, anaemia and a palpable mass, the most likely diagnosis is a caecal carcinoma. An appendix mass will also cause a right iliac fossa mass but the history is likely to be shorter and the patient be septic and unwell. Ovarian carcinoma usually presents with gradual onset of abdominal distension, ascites and no localised mass. The diagnosis can be confirmed by a CT and colonoscopy.

33. B

Anal carcinoma is relatively uncommon but its incidence appears to be increasing. It is more common in homosexuals, especially those with genital warts. Human papilloma virus is an important aetiological factor. Approximately 80% of anal cancer are squamous cell carcinomas. The diagnosis can difficult and many cases are initially misdiagnosed as benign lesions. The inguinal lymph nodes may be enlarged but only 50% of patients with palpable inguinal nodes have metastatic disease. Radiotherapy is often the mainstay of treatment.

34.A

An anal fissure is a break in the skin of the anal canal, often occurring as a result of mucosal ischaemia secondary to muscle spasm of the external anal sphincter. About 90% occur in the posterior midline. Treatment involves relaxing the sphincter either with drugs or surgery. GTN ointment is effective but patients often develop headaches with its use. Surgery produces symptomatic improvement but following internal sphincterotomy about 20% patients develop some degree of incontinence.

Hepatobiliary surgery

35.C

Gallstone are common and are fund in about 12% of men and 24% of women respectively. Many stones remain asymptomatic. Biliary colic arises as a result of intermittent obstruction of the cystic duct due to the presence of a gallstone within Hartmann's pouch. Acute cholecystitis results from persistent obstruction of the cystic duct. Biliary colic presents with intermittent right upper quadrant abdominal pain. Patients remain systemically well and the pain settles rapidly. The symptoms of acute cholecystitis are more prolonged and patients with cholangitis and Mirrizi's syndrome are usually jaundiced.

36.D

The two commonest causes of obstructive jaundice in an elderly patient are gallstones or carcinoma of the head of the pancreas. In both, posthepatic jaundice occurs and both the serum and urinary conjugated bilirubin are raised. An abdominal ultrasound will show the common bile duct to be dilated. In patients with gallstones, the gallbladder is usually fibrosed and will not distend as the pressure in the obstructed biliary tree increases. Therefore, if in the presence of obstructive jaundice the gallbladder is palpable, the underlying cause is unlikely to be gallstones (Courvoisier's Law).

37.D

Clinically, this woman has ascites; free fluid within the abdominal cavity. In the absence of a past history of cardiac, liver or renal disease the most likely cause is an intra-abdominal malignancy. Ovarian carcinoma is the commonest cause of malignant ascites in women. The symptoms are often non-specific and the diagnosis is often delayed. A diagnostic peritoneal tap will show the fluid to be an exudate (high protein content). Malignant cells are often found in the peritoneal fluid. The diagnosis can be confirmed with an abdominal and pelvic CT scan and raised serum CA125.

38.B

Hepatocellular carcinoma (HCC) is a primary malignant tumour of the liver that can present as either a solitary lesion or multiple tumours. It is one of the commonest malignant tumours in Africa and south-east Asia. Its incidence mirrors the population prevalence of Chronic Hepatitis B and C. Important aetiological factors include cirrhosis, viral hepatitis, mycotoxins an anabolic steroids. The possibility of a HCC should be suspected in any patient with cirrhosis who shows evidence of clinical deterioration.

Urology

39.A

Acute cystitis is common in young women and *Escherichia coli* is responsible for 85% of uncomplicated urinary tract infections. *Proteus mirabilis* and enterococci can cause urinary tract infections, particularly in patients with abnormalities of the urinary system or a urinary catheter. *Staphylococcus aureus* is a rare cause of urinary tract infections and usually results from a blood-born infection.

40.D

This man has the typical symptoms of ureteric colic: severe colicky loin to groin pain associated with urinary frequency. Macroscopic haematuria is uncommon but microscopic haematuria is invariably present. A diagnosis of ureteric colic is unlikely in the absence of microscopic haematuria. The diagnosis can be confirmed with a CT-KUB. This will confirm the presence and site of the stone and any evidence of obstruction of the urinary tract. Most stones are small, will pass spontaneously and no surgical intervention is required.

41. D

Testicular tumours usually present with a painless testicular lump. Examination shows a firm and irregular lump that cannot be separated from the underlying testis. It is important to be able to differentiate them from other causes of scrotal swellings. Acute epididymitis and testicular torsion both present with severe scrotal pain with a tender and swollen epididymis and testis, respectively. A hydrocele causes a painless scrotal swelling. The testis cannot be separated from the swelling and transillumination is a typical physical sign. A varicocele consists of dilated veins of the pampiniform plexus and feels like a 'bag of worms' within the scrotum.

42.E

Renal cell carcinomas are uncommon. The classical triad of clinical features is haematuria, loin pain and a renal mass; a sign of advanced disease. Many patients present with painless haematuria and some tumours are identified on CT scan performed for another reason. Renal cell carcinomas occasionally produce hormones that influence the clinical presentation. Polycythaemia can occur due to erythropoietin production. Hypercalcaemia can occur due to production of a PTH-like hormone.

43. A

Bladder outflow obstruction in elderly men is usually due to benign prostatic hyperplasia. If affects 50% men older than 60 years and 90%

of men older than 90 years. The assessment of bladder outflow obstruction requires measurement of urinary flow followed by a clinical, radiological and pathological assessment of the patient to identify the underlying cause. An ultrasound scan should be performed to exclude hydronephrosis and a serum PSA should be measure to exclude prostate carcinoma.

44.C

Testicular torsion is a common surgical emergency in adolescent boys. It results from twisting of the testicle on its blood supply. It usually presents with acute scrotal pain. However, it may present with acute abdominal pain and no testicular symptoms. Therefore, it is essential to examine the scrotum in all boys who present with acute abdominal pain. Urinary symptoms are uncommon. Examination shows an exquisitely tender high-riding testis.

Vascular surgery

45.A

The patient has typical symptoms and signs of intermittent claudication. The diagnosis can be confirmed by measurement of the ankle-brachial pressure index. Extensive investigation is usually not required but assessment of risk factors and life style modification is important. Blood should be taken to measure blood sugar, lipids and cholesterol. Patients should be encouraged to exercise and lose weight. Stopping smoking will reduce the risk of disease progression. Surgical intervention is rarely required.

46.D

The patient has acute limb ischaemia. She has no risk factors for peripheral vascular disease. She has no symptoms of intermittent claudication nor signs of chronic limb ischaemia. Her pulses are normal in the contralateral leg. Clinically she appears to have an acute embolus. She is in atrial fibrillation and the most likely source of the embolus is the left atrium of her heart.

47. C

Clinically, the patient seems to have a leaking abdominal aortic aneurysm. His symptoms have occurred as a result of hypovolaemia due to blood leaking in to either the retroperitoneum or peritoneal cavity. The diagnosis can be confirmed by an abdominal CT scan. The patient should be rapidly resuscitated with blood and emergency surgery performed. Despite rapid surgical intervention, the mortality associated with emergency surgery is approximately 50%.

48.C

The patient has varicose veins in the distribution of the long saphenous veins. These occur on the medial aspect of the leg. Short saphenous varicose veins occur on the posterior and lateral aspect of the calf. Varicose veins occur as a result of incompetence of the venous valves. Most cases are idiopathic but some arise following deep venous thrombosis. The indications for surgical intervention are lipodermatosclerosis or venous ulceration, recurrent thrombophlebitis or bleeding from a saphena varix.

49.B

The muscles of the lower limb are enclosed with fascial planes that divide the limbs into compartments. A compartment syndrome occurs when the circulation and function of the tissues within the closed space is compromised by an increase in pressure. Venous drainage is impeded before the arterial inflow. Compartment syndromes usually present within 24 hours of the precipitating insult. The pain clinical feature is increasing pain and altered sensation in the distribution of nerves that pass through the compartment. Muscle swelling, tenderness and pain on passive movement may be seen.

50.C

Foot problems are common in diabetics due to a combination of a peripheral neuropathy and peripheral vascular disease. Patients should be monitored and educated about washing, care of corns and calluses, toenail cutting and suitable footwear. In those with ulceration, assessment should be made of potential infection and vascular insufficiency. Antibiotics should be prescribed based on the sensitivities of the organism present. Plain radiography or MRI may demonstrate the extent of the infection.

51.B

A true aneurysm consists of one or more of the vessel wall layers. The wall of a false aneurysm is made up of connective tissue and is usually the result of trauma or surgery. A false aneurysm most commonly occurs following catheterisation of the femoral artery and usually presents with pain, bruising and a pulsatile swelling at the site of the puncture. The diagnosis can be confirmed by Doppler ultrasound. It may be possible to obliterate the aneurysm by ultrasound-guided compression therapy. Suturing of puncture site or a vein patch may be required.

Surgical emergencies

52.E

In a patient whom has previously drunk heavily, is known to have alcoholic liver disease and now has hypovolaemic shock from an upper gastrointestinal bleed, then the most likely diagnosis is bleeding oesophageal varices. A bleeding

Meckel's diverticulum presents, often in child-hood or adolescence with the passage of fresh blood per rectum. A Mallory Weiss tear occurs in the lower oesophagus following vomiting and usually presents with altered blood in the vomit.

53. A

The patient has a good history for acute appendicitis with migratory abdominal pain and features of sepsis. However, the diagnosis of acute appendicitis can be difficult, particu-larly in young women. An appendix abscess is unlikely in view of the short history and the absence of a palpable abdominal mass. A urinary tract infection is unlikely when the urinalysis is clear. The most difficult differential diagnosis is between acute appendicitis and an acute gynaecological problem such as acute salpingitis or ruptured ovarian cyst. In these patients a diagnostic laparoscopy is often a use-ful investigation.

54. B

This patient has the cardinal features of intestinal obstruction – colicky abdominal pain, vomiting, distension and constipation. The early onset of pain and vomiting and the subsequent develop-ment of constipation favours a diagnosis of small bowel obstruction. In the absence of previous surgery adhesional obstruction is unlikely. Small bowel obstruction can result from an occult groin hernia, but the presence of a right iliac fossa mass suggests an obstruction caecal carcinoma. The diagnosis can be confirmed by an abdominal CT scan and appropriate surgery planned.

55. C

This patient appears to have acute pancreati-tis evidenced by the clinical features and the presence of a raised serum amylase. The two commonest causes of acute pancreatitis in the United Kingdom are gallstones and alcohol excess. The onset of his symptoms soon after a period of alcohol excess suggests the latter, but other causes need to be considered. Serum amylases has a low sensitivity and specificity for the diagnosis of acute pancreatitis. It can be increased in patients with other causes of acute abdominal pain such as perforated peptic ulcer, mesenteric ischaemia and a leaking abdominal aortic aneurysm.

56. D

Acute mesenteric ischaemia should be consid-ered as part of the differential diagnosis of any patient presenting with sudden onset of abdomi-nal pain. No single clinical feature provides conclusive evidence of the diagnosis. As a result, the diagnosis is difficult and often delayed. Early diagnosis requires a high index of suspicion. The diagnosis may be suggested by the presence of a metabolic acidosis and a raised serum lactate. The serum amylase and white cell count may also be raised. An abdominal X-ray may be normal early in the disease process. A late radiological feature is 'thumb printing' of the bowel wall due to mucosal oedema.

57. B

An acute lower gastrointestinal bleed in the absence of other symptoms in an elderly patient is most likely to be due to diverticular disease. Despite the alarm caused by the symptoms, the volume of blood lost is usually limited. Patients often remain cardiovascularly stable and a blood transfusion can often be avoided. Most bleeding settles spontaneously and can be investigated electively by a colonoscopy.

58. A

Generalised peritonitis is often due to gastroin-testinal perforation and requires rapid assessment and urgent resuscitation. Patients should be given oxygen and resuscitated with intravenous fluids. The adequacy of resuscitation can be assessed by the measurement of vital signs and measurement of the urine output through a urinary catheter. Adequate opiate analgesia should be adminis-tered as there is no evidence that it masks clinical signs. Patients should proceed to surgery once adequate resuscitation has been performed.

59. E

The management of major trauma patients should follow a systematic and concise approach. This will allow the recognition and immediate management of life threatening inju-ries and ensures that all other non-threatening injuries are subsequently identified. During the primary survey the initial assessment is of the airway, breathing, circulation and neurological dysfunction. The patient is subsequently exposed and a head-to-toe examination performed as part of the secondary survey.

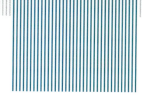

Index

Note: Page numbers in **bold** or *italic* refer to tables or figures, respectively.

A

Abdominal aortic aneurysm 210, *210*
  aetiology 210
  clinical features 210–211
  conservative management 211
  diagnostic approach 211
  endovascular aneurysm repair 212
  epidemiology 210
  investigations 211, *211*
  open aneurysm surgery 212
  prognosis 212
  ruptured 211
Abdominal distension 31–32
Abdominal examination 29
  auscultation 30–31
  palpation 29, *30*
  percussion 30, *31*
Abdominal incision 39, *39*
Abdominal masses 32–33, **33**
Abdominal pain 24
  in colorectal disease 119
  nature of 25
  onset of 24
  site of 24, *24*, **25**, *25*
Abdominal wall hernias 121
  femoral hernias 122–123
  incisional hernias 123
  inguinal hernia 121–122
  obturator hernia 124
  spigelian hernias 123
  umbilical hernia 123
Abscesses 33–34
Accessory nipples 54
Achalasia 101
  balloon dilatation 102
  cardiomyotomy 102
  clinical features 101–102
  diagnostic approach 102, *102*
Acute limb ischaemia 205
  aetiology 205

clinical features 205
diagnostic approach 205
emergency embolectomy 206
epidemiology 205
intra-arterial thrombolysis 206
investigations 206
prognosis 206
Adenomatous polyps 131
Adjuvant therapy 133
Adrenalectomy 85
Adrenal glands, anatomy and physiology 73, *73*
Adrenocorticotrophic hormone (ACTH) 72
Advanced care directive 2
Airway calibre 6, *6*
Aldosterone 68, 73, 88, 172
5-Aminosalicyclic acid (5-ASA), in inflammatory bowel disease 127–128
Anal carcinoma 133–134
Anal dilatation 136
Anal fissure 136
Anaplastic signet-ring tumours 107
Angiodysplasia 228
Angiography 202, **202**
Ankle–brachial pressure index (ABPI) 201
Anorectal sepsis 134
  abscesses and fistulae 134
  clinical features 134
  Goodsall's rule 134, *135*
  management 134–135
Antidiuretic hormone (ADH) 68, 73, 171–172
Appendiceal carcinoid tumours 89
Appendicitis, acute 222–223
Appendix abscess 223
Appendix mass 223
Arterial blood gases 35–36, **36**
Arteriosclerosis 196–197

Ascites 147, 159
  aetiology 159, **159**
  clinical features 159
  diagnostic approach 159
  management 159
Aspiration pneumonitis 19, *19*
Atelectasis 19
Atheroma 196
  aetiology *196*, 196–197
  complicated plaques 197
  complications *196*
  fatty streaks and fibrous plaques *196*, 197
  risk factors **196**
Axillary surgery, in breast cancer 59–60, **60**

B

Bacteraemia **17**
Barrett's oesophagus 106
Benign prostatic hyperplasia 184–185
Bile 144–145
Biliary apparatus
  extrahepatic 142, *143*
  intrahepatic 144–145
Biliary colic 151–152
Bilirubin 145
Bladder 169, *169*
  nerve supply 169–170
  sphincters 169
Bladder calculi 180
Bladder cancers 182–183, **183**, *183*
Bleeding peptic ulcer 226
Blood tests, in surgical patients 35, **35**
Body mass index (BMI) 6
Bowel habit, change in 113–115, 119 *see also* Colorectal diseases
Bradycardia 27
Breast 45
  anatomy *48*, 48–49, *49*

blood supply 48–49, *49*
development of 48
embryology 47–48, *48*
lactation 49–50
lump in 46–47
lymphatic drainage 49
physiology 49–50
premenopausal 49
sensory innervation 49
Breast cancer 57, 58
aetiology 58
axillary surgery 59–60, **60**
biological therapy 61
BRCA1/BRCA2 gene, mutation
   in 58
chemotherapy 60
clinical features 59
epidemiology 58
hormonal treatment 60–61
investigations 59
pathogenesis 58
prognosis 60, **60**
radiotherapy 61
screening 58
surgical treatment 59, *59*
Breast-conserving surgery 59, *59*
Breast disease 50, 57
accessory breast tissue 54
accessory nipples 54
benign **54**, 54–56
breast pain (see Mastalgia)
cysts 55
ductal carcinoma in situ (DCIS)
   58
examination (see Breast
   examination)
fat necrosis 56
fibroadenomas 54–55
galactorrhoea 56, **56**
gynaecomastia **62**, *62*, 62–63
invasive breast cancer 58–61
   (see also Breast cancer)
lactational breast abscess 55
male breast cancer 62
non-lactational breast abscess
   55–56, *56*
Paget's disease of nipple *61*,
   61–62, **62**
papillomas 55
phyllodes tumours 55
symptoms and signs **50**
triple asssessment 50–53
types 57–58
Breast disease, investigation in
   52
core biopsy 53, *53*
fine-needle aspiration 53
mammography 52, *52*

MRI 53
ultrasound 52–53, *53*
Breast examination 50
axillary nodes, position of
   51, *52*
benign and malignant lumps,
   features of **51**
inspection 50–51
palpation 51, *51*
quadrants of breast *51*
Bromocriptine 57
Buerger's angle 200
Bupivacaine 16

C

Calcitonin 70
Carbimazole 77
Carcinoid tumours 89
Cardiac function tests,
   preoperative 4
Cardiovascular complications,
   postoperative 19–20
Carotid artery disease 208
aetiology 208, *208*
carotid angioplasty and
   stenting 210
carotid endarterectomy 209
clinical features 208, **208**
diagnostic approach 209
epidemiology 208
investigations 209, *209*
medical management 209
Catheter-related urinary tract
   infections 20
Charcot's triad 152
Chemotherapy, in breast cancer
   60
Chest radiograph, preoperative 4
Cholangiocarcinoma 156
Cholangitis, acute 152
Cholecystitis, acute 151–152
Cigarette smoking 5
Circumscribed masses, on
   mammography 52
Colloids 11
Colorectal cancer 131
aetiology 131
chemotherapy 133
clinical features 132
diagnostic approach 132
Duke's classification 133, *133*
epidemiology 131
familial 131
investigations 132
laparoscopic surgery 133
pathogenesis 132
prevention 131–132
prognosis 133

radiotherapy 133
surgical management *132*,
   132–133
Colorectal diseases 111, 118
abdominal CT and MRI 120
abdominal wall hernias
   121–124
anal carcinoma 133–134
anal fissure 136
anorectal sepsis 134–136
blood tests 120
colonoscopy 121
colorectal cancer 131–133
colorectal polyps 130–131
diverticular disease 129–130
enterocutaneous fistulae
   124–125
examination 119–120
femoral sheath and canal
   116, *116*
history 119
inflammatory bowel disease
   125–129
inguinal canal and *115*,
   115–116, **116**
intestinal stomas 124
large intestine and 116–118
pilonidal sinus 136–137
plain radiographs 120
rectal prolapse 137
symptoms and signs of **119**
Colorectal malignancy, lower
   gastrointestinal bleed and 229
Colorectal polyps 130, **131**
adenomatous polyps 131
juvenile polyps 131
metaplastic polyps 131
Peutz–Jegher's syndrome 131
Colostomy 124
Compartment syndrome 206,
   206
clinical features 206
management 207
Confusion, postoperative 20–21,
   21
Conn's syndrome 88
Constipation 119
Core biopsy, breast 53, *53*
Corticosteroids, in inflammatory
   bowel disease 128
Crohn's disease 125–129 *see
also* Inflammatory bowel
   disease
Crystalloid solutions 11, *11*
CT angiography 202
CT scanning 36
Cushing's disease 85
Cushing's syndrome 85

algorithm for investigation of
87, *87*
causes **86**
clinical features 85–87, **86**,
86
diagnostic approach 87
imaging 87
management 87
Cysts, breast 55

D

Danazol 57, 63
Diabetic foot 207
Diarrhoea 119
Diathermy 40
bipolar 41, *41*
monopolar *40*, 40–41
Diverticular disease 129–130,
129–130
acute lower gastrointestinal
bleed and 228–229
Drains, surgical 41–42
active/passive 42
open/closed 42
Ductal carcinoma in situ (DCIS)
58
Duplex ultrasonography
201–202, *202*
Dyspepsia 98
Dysphagia 98, **98**

E

Embolism 198, **198**
Empyema of gallbladder 152
Endocrine diseases 65 *see also*
Parathyroid glands; Pituitary
gland; Thyroid gland
carcinoid tumours 89
Conn's syndrome 88
Cushing's syndrome 85–87
endocrine physiology and 68
endocrine system and 65, *66*
examination 75–76
history taking **74**, 74–75
hyperparathyroidism 83–84
hypothyroidism 78
multiple endocrine neoplasia
88
phaeochromocytomas 85
signs of **74**
solitary thyroid nodule
66–67, 79–80, *80*
symptoms of **74**
thyroglossal cysts 78–79
thyroiditis 82–83
thyroid neoplasms 80–82
thyrotoxicosis 76–78

Endoscopic laser ablation 106
Endoscopic retrograde
cholangiopancreatography
(ERCP) 147–148
Endoscopic ultrasound 99
Enteral nutrition 12–13
Enterocutaneous fistulae
124–125
Epididymitis 188
Epidural anaesthesia 16, **16**, *16*
Erectile dysfunction 190–191
Erythropoietin 68
Examination 26
abdominal 29–31
abdominal distension 31–32
abdominal masses 32–33, **33**
abscesses 33–34
body temperature 26–27, **27**
dehydration, signs of **27**
'end-of-the-bed-o-gram' 26,
27
general appearance 26, *27*
hernias 33, **33**, *33*
lump, description of 28–29
pulse and blood pressure
27–28, **28**
rectal 31, *32*
respiratory rate 28, **28**
surgical sieve 35
ulcers 34, *34*
variables and scores of early
warning system **28**
Expiratory reserve volume (ERV)
6

F

Fat necrosis 56
Femoral embolectomy 195, *195*
Femoral hernias 122
clinical features 122–123
management 123
Femoral sheath and canal 116,
116
Fibroadenomas 54–55
giant 55
simple 55
Fine-needle aspiration 53
Fluid balance, in perioperative
period 9
assessment of fluid therapy 11
body fluid compartments 9,
10
fluid replacement therapy
11, *11*
maintenance requirements
9–10
pre-existing and ongoing
losses **10**–11

Follicle stimulating hormone
(FSH) 68, 73

G

Galactorrhoea 56, **56**
Gallbladder 142–143
enlargement 146, **146**
fundus of 143
Gallstone ileus 152
Gallstones 150–151
Gangrene 198, **198**
Gastric cancer 106
aetiology 107, *107*
clinical features 107
diagnostic approach 107
epidemiology 106–107
partial gastrectomy with Polya
reconstruction 107, *108*
prognosis 108
surgical management
107–108, *108*
total gastrectomy with roux-
en-Y reconstruction 107,
108
Gastric lymphoma 108
Gastrinomas 155
Gastrointestinal haemorrhage
lower 227–229
upper 225–227
Gastrointestinal perforation
232–234
Gastrointestinal stromal tumours
108
Gastrointestinal tract
embryology 94
functions 97, **97**
oesophagus, anatomy of
94–95
physiology 97, **97**
small intestine, anatomy of
96–97
stomach, anatomy of *95*,
95–96
wall of 94, *94*
Gastro-oesophageal reflux
disease (GORD) 99, 100
aetiology 100
clinical features 100
diagnostic approach 100
drug therapy 101
epidemiology 100
fundoplication 101, *101*
investigations 100, *100*
lifestyle modifications 100
Gillick competence 3
Glucagonomas 155
Glyceryl trinitrate 136
Goitre **75**, 76

Pancreatic adenocarcinoma 152
  aetiology 153
  clinical features 153
  epidemiology 153
  investigation 153, *153*
  palliative treatment 154
  prognosis 154
  Whipple's procedure
    153–154, *154*
Pancreatitis, acute 234–237
  abdominal CT scan 235,
    236
  APACHE II score 236, **237**
  causes **235**
  complications 237, **237**
  MACHINES mnemonic 236
  Ranson's prognostic criteria
    236
Papillomas, breast 55
Paracetamol 15
Parathyroid glands 70
  anatomy 71
  embryology 70–71, *71*
  physiology 71
Parathyroid hormone 68, 71
Parenteral nutrition 13, **13**
Penile cancer 189
Peptic ulcer disease 102–104,
  103, 104
Perioperative hypothermia 9
Perioperative period 8
  fluid balance 9–11, **10,** *11*
  hypothermia, risk of 9
  infection, prevention of
    11–12
  preoperative fasting 9
  Safe Surgery Checklist 9,
    9, *10*
  surgical nutrition 12–13
Peripheral pulses 199, *199*
Peripheral vascular disease 202
  see also Vascular disease
Peritoneal inflammation, signs
  of 29
Peutz–Jegher's syndrome 131
Phaeochromocytomas 85
Phlegmasia alba dolens 201
Phlegmasia cerulea dolens 201
Phyllodes tumours 55
Pilonidal sinus *136,* 136–137
Pituitary gland 71
  anatomy 71, *72*
  anterior pituitary physiology
    71–73, *72*
Plain radiography 36
Polyps, colorectal 130–131, **131**
Portal hypertension 157–159,
  158

Postoperative pain, management
  of 15, **15**
  adverse effects of pain **15**
  analgesia 15
  assessment of pain 15
  local and regional anaesthesia
    16
  non-steroidal anti-
    inflammatory agents 15
  opiates 15
  spinal and epidural
    anaesthesia 16, **16,** *16*
Postoperative period 13
  cardiovascular complications
    19–20
  pain management 13–16
  postoperative confusion
    20–21, **21**
  postoperative pyrexia 16–17
  renal complications 20
  respiratory complications
    18–19
  sepsis 17, **17**
  wound dehiscence 18
  wound infections 18, **18**
Preoperative assessment 3, **3**
  American Society of
    Anesthesiologists grading
    system 3, **3**
  cardiovascular disease 4
  chronic renal failure 7
  diabetes mellitus 6
  obesity 6
  preoperative investigations
    3–4
  respiratory disease 5–6
Preoperative phase 1
  consent for surgery 1–3 (*see
    also* Informed consent)
  deep vein thrombosis,
    prophylaxis of 7–8
  patient assessment for surgery
    3–7
Pretibial myxoedema 77
Priapism 190
Prostate cancer 185
  aetiology 185
  clinical features 185
  diagnostic approach 185
  epidemiology 185
  hormonal therapy 186
  investigations 185–186
  radical prostatectomy 186
Prostate gland 170, *170*
  assessment of 174, **174**
Prostate-specific antigen (PSA) 186
Pyloric stenosis 104
Pyrexia, postoperative 16–17, **17**

R
Radical cystectomy 183
Radiotherapy, in breast cancer
  61
Rapid urease test 103
Raynaud's disease
  primary 218–219
  secondary 219
Rectal bleeding 119
Rectal examination 31, *32*
Rectal prolapse 137, *137*
Renal cell carcinomas 180–181
Renal complications,
  postoperative 20
  renal failure 20, **20**
  urinary tract infections 20
Renal function tests, preoperative
  7
Renal tract 167 *see also* Urinary
  disease
  bladder *169,* 169–170
  juxtaglomerular apparatus
    171
  kidneys 167–168, **168,** *168,*
    170–171
  male urethra 170
  nephron 168, *168,* 171
  prostate 170, *170*
  renal function, control of
    171–172
  testes 170, *170*
  ureters 168–169, **169**
Respiratory complications,
  postoperative 18
  aspiration pneumonitis 19,
    19
  atelectasis 19
  hypoxia 18–19, **19**
Respiratory function tests,
  preoperative 5–6
Respiratory rate 28, **28**
Robotic surgery 40

S
Safe Surgery Checklist 9, **9,** *10*
Saphena varix 214
Schistosoma haematobium
  infection 182
Screening programmes 38
  criteria for **38**
  IATROGENIC mnemonic 38
  outcomes of test **39**
  potential biases within **39**
  sensitivity and specificity
    38–39, **39**
  success of 38
  UK National Health

Service cancer screening programmes **38**
Scrotum, examination of 174, *174*
Seldinger technique 202
Sengstaken–Blakemore tube 226, *227*
Sentinel lymph node biopsy 60
Sepsis, postoperative 17, **17**
Septic shock **17**
Seton 135
Severe sepsis **17**
Sigmoid volvulus 231–232
Signs of surgical diagnoses *see* Examination
Sister Mary Joseph nodule 108
Small intestine 96
  duodenum 96
  histology 97
  jejunum and ileum 96–97
Solitary thyroid nodules 79
  aetiology 79
  algorithm for assessment and management of *80*
  biochemical assessment 79
  clinical features 79
  diagnostic approach 79
  epidemiology 79
  fine-needle aspiration cytology 80
  isotope scanning 80
  ultrasound 79–80
Sphincterotomy 136
Spiculate mass, on mammography 52, *52*
Spigelian hernias 123
Spinal anaesthesia 16, **16**, *16*
Spirometry *5*, 5–6
Spleen 144, 145
  disorders 160
  palpation of 146, *146*
Splenic rupture 160
Splenomegaly 160, **160**
Staphylococcus aureus 18, 55
Stellate lesions, on mammography 52
Stomach *see also* Upper gastrointestinal disease
  anatomical regions 95, *95*
  blood supply *95*, 95–96
  histology 96
  lymphatic drainage 96
  vagus nerve 96
Stomas 124, **124**
Supernumerary breasts 54
Surgical emergencies 221
  abdominal pain and 221, *221*
  acute appendicitis 222–223

acute mesenteric ischaemia 224–225
  acute pancreatitis 234–237
  gastrointestinal perforation 232–234
  intestinal obstruction 229–231
  lower gastrointestinal haemorrhage 227–229
  sigmoid volvulus 231–232
  upper gastrointestinal haemorrhage 225–227
Surgical sieve 35
Surgical techniques 39
  diathermy *40*, 40–41, *41*
  drains 41–42
  nasogastric tubes 42
  surgical incisions *39*, 39–40
  tourniquets 41
  urinary catheters *42*, 42–43, **43**
  wound closure 43
Sutures 43
Symptoms of surgical diagnoses 23–24
  inflammation 25–26, **26**
  pain *24*, 24–25, **25**, *25*
  ulceration 26, **26**
Systemic inflammatory response syndrome (SIRS) **17**

T

Tachycardia 27
Tamoxifen 60
Tenesmus 119
Testicular torsion 188
Testicular tumours 186
  adjuvant therapy 187–188
  aetiology 186
  clinical features 187, *187*
  diagnostic approach 187
  epidemiology 186
  investigations 187
  prognosis 188
  surgical treatment 187
Testis 170, *170*
Thrombosis 197–198
Thyroglossal cysts 78
  clinical features 78, *78*
  management 79
Thyroid acropachy 77
Thyroidectomy 82
Thyroid gland 68
  anatomy *69*, 69–70, *70*
  embryology 68, *69*
  examination 75
  fine-needle aspiration cytology 76

goitre **75**, 76
  inspection 75
  palpation *75*, 75–76
  physiology 70
  radioisotope scanning 76
  symptoms of disorders of **74**, 74–75
  thyroid function tests 76
  thyroid swellings 74–75
  thyroid ultrasound 76
Thyroiditis 82
  acute suppurative 83
  de Quervain's 82–83
  Hashimoto's 83
  Riedel's 83
Thyroid neoplasms 80, **81**
  anaplastic carcinoma 82
  benign 80–81
  follicular adenoma 81
  follicular tumours **81**, 81–82
  malignant 81–82
  medullary carcinoma 82
  papillary tumours 81, **81**
  surgical management 82
  thyroid lymphoma 82
  toxic adenoma 81
Thyroid stimulating hormone 72
Thyroid storm 78
Thyrotoxicosis 76–77
  anti-thyroid drugs 77
  clinical features 77
  diagnostic approach 77
  investigations 77
  management 77–78
  radioactive iodine 77
  surgical treatment 77–78
Thyroxine 68, 70
Tourniquets 41
  complications 41
  contraindications to use of 41
Transitional cell carcinomas 182
  see also Bladder cancers
Transjugular intrahepatic portosystemic shunting (TIPSS) 158
Transurethral resection of the prostate (TURP) 184–185
Transurethral resection syndrome 185
Trastuzumab (Herceptin) 61, *61*
Triiodothyronine 70
Tylosis 105

U

UK's National Health Service Breast Screening Programme 58

Ulcerative colitis 125–129 see
  also Inflammatory bowel
  disease
Ulcers 26, **26**
  BEDS mnemonic 34
  examination of 34, *34*
Ultrasound 36
  breast 52–53, *53*
  thyroid 76
Umbilical hernia 123
Upper gastrointestinal
  disease 91–93, 98 see also
  Gastrointestinal tract
    achalasia 101–102
    Barrett's oesophagus 106
    endoscopic ultrasound 99
    examination 98
    gastric cancer 106–108
    gastric lymphoma 108
    gastrointestinal stromal
      tumours 108
    gastro-oesophageal reflux
      100–101
    investigation 98–99
    manometry 99
    oesophageal cancer 104–106
    oesophageal pH studies 99
    peptic ulcer disease 102–104
    pyloric stenosis 104
    Sister Mary Joseph nodule
      108
    symptoms and signs **98**
    upper gastrointestinal
      endoscopy 99
Ureteric calculi 178
  abdominal examination 178
  aetiology 178
  clinical features 178
  conservative management
    179, **179**
  diagnostic approach 178
  differential diagnosis **178**
  epidemiology 178
  investigations 178–179, *179*
  lithotripsy 179
  surgery 179, 179–180
Ureters 168–169, **169**
Urethral strictures 183–184, **184**
Urethritis 189–190
Urinary catheter 42, *42*
  complications 43
  contraindication to 42–43
  indications for **43**
  suprapubic catheterisation 43
Urinary disease 163, 172
  abdominal and prostate
    examination *173*, 173–174,
    174

anatomy related to 167–170
benign prostatic hyperplasia
  184–185
bladder calculi 180
bladder cancer 182–183
bladder outflow obstruction
  183–185
computed tomography 175
cystoscopy 175
epididymitis 188
erectile dysfunction 190–191
filling/irritative symptoms 173
haematuria 172, **172**
kidney–ureter–bladder
  radiograph 175
loin pain 172
lower urinary tract symptoms
  173, **173**
obstructive urinary tract
  symptoms 173
penile cancer 189
priapism 190
prostate cancer 185–186
prostate gland, assessment
  of **174**
radioisotope renography 175,
  176
renal cancer 166–167,
  180–182
renal physiology and
  170–172
renal ultrasonography 175
scrotum, examination of 174,
  174
symptoms and signs **172**
testicular torsion 188
testicular tumours 186–188
ureteric calculi 164–165,
  178–180
urethral stricture 183–184
urethritis 189–190
urinalysis 174, **174**
urinary tract infection
  165–166, 176–177
urine cytology 175
urine microscopy and culture
  174
urodynamic studies 175, *176*
varicocele 188–189
Urinary diversion 183, **183**
Urinary tract infection (UTI)
  176–177

V

Vagus nerve 96
Varicocele 188–189, *189*
Varicose veins 213
  aetiology 213

clinical features 213–214,
  214
diagnostic approach 214
endovascular laser treatment
  214
epidemiology 213
investigations 214
radiofrequency ablation
  214
sclerotherapy 214–215
surgery for 215
tests of valvular incompetence
  in **200**
Vascular angle 200
Vascular disease 193
  abdominal aortic aneurysm
    210–212
  acute limb ischaemia
    194–195, 205–206
  anatomy related to *195*,
    195–196
  angiography 202, **202**
  arteriosclerosis 196–197
  carotid artery disease
    208–210
  compartment syndromes
    206–207
  CT angiography 202
  diabetic foot 207
  duplex ultrasonography
    201–202, *202*
  embolism 198, **198**
  examination *199*, 199–200,
    200
  gangrene 198, **198**
  hand-held Doppler scanning
    201, *201*
  intermittent claudication
    and chronic limb ischaemia
    203–205
  investigation 200–202
  ischaemia and infarction 198,
    198
  lymphadenopathy 217–218
  lymphoedema 216–217
  magnetic resonance
    angiography (MRA) 202
  Marjolin ulceration 216
  primary Raynaud's disease
    218–219
  secondary Raynaud's disease
    219
  symptoms and signs **199**
  thrombosis 197–198
  varicose veins 213–215
  vascular trauma 212–213
  venous hypertension and leg
    ulceration 215–216